Cardiovascular Disease in Pregnancy

Guest Editors

GAGAN SAHNI, MD
URI ELKAYAM, MD

CARDIOLOGY CLINICS

www.cardiology.theclinics.com

Consulting Editor

MICHAEL H. CRAWFORD, MD

August 2012 • Volume 30 • Number 3

SAUNDERS an imprint of ELSEVIER, Inc.

W.B. SAUNDERS COMPANY
A Division of Elsevier Inc.

1600 John F. Kennedy Blvd. • Suite 1800 • Philadelphia, PA 19103-2899

http://www.theclinics.com

CARDIOLOGY CLINICS Volume 30, Number 3
August 2012 ISSN 0733-8651, ISBN-13: 978-1-4557-4890-7

Editor: Barbara Cohen-Kligerman

Cardiology Clinics (ISSN 0733-8651) is published quarterly by Elsevier Inc., 360 Park Avenue South, New York, NY 10010-1710. Months of issue are February, May, August, and November. Business and Editorial Offices: 1600 John F. Kennedy Blvd., Ste. 1800, Philadelphia, PA 19103-2899. Customer Service Office: 3251 Riverport Lane, Maryland Heights, MO 63043. Periodicals postage paid at New York, NY and additional mailing offices. Subscription prices are $305.00 per year for US individuals, $488.00 per year for US institutions, $150.00 per year for US students and residents, $373.00 per year for Canadian individuals, $606.00 per year for Canadian institutions, $432.00 per year for international individuals, $606.00 per year for international institutions and $212.00 per year for Canadian and international students/residents. To receive student/resident rate, orders must be accompanied by name of affiliated institution, data of term, and the *signature* of program/residency coordinator on institution letterhead. Orders will be billed at individual rate until proof of status is received. Foreign air speed delivery is included in all *Clinics* subscription prices. All prices are subject to change without notice. **POSTMASTER:** Send address changes to *Cardiology Clinics*, Elsevier Health Sciences Division, Subscription Customer Service, 3251 Riverport Lane, Maryland Heights, MO 63043. **Customer Service: 1-800-654-2452 (U.S. and Canada); 314-447-8871 (outside U.S. and Canada). Fax: 314-447-8029. E-mail: journalscustomerservice-usa@elsevier.com (for print support); journalsonlinesupport-usa@elsevier.com (for online support).**

Reprints. For copies of 100 or more, of articles in this publication, please contact the Commercial Reprints Department, Elsevier Inc., 360 Park Avenue South, New York, NY 10010-1710. Tel.: 212-633-3812; Fax: 212-462-1935; E-mail: reprints@elsevier.com.

Cardiology Clinics is also published in Spanish by McGraw-Hill Interamericana Editores S. A., P.O. Box 5-237, 06500, Mexico D. F., Mexico; in Portuguese by Reichmann and Alfonso Editores Rio de Janeiro, Brazil; and in Greek by Dimitrios P. Lagos, 8 Pondon Street, GR115-28 Ilissia, Greece.

Cardiology Clinics is covered in *MEDLINE/PubMed (Index Medicus), Excerpta Medica, The Cumulative Index to Nursing and Allied Health Literature* (CINAHL).

Printed and bound by CPI Group (UK) Ltd, Croydon, CR0 4YY

Transferred to Digital Print 2012

Contributors

CONSULTING EDITOR

MICHAEL H. CRAWFORD, MD
Professor of Medicine, University of California,
San Francisco; Lucie Stern Chair in Cardiology
and Chief of Clinical Cardiology, University of
California, San Francisco Medical Center,
San Francisco, California

GUEST EDITORS

GAGAN SAHNI, MD, FACC, FACP
Assistant Professor, Cardiovascular Institute,
Mount Sinai Medical Center, New York,
New York

URI ELKAYAM, MD
Professor of Medicine, Division of Cardiology,
Department of Medicine; Department of
Obstetrics and Gynecology, University of
Southern California Keck School of Medicine,
Los Angeles, California

AUTHORS

DAVID L. AIN, MD
The Zena and Michael A. Wiener
Cardiovascular Institute, Mount Sinai School
of Medicine, New York, New York

VINCENT T. ARMENTI, MD, PhD
Professor, Department of Surgery, Thomas
Jefferson University, Philadelphia, Pennsylvania

WILBERT S. ARONOW, MD, FACC, FAHA
Professor of Medicine, Cardiology Division,
New York Medical College/Westchester
Medical Center, Valhalla, New York

MOHAMAD BARAKAT, MD
Division of Cardiology, Department of Medicine;
Department of Obstetrics and Gynecology,
University of Southern California Keck School
of Medicine, Los Angeles, California

LESLIE S. CHO, MD
Director of the Women's Cardiovascular
Center; Section Head, Preventive Cardiology
and Rehabilitation, Robert and Suzanne
Tomsich Department of Cardiovascular
Medicine, Cleveland Clinic, Cleveland, Ohio

SCOTT W. COWAN, MD
Assistant Professor, Department of Surgery,
Thomas Jefferson University, Philadelphia,
Pennsylvania

JOHN M. DAVISON, MD
Emeritus Professor, Institute of Cellular
Medicine, Newcastle University, Newcastle
upon Tyne, United Kingdom

CATALDO DORIA, MD, PhD
Nicoletti Family Professor of Transplant
Surgery, Department of Surgery, Thomas
Jefferson University, Philadelphia, Pennsylvania

URI ELKAYAM, MD
Professor of Medicine, Division of Cardiology,
Department of Medicine; Department of
Obstetrics and Gynecology, University of
Southern California Keck School of Medicine,
Los Angeles, California

CHRISTINE K. FARINELLI, MD
Clinical Instructor of Obstetrics and Gynecology;
Fellow, Maternal Fetal Medicine, University of
California, Irvine, Orange, California

WAYNE J. FRANKLIN, MD, FACC
Director, Texas Adult Congenital Heart
Disease Program, Texas Children's Hospital;
Departments of Pediatrics and Medicine,
Baylor College of Medicine, Houston, Texas

WILLIAM H. FRISHMAN, MD
Rosenthal Professor and Chair, Professor of
Pharmacology, Department of Medicine,
New York Medical College; Director of Medicine,
Acting Chief of Cardiology, Westchester
Medical Center, Valhalla, New York

MANISHA GANDHI, MD, FACOG
Departments of Obstetrics and Gynecology,
Baylor College of Medicine, Houston, Texas

SOREL GOLAND, MD
Department of Cardiology, Kaplan Medical
Center, Rehovot, Israel

AFSHAN B. HAMEED, MD
Associate Professor of Clinical Obstetrics and
Gynecology, Associate Professor of Clinical
Cardiology, Medical Director, Obstetrics,
Maternal Fetal Medicine, University of
California, Irvine, Orange, California

SAWAN JALNAPURKAR, MD
Division of Cardiology, Department of
Medicine; Department of Obstetrics and
Gynecology, University of Southern California
Keck School of Medicine, Los Angeles,
California

JOHN H. MCANULTY, MD
Medical Director of Legacy Arrhythmia
Services, Legacy Good Samaritan Hospital
and Medical Center; Emeritus Professor,
Oregon Health and Sciences University,
Portland, Oregon

MICHAEL J. MORITZ, MD
Professor, Department of Surgery, Lehigh
Valley Health Network, Allentown,
Pennsylvania

JAGAT NARULA, MD, PhD
Philip J. and Harriet L. Goodhart Chair in
Cardiology, Professor of Medicine, Associate
Dean for Global Health, Mount Sinai School of
Medicine; Director, Cardiovascular Imaging
Program, Zena and Michael A. Wiener
Cardiovascular Institute, and Marie-Josée and
Henry R. Kravis Center for Cardiovascular
Health, Mount Sinai School of Medicine,
New York, New York

JOSEPH G. OUZOUNIAN, MD
Associate Professor, Chief, Maternal-Fetal
Medicine, University of Southern California
Keck School of Medicine, Los Angeles,
California

GAGAN SAHNI, MD, FACC, FACP
Assistant Professor of Medicine,
Cardiovascular Institute, Mount Sinai Medical
Center, New York, New York

PARTHO P. SENGUPTA, MD
The Zena and Michael A. Wiener
Cardiovascular Institute, Mount Sinai School
of Medicine, New York, New York

THOMAS A. TRAILL, BM, FRCP
Professor of Medicine, Division of Cardiology,
Johns Hopkins University School of Medicine,
Baltimore, Maryland

AMANDA R. VEST, MBBS, MRCP
Fellow in Cardiovascular Medicine, Heart
and Vascular Institute, Cleveland Clinic,
Cleveland, Ohio

Contents

> The major adaptations of the maternal cardiovascular system that progress through-
> out gestation may unmask previously unrecognized heart disease and result in sig-
> nificant morbidity and mortality. Most of these changes are almost fully reversed in
> the weeks and months after delivery. Hemodynamic changes during pregnancy
> include increased blood volume, cardiac output (CO), and maternal heart rate;
> decreased arterial blood pressure; decreased systemic vascular resistance. CO
> increases up to 30% in the first stage of labor, primarily because of increased stroke
> volume; maternal pushing efforts in the second stage of labor can increase CO by as
> much as 50%.

> Diagnostic imaging procedures, including echocardiography, chest radiography,
> angiography, CT, and cardiovascular MRI, may be indicated in pregnant patients.
> Concerns related to the safety of these tests must be balanced against the im-
> portance of accurate diagnosis and assessment of a pathologic state. Such
> a calculation requires an understanding of the normal physiology of pregnancy,
> manifestations of pre-existing cardiac disease in pregnant women, and signs and
> symptoms of nascent cardiovascular disease. Additionally cardiologists must un-
> derstand indications for and limitations of each diagnostic imaging test, potential
> harmful effects of various modalities, and precautions that must be taken to protect
> the fetus.

> Chest pain syndromes in pregnancy include numerous catastrophic cardiovascular
> events. Acute myocardial infarction, aortic dissection, pulmonary embolism, and
> amniotic fluid embolism are the most important causes of nonobstetric mortality
> and morbidity in pregnancy. Each of these could result in poor maternal and fetal
> outcomes if not diagnosed and treated in a timely fashion. However, their diagnosis
> and management is limited by fetal risks of diagnostic procedures, dangers of phar-
> macotherapy and interventions that have neither been widely studied nor validated.
> This article reviews the current literature on epidemiology, risk factors, pathogene-
> sis, diagnosis, and management of 4 potentially lethal chest pain syndromes in
> pregnancy.

Among women with valvular heart disease, those with mitral stenosis carry the greatest potential for problems during pregnancy. Asymptomatic women with aortic stenosis and only mild or moderate left ventricular outflow obstruction generally tolerate pregnancy well, as do those with regurgitant lesions. In Marfan syndrome, pregnancy should not be undertaken if the aortic root dimension exceeds 4 cm. Even if the aortic root is normal, a small increased risk of dissection is present. Women with well-functioning bioprosthetic valves and normal hemodynamics may safely undertake a pregnancy, although bioprostheses deteriorate rapidly in young people.

Heart disease is a main cause of maternal mortality in the United States and the United Kingdom. Most deaths are from acquired conditions. However, due to the increased survival of children born with congenital heart disease (CHD) over the past 30 years, the population of adults with congenital heart disease in the U.S. now exceeds 1 million. Thus, there are now more adults with CHD than children with CHD. Many of these adult survivors of pediatric heart disease are of childbearing age and are considering pregnancy. This article reviews the literature concerning pregnancy and CHD.

Pregnancy-associated thrombosis is an important cause of morbidity and mortality during pregnancy. Anticoagulation therapy is an important component of the management of thrombotic complications in pregnancy but may result in fetal and maternal complications. Although evidence-based recommendations are available for the prevention and treatment of venous thromboembolism, the management of pregnant women with mechanical valves still presents a challenge, because there are no controlled clinical trials to provide guidelines for optimal antithrombotic therapy. This review presents information on anticoagulation therapy during pregnancy for thromboembolic prophylaxis in women with various cardiovascular disorders, focusing on patients with mechanical heart valves.

Hypertension in pregnancy is diagnosed on systolic blood pressure greater than or equal to 140 mm Hg and/or diastolic greater than or equal to 90 mm Hg. The classification systems separate chronic and gestational hypertension from preeclampsia. Significant uncertainty regarding optimal management is reflected in the differing major international society recommendations. Blood pressure treatment is designed to minimize maternal end-organ damage. Methyldopa, labetalol, hydralazine, and nifedipine are oral options; angiotensin-converting enzyme inhibitors and angiotensin receptor antagonists are contraindicated. Women with preeclampsia should be closely monitored and receive intravenous magnesium sulfate.

Pregnant women have an increased risk of having the usual arrhythmias seen in women of childbearing age. Most of these are benign sinus tachycardias or bradycardias or atrial and ventricular ectopic beats. Women who have had sustained supraventricular or ventricular tachycardias before pregnancy frequently develop them during pregnancy. These arrhythmias often have enough hemodynamic significance to decrease uterine blood flow, which adds a sense of urgency for treatment. The management is similar to that of nonpregnant women, with nuances important for the protection of the developing fetus.

In 1971, Demakis and colleagues established the term peripartum cardiomyopathy (PPCM) and defined it by criteria based on the clinical profile of their patients. With the recognition that these criteria are arbitrary and that PPCM often presents earlier in pregnancy, the definition of PPCM has been recently updated by a working group on PPCM of the European Society of Cardiology. This article discusses the cause, clinical presentation, prognosis, and treatment of PPCM, as well as other related topics.

More women are reporting pregnancy following heart transplantation. Although successful outcomes have been reported for the mother, transplanted heart, and newborn, such pregnancies should be considered high risk. Hypertension, preeclampsia, and infection should be treated. Vaginal delivery is recommended unless cesarean section is obstetrically necessary. Most outcomes are live births, and long-term follow-up of children show most are healthy and developing well. Maternal survival, independent of pregnancy-related events, should be part of prepregnancy counseling.

Cardiac arrest in pregnancy is not only uncommon but also catastrophic. Early aggressive resuscitation by well-trained health care providers improves the chances of successful outcomes for both the patient and her fetus. Significant physiologic changes that occur normally in pregnancy require several modifications to standard cardiopulmonary resuscitation, and urgent cesarean delivery may be indicated to benefit both the mother and the infant.

Cardiovascular drugs are used in pregnancy to treat maternal and fetal conditions. Mothers may also require drug therapy postpartum. Most cardiovascular drugs taken by pregnant women can cross the placenta and therefore expose the developing embryo and fetus to their pharmacologic and teratogenic effects. These effects are influenced by the intrinsic pharmacokinetic properties of a given drug and by the complex physiologic changes occurring during pregnancy. Many drugs are also transferred into human milk with potential adverse effects on the nursing infant. This article summarizes some of the literature concerning the risks and benefits of using cardiovascular drugs during pregnancy.

CARDIOLOGY CLINICS

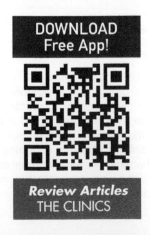

DOWNLOAD
Free App!

Review Articles
THE CLINICS

NOW AVAILABLE FOR YOUR iPhone and iPad

Foreword

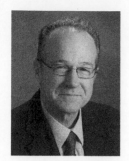

Michael H. Crawford, MD
Consulting Editor

Although the United States spends more on health care than any other nation, health outcomes in the United States are not number 1. One notable area of deficiency compared to many other industrial countries is maternal–fetal health. Thus, I was delighted that Drs Sahni and Elkayan agreed to guest edit an issue of *Cardiology Clinics* on the topic of Cardiovascular Disease in Pregnancy. The issue is particularly timely due to the release of the European Society of Cardiology guidelines on this topic last year. Some of the reasons for our deficiencies in this area are detailed in Dr Sahni and Elkayan's preface, but suffice it to say that a major reason is the health status of pregnant women. Seven of the 12 articles in this issue focus on maternal health issues. There are three articles on therapy and one on diagnostic testing in pregnant women. The final article details the normal physiologic changes during pregnancy, which should not be confused with signs of heart disease.

Although not all primary care physicians or cardiologists see pregnant women, we all see nonpregnant women of reproductive age and their health is the key to reducing maternal–fetal mortality rates in the United States. The better the health of the mother, the more likely there will be a successful pregnancy and a viable fetus. For example, there has been a tendency to view women of reproductive age as immune from atherosclerosis. Although uncommon, pregnant women can have myocardial infarction with disastrous results. Rarely, a myocardial infarction in a pregnant woman is due to aortic dissection. More commonly it is due to the rupture of a non–flow-limiting plaque. Consequently, we must be vigilant about the primary prevention of atherosclerosis in young women as well as in postmenopausal women. This and other important maternal health issues are discussed by an outstanding group of authors who are experts in this field.

Michael H. Crawford, MD
Division of Cardiology
Department of Medicine
University of California
San Francisco Medical Center
505 Parnassus Avenue, Box 0124
San Francisco, CA 94143-0124, USA

E-mail address:
crawfordm@medicine.ucsf.edu

doi:10.1016/j.ccl.2012.06.001
0733-8651/12/$ – see front matter

cardiology.theclinics.com

Preface
Cardiovascular Disease in Pregnancy

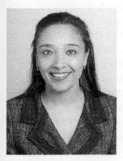 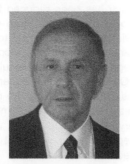

Gagan Sahni, MD   Uri Elkayam, MD
Guest Editors

Cardiac disease complicates only 1 to 4% of pregnancies in the United States, yet is the most important cause of nonobstetric maternal morbidity and mortality.

It was not purely the statistics that prompted us to put together this issue of *Cardiology Clinics* focused on Cardiovascular Disease in Pregnancy. It was the changing epidemiology of pregnant women with heart disease and the challenges that are faced by clinicians, some of whom are not very comfortable treating this special population, that prompted this issue of *Cardiology Clinics*. Higher maternal age of conception, survival of patients with congenital heart disease late into adulthood, and the success of assisted reproductive medicine (even in patients with Turner's syndrome) have changed the profile of women who present to high-risk pregnancy clinics today. Racial and socioeconomic disparities in antenatal care add to the challenging statistics. The Healthy People 2000 objective for maternal mortality of no more than 3.3 maternal deaths per 100,000 live births in the United States was *not achieved* during the twentieth century. In fact there was *worsening* maternal mortality in subpopulations such as African Americans, making the latest maternal mortality rate 12.7 per 100,000 live births as of 2008 a discouraging number, with cardiovascular disease being the most important cause of nonobstetric mortality. These are numbers *we need to change*!

This is the era in which we are faced with the mounting conundrum of patients in whom clinical presentation could be difficult to interpret and differentiate from the normal physiological changes during pregnancy; the diagnostic procedures are either underperformed or performed with caution due to radiation and other fetal hazards; the effects of pharmacotherapeutics have not been extensively studied for teratogenic and other fetal effects; cardiovascular interventional and surgical procedures intimidate many a health care provider due to the higher risks that impact two lives during a single procedure. And what certainly does not make it easier is that this population is grossly underrepresented in clinical trials and research projects, considering that pregnancy is a 9-month condition at best! Novel therapeutics and safe procedures are harder to develop or test in pregnant women due to logistic issues, funding constraints, inadequate registries, and lack of long-term historical data.

If Hollywood has made forays into portraying male pregnancy in reel life, modern medicine is not far behind in finding improved solutions for managing pregnancy and cardiovascular disease in real life! Some plausible concepts include maternal-fetal medicine fellowships that would closely liaison with cardiology fellowship programs in order for this interdisciplinary approach to evolve *early on during training*. This would not only facilitate appropriate training and experience but also develop important databases for research. Developing international registries such as the Study Group on Peripartum Cardiomyopathy (supported by the European Society of Cardiology [ESC]) is

Cardiol Clin 30 (2012) xi–xii
doi:10.1016/j.ccl.2012.05.005
0733-8651/12/$ – see front matter © 2012 Elsevier Inc. All rights reserved.

an example of international collaborative endeavors that would allow sharing of cross-cultural research and efforts. However, the concept of developing "high-risk pregnancy clinics" is *key*, especially in most tertiary care centers: these would comprise an ideal multidisciplinary team of experienced obstetricians, adult and pediatric cardiologists, anesthesiologists, neonatologists, genetic specialists, and preconception counselors working in cohesion for superior outcomes in pregnant women with cardiovascular diseases. A scaled down version of such clinics is very conceivable even in smaller community health care facilities with appropriate referrals to the tertiary care centers as necessary. Community clinicians who care for women could be educated in identifying medical conditions that pose additional risk if pregnancy occurs, be able to offer preconception counseling (including discussion of appropriate contraception), and refer high-risk patients to tertiary care centers with expertise in caring for these patients. This issue of *Cardiology Clinics* strives to guide clinicians to achieve this to some extent across a broad spectrum of cardiovascular diseases. The content ranges from management of hypertension and arrhythmias in pregnancy to the more complex congenital heart diseases; understanding basic drugs that are safe from a pregnancy perspective to the basic physiology of pregnancy; from newer therapies in peripartum cardiomyopathy and coronary artery disease to the difficult management of pregnancy in cardiac transplant recipients.

Hope is already on the horizon; 66 successful deliveries have been reported in heart transplant recipients as of December 2010 as per the National Transplantation Pregnancy Registry. Novel experimental therapies such as bromocriptine and pentoxyfylline have been used in patients with peripartum cardiomyopathy with promising outcomes. Organizations such as the ESC have devised specific guidelines for management of cardiovascular disease in pregnancy in 2011 with ACC/AHA addressing issues of valvular and aortic disease management in pregnancy specifically under each of the broader guidelines. A systematic review of patients with congenital heart disease from 1985–2006 showed that the majority have had successful deliveries and the major adverse cardiovascular event rate was only 2%[1] with the overall cardiac complication rate ranging from 7.6 to 11%.[1,2] The National Institute of Child Health and Human Development reported 13 successful pregnancies in patients with Turner's syndrome in the period between 2000 and 2010. Maternal mortality from acute myocardial infarction in pregnancy has been reduced from a prodigious 38% prior to the year 2000 to about 5–11% in recent reviews,[3,4] owing partly to the increasing use of primary percutaneous coronary intervention in pregnancy with successful outcomes.

Once again, it is not merely about the statistics; it is about extending the rapidly expanding frontiers of cardiovascular medicine to a small yet very special population, where each successful pregnancy will save not one but at least two precious lives.

Gagan Sahni, MD
Cardiovascular Institute
Mount Sinai Medical Center
1 Gustave L. Levy Place, Box 1030
New York, NY 10029-6574, USA

Uri Elkayam, MD
University of Southern California
Keck School of Medicine
2020 Zonal Avenue, IRD Room 331
Los Angeles, CA 90033, USA

E-mail addresses:
gagan.sahni@mountsinai.org (G. Sahni)
Elkayam@usc.edu (U. Elkayam)

REFERENCES

1. Drenthen W, Pieper PG, Roos-Hesselink JW, et al. Outcome of pregnancy in women with congenital heart disease: a literature review. J Am Coll Cardiol 2007;49:2303–11.
2. Drenthen W, Boersma E, Balci A, et al; ZAHARA Investigators. Predictors of pregnancy complications in women with congenital heart disease. Eur Heart J 2010;31(17):2124–32.
3. Roth A, Elkayam U. Acute myocardial infarction associated with pregnancy. J Am Coll Cardiol 2008;52: 171–80.
4. James AH, Jamison MG, Biswas MS, et al. Acute myocardial infarction in pregnancy: a United States population-based study. Circulation 2006;113:1564–71.

Physiologic Changes During Normal Pregnancy and Delivery

Joseph G. Ouzounian, MD*, Uri Elkayam, MD

KEYWORDS

- Pregnancy • Physiology • Hemodynamic changes • Cardiocirculatory • Labor and delivery

KEY POINTS

- The major adaptations of the maternal cardiovascular system that progress throughout gestation may unmask previously unrecognized heart disease and result in significant morbidity and mortality.
- Most of these changes are almost fully reversed in the weeks and months after delivery.
- Hemodynamic changes during pregnancy include increased blood volume, cardiac output (CO), and maternal heart rate; decreased arterial blood pressure; decreased systemic vascular resistance.
- CO increases up to 30% in the first stage of labor, primarily because of increased stroke volume; maternal pushing efforts in the second stage of labor can increase CO by as much as 50%.

INTRODUCTION

Soon after conception, the maternal cardiovascular system undergoes major adaptations that progress throughout gestation. In conjunction with the increased circulatory burden of pregnancy, these changes may unmask previously unrecognized heart disease and result in significant morbidity and mortality. Most of these changes are almost fully reversed in the weeks and months after delivery.

HEMODYNAMIC CHANGES DURING PREGNANCY
Blood Volume

Blood volume increases significantly during pregnancy. The increase starts at around 6 weeks' gestation and reaches a maximal volume of 4700 to 5200 mL by 32 weeks' gestation.[1–20] A rapid increase is typically noted until midpregnancy, with a slower increase thereafter (**Fig. 1**).[6] Overall, a continuous blood volume increase of about 45% (1200–1600 mL), or a mean recorded blood volume ranging from 73 to 96 mL/kg greater than nonpregnant values is typical.[2–12,21]

In addition to blood volume expansion, there is redistribution of fluid during pregnancy.[20] Studies of pregnant women in their third trimester have shown increases of interstitial and plasma volume, with more extracellular fluid volume in the intravascular space in pregnant versus nonpregnant women.[19] In twins, the increase in blood volume after 20 weeks parallels that in singletons, but at a 20% higher volume (**Fig. 2**).[5,13–16,19,22]

This increase in blood volume during pregnancy has important clinical implications. Normal fetal growth and birthweight are directly correlated with the degree of plasma volume expansion.[3,8,16,17,19] In contrast, pathologic conditions like intrauterine growth restriction and small for gestational age newborns, as well as preeclampsia, have been

Disclosures: None.
University of Southern California, Keck School of Medicine, Los Angeles, CA, USA
* Corresponding author. University of Southern California, Keck School of Medicine, 2020 Zonal Avenue, IRD 220 Room 331, Los Angeles, CA 90033.
E-mail address: Joseph.Ouzounian@med.usc.edu

Cardiol Clin 30 (2012) 317–329
doi:10.1016/j.ccl.2012.05.004
0733-8651/12/$ – see front matter © 2012 Elsevier Inc. All rights reserved.

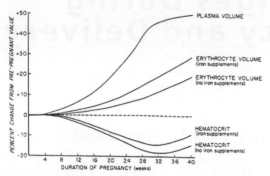

Fig. 1. Changes in plasma volume, erythrocyte volume, and hematocrit during pregnancy. Increase in plasma volume is more rapid than increase in erythrocyte volume, causing the physiologic anemia of pregnancy, which can be partially corrected with iron supplements. (*From* Pitkin RM. Nutritional support in obstetrics and gynecology. Clin Obstet Gynecol 1976;19(3):491; with permission.)

associated with reduced blood volume expansion.[20,23] In cases of concomitant maternal cardiac disease, rapid decompensation may result. An accumulation of approximately 900 mmol of sodium is seen in normal pregnancy, which leads to water accumulation.[20]

Additional changes include increased production of red blood cells leading to a significant increase of 17% to 40% (250 mL–450 mL) in red blood cell mass.[7,18] Red blood cell life remains unchanged.[18] Progesterone, placental chorionic somatomammotropin, and perhaps prolactin are responsible for the increased erythropoiesis.[24] The increased production, in turn, increases maternal demand for iron by 500 mg during pregnancy. In addition, increased pregnancy levels of 2,3-diphosphoglycerate lead to enhanced fetal

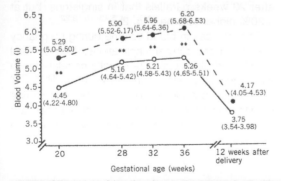

Fig. 2. Changes in blood volume during twin pregnancy (solid circles, N = 10) and singleton pregnancy (open circles, N = 40). (*From* Thomsen JK, Fogh-Andersen N, Jaszczak P. Atrial natriuretic peptide, blood volume, aldosterone, and sodium excretion during twin pregnancy. Acta Obstet Gynecol Scand 1994;73(1):16; with permission.)

oxygen transfer.[25] Despite the increase in red cell mass, plasma volume increases are greater and more rapid, such that hemoglobin concentrations decrease during pregnancy. This phenomenon has been called the physiologic anemia of pregnancy. Hemoglobin and hematocrit levels can be as low as 11 to 12 g/dL and 33% to 38%, respectively.[15,26] Oral iron supplementation helps mitigate this decrease in maternal hemoglobin.[27,28]

Mechanisms of hypervolemia in pregnancy

Although sodium and water retention physiologically protect a pregnant woman from potential hemodynamic instability caused by blood loss at delivery, the specific mechanisms responsible for the hypervolemia remain unclear. Many different factors, including steroid hormones and nitric oxide, act simultaneously to alter maternal fluid balance and increase plasma volume.[29,30] Estrogen promotes sodium retention both by direct renal action and by increased hepatic production of angiotensinogen (renin substrate).[20,31–35]

Estrogen stimulates increased renal renin production, in addition to production in the uterus and liver.[36–39] Increased renin stimulates aldosterone secretion, which in turn increases total body water.[40–42]

Other hormones responsible for increased total body water include deoxycorticosterone, prostaglandins, prolactin, placental lactogen, growth hormone, and adrenocorticotrophic hormone.[26] Increased ureteral pressure secondary to mechanical obstruction may also contribute to sodium retention.[43] However, a fetus is not essential for the development of hypervolemia. A 50% increase in volume has been reported in patients with hydatidiform moles.[18]

Atrial natriuretic peptide and brain natriuretic peptide

Atrial natriuretic peptide (ANP) and brain natriuretic peptide (BNP) are peptide hormones that play important roles in volume homeostasis during pregnancy. ANP is released primarily by the atria in response to atrial stretching from volume expansion. ANP is a peripheral vasodilator and a diuretic hormone.[22,44–46] Genetically altered mice lacking the ANP-receptor show chronically increased plasma volume, hypertension, and cardiac hypertrophy.[47] In early pregnancy, volume expansion contributes to increased ANP release, increased stroke volume, and peripheral vasodilation.[48] ANP levels increase throughout pregnancy and increase further after delivery, implicating its role in postpartum diueresis.[49,50] Patients with preeclampsia have relative volume depletion and endothelial cell injury, but ANP levels are higher than in women without preeclampsia. This finding suggests that the hemodynamic changes with preeclampsia are more complex.[49] Increased ANP and BNP levels are also associated with higher rates of left ventricular dysfunction.[51,52] In preeclamptic women, the degree of ANP and BNP increase has been correlated with the severity of maternal left ventricular dysfunction.[53]

BNP is a peptide similar to ANP and is produced by the cardiac ventricles. Its actions are similar to those of ANP in that it leads to decreased systemic vascular resistance and increased diuresis, thereby increasing cardiac output (CO). In addition to its role in the complex milieu of maternal fluid homeostasis, a link between BNP and myometrial quiescence has also been shown. At least 2 reports have found production of BNP in chorioamniotic membranes with measurable levels in amniotic fluid. Furthermore, BNP was shown to inhibit contractions in preterm (but not term) human myometrium, thereby implicating a broader role for the peptide that extends beyond the mitigation of volume expansion.[54–57]

CO

CO is calculated as the product of stroke volume and heart rate (HR), and can be considered a measure of the functional capacity of the heart. Numerous studies have shown that CO increases as much as 50% in pregnancy.[58–69] CO begins to increase during the first trimester, and peaks between 25 and 35 weeks' gestation.[63–69] The increase in CO early in pregnancy is mostly caused by stroke volume (**Fig. 3**).[64] As pregnancy advances, HR increases and becomes a more

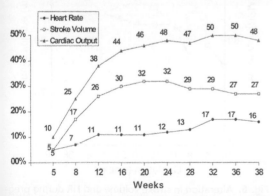

Fig. 3. Percent changes of HR, stroke volume, and CO measured in the lateral position throughout pregnancy compared with prepregnancy values. (*Modified from* Robson SC, Hunter S, Boys RJ, et al. Serial study of factors influencing changes in cardiac output during human pregnancy. Am J Physiol 1989;256:H1060; with permission.)

dominant factor in increasing CO. Stroke volume increases gradually until the end of the second trimester and then remains constant.[64,66]

CO fluctuates with changes in maternal position.[70–72] Compression of the inferior vena cava by the enlarged gravid uterus in the supine position results in decreased venous return to the heart and significant decrease in CO (**Fig. 4**). Evaluation of hemodynamic changes in twin gestations shows a significantly greater increase in CO compared with singletons (approximately 15% at 24 weeks).[65]

Techniques to measure CO in pregnancy

CO may be calculated by invasive heart catheterization using the Fick method, dye dilution, or thermodilution,[60–63] or noninvasively with thoracic electric bioimpedance (impedance cardiography)[73,74] and echocardiography.[64–69] Although assessment of CO by thermodilution remains the gold standard, the technique requires insertion of a pulmonary artery catheter, which precludes its use in most pregnant patients. More recently, M-mode echocardiography and Doppler studies have been shown to correlate well with thermodilution, and are frequently used to assess CO during pregnancy.[75–78] Noninvasive CO measurements with thoracic electrical bioimpedance techniques have correlated well with invasive methods,[73,74,79] although some investigations have reported a poor correlation in certain clinical situations.[80,81]

HR

Maternal HR increases as early as 5 weeks' gestation to a maximal increase of 15 to 20 beats per minute at by 32 weeks' gestation (**Figs. 5** and **6, Table 1**). The magnitude of the increase is greater in twin gestations.[66] Maternal HR decreases slightly with a change from the supine to the left lateral position.[82,83] Note that the increase in HR is gradual with a peak at the third trimester,[64,66] such that maternal tachycardia is primarily responsible for maintaining CO late in pregnancy.

Blood Pressure

Arterial blood pressure (BP) decreases as early as 7 weeks' gestation.[26,64,66,84–87] The decrease in BP reaches a nadir by midpregnancy, when the BP starts a gradual increase, returning to or exceeding prepregnancy levels by term (see **Fig. 5, Table 1**).[66,69]

Several issues related to BP during pregnancy are important. First, reliable measurement of diastolic pressure has been complicated by the absence of a fifth Korotkoff sound in some women. This absence may be related to the hyperdynamic state of maternal circulation, which may cause the fifth Korotkoff sound to be heard even after

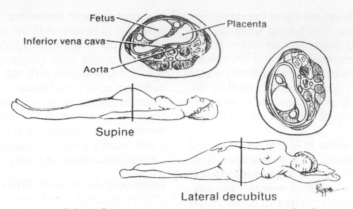

Fig. 4. Venocaval compression of the inferior vena cava and abdominal aorta by the gravid uterus can lead to reduced venous return and thus to decreased CO. (*From* Elkayam U, Gleicher N. Diagnosis and management of maternal and fetal heart disease, 3rd Edition. 1998; New York, Wiley-Liss; with permission.)

complete deflation of the cuff.[88] However, the fifth Korotkoff sound can be heard in most pregnant women and is more accurate than the fourth sound, compared with results obtained from invasive BP measurements.[89,90] The diastolic BP measured with the use of the fourth sound is 5 to 13 mm Hg higher than that measured using the fifth sound and may lead to an erroneous conclusion. The use of the fifth sound is therefore recommended for the measurement of diastolic BP during gestation.[91] The use of automated cuff measurement of BP may avoid many operator-dependent biases associated with measurement of BP by auscultation.[88,92] A second important issue is the patient's position, which may greatly influence levels of recorded BP during pregnancy. In general, BPs, both systolic and diastolic, are approximately 16 mm Hg higher in the sitting

position than in the recumbent position.[93] After midpregnancy, because of potential vena caval occlusion in the recumbent position, BP may be measured in the lateral position. In either case, consistency in position during successive BP measurements is critical for accurate determination of BP trends. Both increasing maternal age and parity seem to be associated with higher systolic and diastolic BPs during pregnancy.[86,87]

Chronic hypertension in pregnancy is defined as a maternal BP greater than or equal to 140/90 mm Hg diagnosed before 20 weeks' gestation.[94,95]

A decrease in CO caused by a change in posture is typically followed by a compensatory increase in

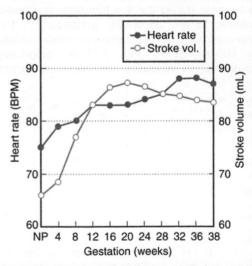

Fig. 6. Alteration in stroke volume and HR during pregnancy. Stroke volume increases during the first half of gestation, with a slight decrease thereafter until term. A mild increase in HR begins in early pregnancy continues until term. (*Adapted from* Robson SC, Hunter S, Boys RJ, et al. Serial study of factors influencing changes in cardiac output during human pregnancy. Am J Physiol 1989;256:H1060; with permission.)

Sodium Excretion
  Aldosterone
  Deoxycorticosterone
  Estrogen
  Prolactin
  Human placental lactogen
  Uretroplacental shunt (i.e. a large arteriovenous fistula)
  Upright and supine posture
  Increased ureteral pressure

↑ Human chorionic somatotropin

↑ Prolactin

↓

Na+ & water retention

Erythropoiesis

↓

↑ **Extracellular fluid volume**

↑ **Red blood cell mass**

↓

↑ Blood volume

Fig. 5. Potential mechanisms of hypervolemia during pregnancy.

Table 1
Circulatory changes during normal pregnancy

Parameter	Changes at Various Times (wk)					
	5	12	20	24	32	38
HR	↑	↑↑↑	↑↑↑	↑↑↑	↑↑↑↑	↑↑↑↑
Systolic blood pressure	↔	↓	↓	↔	↑	↑↑
Diastolic blood pressure	↔	↓	↓↓	↓	↔	↑↑
Stroke volume	↑	↑↑↑↑↑	↑↑↑↑↑↑	↑↑↑↑↑↑	↑↑↑↑↑	↑↑↑↑↑
CO	↑↑	↑↑↑↑↑↑↑	↑↑↑↑↑↑↑	↑↑↑↑↑↑↑	↑↑↑↑↑↑↑	↑↑↑↑↑↑↑
Systemic vascular residence	↓↓	↓↓↓↓↓	↓↓↓↓↓↓	↓↓↓↓↓↓	↓↓↓↓↓↓	↓↓↓↓↓
Left ventricular ejection fraction	↑	↑↑	↑↑	↑↑	↑	↑

↑, ≤5%; ↑↑, 6–10%; ↑↑↑, 11–15%; ↑↑↑↑, 16–20%; ↑↑↑↑↑, 21–30%; ↑↑↑↑↑↑, >30%; ↑↑↑↑↑↑↑, >40%.
Data from Robson SC, Hunter S, Boys RJ, et al. Serial study of factors influencing changes in cardiac output during human pregnancy. Am J Physiol 1989;256:H1061.

peripheral resistance, with no overall significant change in systemic BP or HR.[96] However, a significant increase in HR with a decrease in BP is sometimes noted, resulting in symptoms such as weakness, lightheadedness, nausea, dizziness, and even syncope.[96–102] This phenomenon occurs in 0.5% to 11.2% of pregnancies, and is described as the supine hypotensive syndrome of pregnancy. Symptoms usually resolve quickly with appropriate maternal positioning.[100,103]

Systemic Vascular Resistance

A significant decrease in systemic vascular resistance (SVR) occurs during pregnancy (see **Table 1**), with concomitant decrease in BP (primarily the diastolic component) and a widened pulse pressure. These changes begin as early as 5 weeks' gestation, and result from a variety of factors including the vasodilatory effects of progesterone and prostaglandin, as well as the contribution of the low-resistance flow of the uteroplacental unit.[29,104–106] An approximate 10% decrease in SVR has been shown to occur in the first trimester, with a nadir of about 35% less than baseline at 20 weeks' gestation. Thereafter, SVR remains constant until around 32 weeks, with a small increase noted from week 32 to term.[63,64,69] As SVR decreases, vascular compliance increases.[107]

Differing mechanisms related to the decreased SVR in pregnancy have been studied. Estrogen, progesterone, prostaglandins, and prolactin play a role in SVR reduction.[105,108–111] Furthermore, prostacyclin attenuates the vasoconstrictor effect of angiotensin II described during pregnancy. Resistance to the pressor effect of angiotensin and noradrenaline may also contribute to a decreased SVR.[112–115]

Recent evidence suggests that nitric oxide (NO) may also be related to gestational vasodilation.[116] Nitric oxide is produced from L-arginine and is a potent endothelium-derived relaxing factor. Increased production of NO in pregnancy acts to maintain vascular relaxation, in part to counteract the vasoconstrictive effects of thromboxane.[117] NO targets guanylate cyclase, leading to increased formation of cyclic guanosine monophosphate (cGMP). The cGMP, in turn, helps maintain dephosphorylated myosin light chains, thus causing relaxed vascular smooth muscle.[118] Doppler studies in pregnant women treated with NO donors showed decreased peripheral resistance and pulsatility indices in women treated with glyceryl trinitrate.[119] Similar results were shown in a study of isosorbide dinitrate infusion in the second trimester.[120] Thus, it seems that NO plays a key role in maternal vascular dynamics and SVR.

Another important hormone in the regulation of SVR in pregnancy is relaxin. Relaxin is a heterodimer of 2 peptide chains, with peak levels in the first trimester and at delivery. In addition to its effects on SVR, in pregnant women relaxin contributes to changes in connective tissue composition, myometrial activity, and labor.[121,122] Relaxin causes reduced arterial load by decreasing SVR and reduced plasma osmolality. The net effect is an increase in CO. Recent reports have shown relaxin expression in myocardial muscle, where its production attenuates endothelial-derived vasoconstrictors.[123] Thus, relaxin is essential for SVR and osmoregulatory changes in early and mid-pregnancy and likely plays a role in the transition of the maternal cardiovascular system from the nonpregnant to the pregnant state. At term, relaxin helps soften the maternal pubic symphysis to help facilitate delivery.[124,125]

Effect of the Gravid Uterus on the Circulation

The gravid uterus causes femoral vein and inferior vena caval obstruction in up to 90% of women.[96,97,126,127] These effects can be relieved with a lateral recumbent position (see **Fig. 4**).[96] In addition, paravertebral and collateral circulation facilitate venous return from the legs and the pelvic organs limited by a compressed inferior vena cava.[127] Various studies have shown that the enlarged uterus also compresses the arterial system. Angiography has shown compression and reduced flow in the aorta and iliac vessels and other smaller vessels (right renal artery, ovarian artery, lumbar artery).[97,98]

Other Changes in Blood Flow

Along with the changes described earlier for maternal BP, CO, and HR, many other organs have changes in blood flow during normal pregnancy. These changes are summarized in **Table 2**.[106,128–155] The effect of pregnancy on coronary blood flow is still unknown. However, an increase caused by the augmentation in CO is likely.

Oxygen Consumption

Oxygen consumption, commonly estimated by measurement of oxygen extracted by the lungs over a given time period, reflects the rate of the body's metabolism. In pregnancy, there is a progressive increase in resting oxygen consumption, with a peak increase of 20% to 30% near term.[156] However, in early gestation, there is a rapid increase in CO that is proportionally greater than the increase in oxygen consumption to ensure a well-oxygenated blood supply during organogenesis.[157]

The continuous increase in oxygen consumption in the later phases of pregnancy, when CO increase is slow and small, results in a widening of the arterial venous oxygen difference to nonpregnant levels.

The arterial venous oxygen difference is, therefore, small in early pregnancy, increases gradually throughout pregnancy, and reaches nonpregnant levels in the later part of gestation.

Functional and Anatomic Cardiac Changes During Pregnancy

Ventricular wall muscle mass and end-diastolic volume increase in pregnancy, although end-systolic volume and end-diastolic pressure remain unchanged.[158–160] Because this increases cardiac compliance, a physiologically dilated maternal heart results, without a decrease in ejection fraction (see **Table 1**).[64–66,68] Using invasive hemodynamic monitoring with a pulmonary artery catheter at 36 to 38 weeks of gestation, no difference was shown in the level of left ventricular filling pressure and left ventricular stroke work index compared with 11 to 13 weeks postpartum.[63]

Overall, left ventricular systolic function improves early in pregnancy and progresses gradually until 20 weeks' gestation. Because left ventricular systolic function directly correlates with changes in SVR, improvement in systolic function is most likely caused by left ventricular afterload reduction.

CARDIOCIRCULATORY CHANGES DURING LABOR AND DELIVERY

Women with cardiac disease require close monitoring during labor and delivery. Uterine contractions alone can transfer 300 to 500 mL of blood from the uterus to the general circulation and lead to significant circulatory stress.[161–164]

Effects on CO

CO increases up to 30% in the first stage of labor primarily because of increased stroke volume.[164,165] Maternal pushing efforts in the second stage of labor can increase CO by as

Table 2		
Changes in regional blood flow during normal pregnancy		
Organ	**Change**	**Comments**
Uterus	Increased	Increase from 50 mL/min at 10 wk to 1200 mL/min at term
Kidneys	Increased	30%–80% increase with 50% increase in GFR. Returns to nonpregnant state at term
Extremities	Increased	Flow to hands greater than flow to feet
Skin	Increased	Results in warm skin, clammy hands, nasal congestion
Liver	Unchanged	—
Brain	Unchanged	—
Breast	Increased	May cause flow murmurs

Abbreviation: GFR, glomerular filtration rate.

much as 50%. Laboring in the left lateral decubitus position or with epidural anesthesia reduces, but does not eliminate, this increase.[166,167]

Compression of the uterus with contractions results in an increase in circulating blood volume and venous return to the heart, with concomitant increase in stroke volume. Pulmonary arterial venous oxygen difference also increases with contractions, corroborating a flow of blood from the maternal uterine vascular bed into the systemic circulation.[168] Pain and anxiety leads to increased sympathetic tone with increased BP and HR, which also contributes to the increased CO.[161,163]

Effects on Maternal HR

In contrast with CO, the effects of contractions on maternal HR seem to be more variable. The observed differences in reported HR responses to uterine contractions relate to differences in maternal position and pain control during labor, as well as individual variation.[163,165–172]

Effects on Maternal BP

Both systolic and diastolic BPs increase with uterine contractions,[161–165,173,174] and this increase seems to precede a contraction by up to 8 seconds. The maximal increase occurs in the second stage of labor. Because peripheral resistance changes only slightly during labor, the increase in BP is attributed to increased CO.[163] As expected, the hemodynamic effects of uterine contractions are less pronounced in the left lateral recumbent position.[171] Oxygen consumption increases about 3-fold during uterine contractions, with its mean value increasing gradually to levels 100% higher than those before labor.[175,176]

Effects of Maternal Anesthesia

With local anesthesia, tachycardia may develop during the second stage of labor, which can be additive to the effect of uterine contractions. Both the systolic and diastolic BPs show a mild gradual increase during the first stage of labor and a significant increase during the second stage. These changes are associated with a progressive increase in stroke volume toward a peak immediately following delivery. In contrast, regional anesthesia is not associated with a significant change in HR or BP. Many patients with regional anesthesia have transient hypotension early on, which can be mitigated with preinduction volume load. Unlike local anesthesia, stroke volume with regional anesthesia remains constant throughout labor but increases rapidly after delivery. Mean blood loss does not seem to be affected by type of anesthesia at delivery.[164]

In patients with underlying cardiac disease, anesthesia during labor and delivery can pose unique challenges. Continuous lumbar epidural anesthesia with or without local anesthetics or narcotics, is frequently optimal. Limited sympathetic blockade and its effects on preload and afterload can be helpful in patients with mitral valve lesions. In patients with more complex lesions, anesthesia options must be considered on a case-by-case basis using a multidisciplinary approach.

HEMODYNAMIC EFFECTS OF CESAREAN SECTION

Transient maternal hypotension can occur in up to 30% of women undergoing regional anesthesia for cesarean section,[74] but most women undergoing cesarean section under epidural anesthesia remain stable hemodynamically. BP typically declines moderately after anesthesia induction, but then remains constant. In addition, HR, CO, and stroke volume remain constant. Following delivery, CO increases about 25% more than baseline, with a stable HR. In contrast, cesarean section under spinal anesthesia is associated with significant cardiovascular changes and should be used with extreme caution in patients with heart disease.[177–180]

Hemodynamic fluctuations during cesarean section were less with thiopental, nitrous oxide, and succinylcholine anesthesia.[178] Thus, balanced anesthesia with thiopental, nitrous oxide, and succinylcholine, or epidural anesthesia without epinephrine, are preferred in patients with limited cardiac reserves.

HEMODYNAMIC CHANGES POSTPARTUM

A 60% to 80% increase in CO occurs immediately after delivery, followed by a rapid decrease within 10 minutes to values approaching normal 1 hour postpartum. In addition, SVR decreases.[163,164,178,181,182] This high output state is likely caused by the transfer of blood from the uterus into the systemic circulation (autotransfusion) in conjunction with improved venous return caused by decreased vena caval compression and the rapid mobilization of extracellular fluid. Placental separation in the third stage of labor does not seem to cause any further hemodynamic changes. These changes are summarized in **Fig. 7**.

Even though childbirth can result in a mean blood loss of 1000 mL or more, patients are protected by the significant blood volume expansion

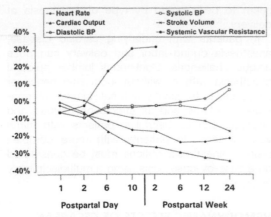

Fig. 7. Percent postpartum changes in hemodynamic parameters compared with 38 weeks of gestation. (*From* Robson SC, Hunter S, Moore M, et al. Haemodynamic changes during the puerperium: a Doppler and M-mode echocardiographic study. Br J Obstet Gynaecol 1987;94(11):1037; with permission.)

during pregnancy. In women with postpartum hemorrhage, stroke volume decreases and HR increases, whereas BP and CO remain stable.[183] Equally important, levels of ANP and BNP increase postpartum. Both ANP and BNP have potent diuretic effects, and help mediate the diuresis noted in the early postpartum period.[184]

REFERENCES

1. Dieckmann WJ, Wegner CR. The blood in normal pregnancy. I. Blood and plasma. Arch Intern Med 1934;53:71–86.
2. Berlin NI, Goetsch C, Hyde GM, et al. The blood volume in pregnancy as determined by P-32 labelled red blood cells. Surg Gynecol Obstet 1953;97:173–6.
3. Hytten FE, Pfaintain DB. Increase in plasma volume during normal pregnancy. J Obstet Gynaecol Br Commonw 1963;70:402–7.
4. Rovinsky JJ, Jaffin H. Cardiovascular hemodynamics in pregnancy. I. Blood and plasma volumes in multiple pregnancies. Am J Obstet Gynecol 1965;93:1–15.
5. Pritchard JA, Rowland RC. Blood volume changes in pregnancy and the puerperium. III. Whole body and large vessel hematocrits in pregnant and nonpregnant women. Am J Obstet Gynecol 1964; 88:391–5.
6. Lund CJ, Donovan JC. Blood volume during pregnancy. Am J Obstet Gynecol 1967;98:393–403.
7. Chesley LC. Plasma and red cell volumes during pregnancy. Am J Obstet Gynecol 1972;112:440–50.
8. Ueland K. Maternal cardiovascular dynamics. VII. Intrapartum blood volume changes. Am J Obstet Gynecol 1976;126:671–7.
9. Thomson KJ, Hirsheimer A, Gibson JC, et al. Studies on the circulation in pregnancy. III. Blood volume changes in normal pregnant women. Am J Obstet Gynecol 1938;36:48–59.
10. Roscoe MH, Donaldson GM. The blood in pregnancy. II. The blood volume, cell volume and haemoglobin mass. J Obstet Gynaecol Br Emp 1946; 53:527–38.
11. McLennan CE, Thouin LG. Blood volume in pregnancy. A critical review and preliminary report of result with a new technique. Am J Obstet Gynecol 1948;55:189–200.
12. Caton WL, Roby CC, Reid DE, et al. Plasma volume and extravascular fluid volume during pregnancy and the puerperium. Am J Obstet Gynecol 1949; 57:471–81.
13. Adams JQ. Cardiovascular physiology in normal pregnancy: studies with the dye dilution technique. Am J Obstet Gynecol 1954;67:741–59.
14. Rovinsky JJ. Blood volume and the hemodynamics of pregnancy. In: Philipp EE, Parnes J, Newton M, editors. Scientific foundation of obstetrics and gynaecology. Philadelphia: FA Davis; 1970. p. 332–40.
15. Hytten FE, Thomson AM. Maternal physiological adjustments. In: Assali NS, editor. Biology of gestation. New York: Academic Press; 1968. p. 449.
16. Pirani BB, Campbell DM, MacGillivary I. Plasma volume in normal first pregnancy. J Obstet Gynaecol Br Commonw 1973;80:884–7.
17. Goodlin RC, Dobry CA, Anderson JC, et al. Clinical signs of normal plasma volume expansion during pregnancy. Am J Obstet Gynecol 1983;145:1001–7.
18. Pritchard JA. Changes in the blood volume during pregnancy and delivery. Anesthesiology 1965;26: 393–9.
19. Brown MA, Zammit VC, Mitar DM. Extracellular fluid volumes in pregnancy induced hypertension. J Hypertens 1992;10:61–8.
20. Brown MA, Gallery ED. Volume homeostasis in normal pregnancy and preeclampsia: physiology and clinical implications. Baillieres Clin Obstet Gynaecol 1994;8:287–310.
21. Miller JR, Keith NM, Rownreel LG. Plasma and blood volume in pregnancy. JAMA 1915;65:779–82.
22. Thomsen JK, Fogh-Andersen N, Jaszczak P. Atrial natriuretic peptide, blood volume, aldosterone, and sodium excretion during twin pregnancies. Acta Obstet Gynecol Scand 1994;73:14–20.
23. Salas SP, Rosso P, Espinoza R, et al. Maternal plasma volume expansion and hormonal changes in women with idiopathic fetal growth retardation. Obstet Gynecol 1993;81:1029–33.
24. Jepson JH. Endocrine control of maternal and fetal erythropoiesis. Can Med Assoc J 1968;98:884.
25. Bille-Brahe NE, Rorth M. Red cell 2,3,-diphosphoglycerate in pregnancy. Acta Obstet Gynecol Scand 1979;58:19.

26. Duvekot JJ, Peeters LL. Renal hemodynamics and volume hemostasis in pregnancy. Obstet Gynecol Surv 1994;49:830–9.
27. Butler EB. The effect of iron and folic acid on red cell and plasma volume in pregnancy. J Obstet Gynaecol Br Commonw 1968;75:497–510.
28. Pritchard JA. Anemias complicating pregnancy and the puerperium. In: Committee on Maternal Nutrition/Food and Nutrition Board, National Research Council, editors. Maternal nutrition and the course of pregnancy. Washington, DC: National Academy of Sciences-National Research Council; 1970–1974. p. 1–21.
29. Carbillon L, Uzan M, Uzan S. Pregnancy, vascular tone, and maternal hemodynamics: a crucial adaptation. Obstet Gynecol Surv 2000;55(9):574–81.
30. Longo LD. Maternal blood volume and cardiac output during pregnancy: a hypothesis of endocrinologic control. Am J Physiol 1983;245:R720–9.
31. Friedlander M, Laskey N, Silbert S. Effect of estrogenic substance on blood volume. Endocrinology 1936;20:329–32.
32. Walters WA, Lim YL. Haemodynamic changes in women taking oral contraceptives. J Obstet Gynaecol Br Commonw 1970;77:1007–12.
33. Luotola H, Pyorala T, Lahteenmaki P, et al. Haemodynamic and hormonal effects of short-term oestradiol treatment in post-menopausal women. Maturitas 1979;1:287–94.
34. Varenhost E, Karlberg BE, Wallentin L, et al. Effects of oestrogens, orchidectomy and cyproterone acetate on salt and water metabolism in carcinoma of the prostate. Eur Urol 1981;7:231–6.
35. Bateman JC. A study of blood volume and anemia in cancer patients. Blood 1951;6:639–51.
36. Broughton Pipkin F. The renin-angiotensin system in normal and hypertensive pregnancies. In: Rubin PC, editor. Handbook of hypertension. 10. Hypertension in pregnancy. Amsterdam: Elsevier; 1988. p. 118–67.
37. Crane MG, Harris JJ. Plasma rennin activity and aldosterone excretion rate in normal subjects. II. Effect of oral contraceptive agents. J Clin Endocrinol Metab 1969;29:558–62.
38. Huseh WA, Luetscher JA, Carlson EJ, et al. Changes in active and inactive renin throughout pregnancy. J Clin Endocrinol Metab 1982;54:1010–6.
39. Tapia HR, Johnson CE, Strong CG. Effect of oral contraceptive therapy on the rennin-angiotensin system in normotensive and hypertensive women. Obstet Gynecol 1973;41:643–9.
40. Seitchik J. Total body water and total body density of pregnant women. J Obstet Gynecol 1967;29:155–66.
41. Preedy JR, Aitken EH. The effect of estrogen on water an electrolyte metabolism. I. The normal. J Clin Invest 1956;35:423–9.
42. Biglier EG, Forsham PH. Studies on the expanded extracellular fluid and the responses to various stimuli in primary aldosteronism. Am J Med 1961;30:564–76.
43. Dafnis E, Sabatini S. The effect of pregnancy on renal function: physiology and pathophysiology. Am J Med Sci 1992;303:184–205.
44. Fournier A, Gregoire I, El-Esper N, et al. Atrial natriuretic factors in pregnancy and pregnancy-induced hypertension. Can J Physiol Pharmacol 1991;69:1601–8.
45. Thomsen JK, Fogh-Andersen N, Jasczak P, et al. Atrial natriuretic peptide (ANP) decrease during normal pregnancy as related to hemodynamic changes and volume regulation. Acta Obstet Gynecol Scand 1993;72:103–10.
46. Levin ER, Gardner DG, Samson WK. Natriuretic peptides. N Engl J Med 1998;339:321.
47. Sabrane K, Kruse MN, Fabritz L, et al. Vascular endothelium is critically involved in the hypotensive and hypovolemic actions of atrial natriuretic peptide. J Clin Invest 2005;115:1666.
48. Sala C, Campise M, Ambroso G, et al. Atrial natriuretic peptide and hemodynamic changes during normal human pregnancy. Hypertension 1995;25:631–6.
49. Castro LC, Hobel CJ, Gornbein J. Plasma levels of atrial natriuretic peptide in normal and hypertensive pregnancies: a metaanalysis. Am J Obstet Gynecol 1994;171(6):1642–51.
50. Irons DW, Baylis PH, Davison JM. Atrial natriuretic peptide in normal and pre-eclamptic human pregnancy. Fetal Matern Med Rev 1997;9(4):209–21.
51. Adam B, Malatyalio Igbrevelu E, Alvur M, et al. Plasma atrial natriuretic peptide levels in preeclampsia and eclampsia. J Matern Fetal Investig 1998;8:85–8.
52. Stein BC, Levin RI. Natriuretic peptides: physiology, therapeutic potential, and risk stratification in ischemic heart disease. Am Heart J 1998;135:914–23.
53. Borghi C, Esposti DD, Immordino V, et al. Relationship of systemic hemodynamics, left ventricular structure and function, and plasma natriuretic peptide concentrations during pregnancy complicated by preeclampsia. Am J Obstet Gynecol 2000;183:140–7.
54. Carvajal JA, Delpiano AM, Cuello MA, et al. Brain natriuretic peptide (BNP) produced by the human chorioamnion may mediate pregnancy myometrial quiescence. Reprod Sci 2009;16(1):32–42.
55. Lev-Sagie A, Bar-Oz B, Salpeter L, et al. Plasma concentrations of N-terminal pro-B-type natriuretic peptide in pregnant women near labor and during early puerperium. Clin Chem 2005;51:1909–10.
56. Bar-Oz B, Lev-Sagie A, Arad I, et al. N-terminal pro-B-type natriuretic peptide concentrations in mothers just before delivery, in cord blood, and in newborns. Clin Chem 2005;51:926–7.

57. Flemin SM, O'Byrne L, Grimes H, et al. Amino-terminal pro-brain natriuretic peptide in normal and hypertensive pregnancy. Hypertens Pregnancy 2001;20(2):169–75.

58. Chesley LC, Duffus GM. Posture and apparent plasma volume in late pregnancy. J Obstet Gynaecol Br Commonw 1971;78:406–12.

59. Lindhard J. Über das Minutenvolumen des Herzens bei Ruhe und bei Muskelarbeit. Pfluegers Arch 1915;161:233–383 [in German].

60. Bader RA, Bader MG, Rose DJ, et al. Hemodynamics at rest and during exercise in normal pregnancy as studied by cardiac catheterization. J Clin Invest 1955;34:1524–36.

61. Walters WA, MacGregor WG, Hills M. Cardiac output at rest during pregnancy and the puerperium. Clin Sci 1966;30:1–11.

62. Lees MM, Taylor SH, Scott DB, et al. A study of cardiac output at rest throughout pregnancy. J Obstet Gynaecol Br Commonw 1967;74:319–28.

63. Clark SL, Cotton DB, Lee W, et al. Central hemodynamic assessment of normal term pregnancy. Am J Obstet Gynecol 1989;161:1439–42.

64. Robson SC, Hunter S, Boys RJ, et al. Serial study of factors influencing changes in cardiac output during human pregnancy. Am J Physiol 1989;256:H1060–5.

65. Robson SC, Hunter S, Boys RJ, et al. Hemodynamic changes during twin pregnancy: a Doppler and M-mode echocardiographic study. Am J Obstet Gynecol 1989;161:1272–8.

66. Mabie WC, DiSessa TG, Crocker LG, et al. A longitudinal study of cardiac output in normal human pregnancy. Am J Obstet Gynecol 1994;170:849–56.

67. Vered Z, Poler SM, Gibson P, et al. Noninvasive detection of the morphologic and hemodynamic changes during normal pregnancy. Clin Cardiol 1991;14:327–34.

68. Capeless EL, Clapp JF. Cardiovascular changes in early phase of pregnancy. Am J Obstet Gynecol 1989;161:1449–53.

69. Easterling TR, Benedetti TJ, Schmucker BC, et al. Maternal hemodynamics in normal and preeclamptic pregnancies: a longitudinal study. Obstet Gynecol 1990;76:1061–9.

70. Ueland K, Novy MJ, Peterson EN, et al. Maternal cardiovascular dynamics. IV. The influence of gestational age on the maternal cardiovascular response to posture and exercise. Am J Obstet Gynecol 1969;104:856–65.

71. Kerr MG. Cardiovascular dynamics in pregnancy and labour. Br Med Bull 1968;24:19–24.

72. Lees HM, Taylor SH, Scott BD, et al. The circulatory effect of recumbent postural change in late pregnancy. Clin Sci 1967;32:453–65.

73. Masaki DI, Greenspoon JG, Ouzounian JG. Measurement of cardiac output in pregnancy by thoracic electrical bioimpedance and thermodilution. Am J Obstet Gynecol 1989;161:680–4.

74. Ouzounian JG, Masaki DI, Abboud TA, et al. Systemic vascular resistance index determined by thoracic electrical bioimpedance predicts the risk for maternal hypotension during regional anesthesia for cesarean delivery. Am J Obstet Gynecol 1996;174:1019.

75. Mashini IS, Albazzaz SJ, Fadel HE, et al. Serial noninvasive evaluation of cardiovascular hemodynamics in pregnancy. Am J Obstet Gynecol 1987;156:1208.

76. Ihlen H, Amlie JP, Dale J, et al. Determination of cardiac output by Doppler echocardiography. Br Heart J 1984;54:51.

77. Easterling TR, Watts H, Schmucker BC, et al. Measurement of cardiac output during pregnancy: validation of Doppler technique and clinical observations in preeclampsia. Obstet Gynecol 1987;69:845.

78. Easterling TR, Carlson KL, Schmucker BC, et al. Measurement of cardiac output in pregnancy by Doppler technique. Am J Perinatol 1990;7:220.

79. Castor G, Klocke K, Stoll M, et al. Simultaneous measurement of cardiac output by thermodilution, thoracic electrical bioimpedance, and Doppler ultrasound. Br J Anaesth 1994;72:133–8.

80. Gotshall RW, Wood VC, Miles DS. Comparison of two impedance cardiographic techniques for measuring cardiac output in critically ill patients. Crit Care Med 1989;17:806–11.

81. Young JD, McQuillan P. Comparison of thoracic electrical bioimpedance and thermodilution for the measurement of cardiac index in patients with severe sepsis. Br J Anaesth 1993;70:58–62.

82. Kim YI, Chandra P, Marx GF. Successful management of severe aortocaval compression in twin pregnancy. Obstet Gynecol 1975;46:362–4.

83. Ueland K, Metcalfe J. Circulatory changes in pregnancy. Clin Obstet Gynecol 1975;18:41–50.

84. Rubler S, Prabodhkumar MD, Pinto ER. Cardiac size and performance during pregnancy: estimates with echocardiography. Clin Obstet Gynecol 1977;40:534–40.

85. Katz R, Karliner JS, Resnik R. Effects of a natural volume overload state (pregnancy) on left ventricular performance in normal human subjects. Circulation 1978;58:434–41.

86. Christianson RE. Studies on blood pressure during pregnancy. I. Influence on parity and age. Am J Obstet Gynecol 1976;125:509–13.

87. MacGillivary I. Hypertension in pregnancy and its consequences. J Obstet Gynaecol Br Commonw 1961;68:557–69.

88. Lee W. Cardiorespiratory alterations during normal pregnancy. Crit Care Clin 1991;7:763–75.

89. Shenan A, Gupta M, Halligan A, et al. Lack of reproducibility in pregnancy of Korotkoff phase IV as measured by mercury sphygmomanometry. Lancet 1996;347:139–42.

90. Brown MA, Recter L, Smith B, et al. Measuring blood pressure in pregnant women: a comparison of direct and indirect methods. Am J Obstet Gynecol 1994;171:661–7.

91. Blank SG, Helseth G, Pickering TG, et al. How should diastolic blood pressure be defined during pregnancy? Hypertension 1994;24:234–40.

92. Sherman AH, Kissane J, deSwiet M. Validation of the Spacelab 90207 ambulatory blood pressure monitor for use in pregnancy. Br J Obstet Gynaecol 1993;100:904–8.

93. Easterling TR. Cardiovascular physiology of the normal pregnancy. In: Gleicher N, editor. Principles and practice of medical therapy in pregnancy. 3rd edition. Norwalk (CT): Appleton & Lange; 1992. p. 762–6.

94. Lindheimer MD. Hypertension in pregnancy. Hypertension 1993;22:127–37.

95. Gifford R. Working group report on high blood pressure in pregnancy. Bethesda (MD): NIH Publications; 2000. No. 00-3029.

96. Kerr MG. The mechanical effects of the gravid uterus in late pregnancy. J Obstet Gynaecol Br Commonw 1965;72:513–29.

97. Bieniarz J, Mapueda E, Caldeyro-Barcia R. Compression of aorta by the uterus in late human pregnancy. I. Variations between femoral and brachial artery pressure with changes from hypertension to hypotension. Am J Obstet Gynecol 1966;95:795–808.

98. Bieniarz J, Crottongini JJ, Curuchet E, et al. Aortocaval compression by the uterus in late human pregnancy. II. An angiographic study. Am J Obstet Gynecol 1968;100:203–17.

99. Holmes F. Incidence of the supine hypotensive syndrome in late pregnancy. A clinical study in 500 subjects. J Obstet Gynaecol Br Emp 1960;67:254–8.

100. Pirhonen JP, Erkkola RU. Uterine and umbilical flow velocity waveforms in the supine hypotensive syndrome. Obstet Gynecol 1990;76:176–9.

101. Kinsella SM, Lohmann G. Supine hypotensive syndrome. Obstet Gynecol 1994;83:774–88.

102. Arbitol MM. Inferior vena cava compression in the pregnant dog. Am J Obstet Gynecol 1978;130:194–8.

103. Hirabayashi Y, Saitoh K, Fukuda H, et al. An unusual supine hypotensive syndrome during cesarean section: the importance of trying right tilt if there is a poor response to left tilt. Masui 1994;43:1590–2.

104. Gilson GJ, Samaan S, Crawford MH, et al. Changes in hemodynamics, ventricular remodeling, and ventricular contractility during normal pregnancy: a longitudinal study. Obstet Gynecol 1997;89:957.

105. Greiss FC, Anderson SG. Effect of ovarian hormones on the uterine vascular bed. Am J Obstet Gynecol 1970;107:829–36.

106. Duvekot JJ, Cheriex EC, Pieters FA, et al. Early pregnancy changes in hemodynamics and volume homeostasis are consecutive adjustments triggered by a primary fall in systemic vascular tone. Am J Obstet Gynecol 1993;169:1382–92.

107. Spaanderman ME, Willekes C, Hoeks APG, et al. The effect of pregnancy on the compliance of large arteries and veins in healthy parous control subjects and women with a history of preeclampsia. Am J Obstet Gynecol 2000;183:1278.

108. Walters WA, Lim YL. Cardiovascular dynamics in women receiving oral contraceptive therapy. Lancet 1969;2:879–81.

109. Bryant EE, Douglas BH, Ashburn AD. Circulatory changes following prolactin administration. Am J Obstet Gynecol 1973;115:53–7.

110. Gerber JG, Payne NA, Murphy RC, et al. Prostacyclin produced by the pregnant uterus in the dog may act as a circulating vasodepressor substance. J Clin Invest 1981;67:632–6.

111. Van Assche FA. The role of prostacyclin and thromboxane in pregnancy. Verh K Acad Geneeskd Belg 1990;52:105–25.

112. Schrier RW, Briner VA. Peripheral arterial vasodilation hypothesis of sodium and water retention in pregnancy: implications for pathogenesis of preeclampsia-eclampsia. Obstet Gynecol 1991;77:632–9.

113. Allen R, Castro L, Arora C, et al. Endothelium-derived relaxing factor inhibition and the pressor response to norepinephrine in the pregnant rat. Obstet Gynecol 1994;83:92–6.

114. Brown GP, Venuto RC. Angiotensin II receptor alterations during pregnancy in rabbits. Am J Physiol 1986;251:E58–64.

115. Paller MS. Mechanisms of decreased pressor responsiveness to ANG II, NE and vasopressin in pregnant rats. Am J Physiol 1984;247:H100–8.

116. Podjarney E, Mandelbaum A, Bernheim J. Does nitric-oxide play a role in normal pregnancy and pregnancy-induced hypertension? Nephrol Dial Transplant 1994;9:1527–40.

117. Ylikorla O, Makila UM. Prostacyclin and thromboxane in gynecology and obstetrics. Am J Obstet Gynecol 1985;152:318–29.

118. Anggard EE. Nitric oxide: mediator, murderer, and medicine. Lancet 1994;343:1199–206.

119. Ramsay B, De Belder A, Campbell S, et al. A nitric oxide donor improves uterine artery diastolic blood flow in normal early pregnancy and in women at high risk for preeclampsia. Eur J Clin Invest 1994;24:76–8.

120. Thaler I, Amit A, Jakobi P, et al. The effect of isosorbide dinitrate on uterine artery and umbilical artery

flow velocity waveforms at mid-pregnancy. Obstet Gynecol 1996;88:838–43.

121. McGuane JT, Debrah JE, Debrah DO, et al. Role of relaxin in maternal systemic and renal vascular adaptations during gestation. Ann N Y Acad Sci 2009;1160:304–12.

122. Dschietzig T, Bartsch C, Richter C, et al. Relaxin, a pregnancy hormone, is a functional endothelin-1 antagonist. Circ Res 2003;92:32–40.

123. Dschietzig T, Richter C, Bartsch C, et al. The pregnancy hormone relaxin is a player in human heart failure. FASEB J 2001;15:2187–95.

124. Bryant-Greenwood GD, Schwabe C. Human relaxins: chemistry and biology. Endocr Rev 1994;15:5–26.

125. Lanni SM, Tillinghast J, Silver HM. Hemodynamic changes and baroreflex gain in the supine hypotensive syndrome. Am J Obstet Gynecol 2002; 187:1636–41.

126. Howard BK, Goodson JH, Mengert WF. Supine hypotensive syndrome in late pregnancy. Obstet Gynecol 1953;1:371–7.

127. Kerr MG, Scott DB, Samuel E. Studies of the inferior vena cava in late pregnancy. Br Med J 1964; 1:532–3.

128. Assali NS, Rauramo L, Peltonen T. Measurement of uterine blood flow and uterine metabolism. VIII. Uterine and fetal blood flow and oxygen consumption in early human pregnancy. Am J Obstet Gynecol 1960;79:86–98.

129. Metcalfe J, Romney SL, Ramsey LH, et al. Estimation of uterine blood flow in normal human pregnancy at term. J Clin Invest 1955;34:1632–8.

130. Jurkovic D, Jauniaux E, Kurjak A, et al. Transvaginal color Doppler assessment of the uteroplacental circulation in early pregnancy. Obstet Gynecol 1991;77:365–9.

131. Jaffe R, Warsof SL. Transvaginal color Doppler imaging in the assessment of uteroplacental blood flow in the normal. First-trimester pregnancy. Am J Obstet Gynecol 1991;164:781–5.

132. Kaminopetros P, Higueras MT, Nicolaides KH. Doppler study of uterine artery blood flow; comparison of findings in the first and second trimesters of pregnancy. Fetal Diagn Ther 1991;6:58–64.

133. Bewley S, Cooper P, Campbell S. Doppler investigation of uteroplacental blood flow resistance in the second trimester: a screening study for preeclampsia and intrauterine growth retardation. Br J Obstet Gynaecol 1991;98:871–9.

134. Palmer SU, Zamudio S, Coffin C, et al. Quantitative estimation of human uterine artery blood slow and pelvic blood flow redistribution in pregnancy. Obstet Gynecol 1992;80:1000–6.

135. Kofinas AD, Espeland MA, Penry M, et al. Uteroplacental Doppler flow velocity waveform indices in normal pregnancy: a statistical exercise and the development of appropriate reference values. Am J Perinatol 1992;9:94–101.

136. Boura AL, Walters WA, Read MA, et al. Autacoids and control of human placental blood flow. Clin Exp Pharmacol Physiol 1994;21:737–48.

137. Ferris TF, Stein JH, Kauffman J. Uterine blood flow and uterine rennin secretion. J Clin Invest 1972;51:2827–33.

138. Myers SA, Sparks JW, Makowski EC. Relationship between placental blood flow and placental and fetal size in guinea pig. Am J Physiol 1982;243: H404–9.

139. Hohimer AR, Bissonnette JM, Metcalfe J, et al. Effect of exercise on uterine blood flow in the pregnant pygmy goat. Am J Physiol 1984;246:H207–12.

140. Erkokola RN, Pirhonen JP, Kivijarvi AK. Flow velocity waveform in uterine and umbilical arteries during submaximal bicycle exercise in normal pregnancy. Obstet Gynecol 1992;79:611–5.

141. Nunlap W. Serial changes in renal hemodynamics during normal human pregnancy. Br J Obstet Gynaecol 1981;88:1–9.

142. Lindheimer MD, Katz AI. The kidney in pregnancy. In: Brenner RM, Rector FC, editors. The kidney. 4th edition. Philadelphia: WB Saunders; 1988. p. 1253.

143. Krutzen E, Olofsson P, Back SE, et al. Glomerular filtration rate in pregnancy: a study in normal subjects and in patients with hypertension, preeclampsia, and diabetes. Scand J Clin Lab Invest 1992;52:387–92.

144. Davidson JM, Dunlop W. Changes in renal hemodynamics and tubular function induced by normal human pregnancy. Semin Nephrol 1984;4: 198–207.

145. Fainstat T. Ureteral dilatation in pregnancy: a review. Obstet Gynecol Surv 1963;18:845–60.

146. Gallery ED, Ross M, Grigg R, et al. Are the renal functional changes of human pregnancy caused by prostacyclin? Prostaglandins 1985;30:1019–29.

147. Ginsburg J, Duncan SL. Peripheral blood flow in normal pregnancy. Cardiovasc Res 1967;1:132–7.

148. Katz M, Sokal MM. Skin perfusion in pregnancy. Am J Obstet Gynecol 1980;137:30–3.

149. Beinder E, Huch A, Huch R. Peripheral skin temperature and microcirculatory reactivity during pregnancy. A study with thermography. J Perinat Med 1990;18:383–90.

150. Bean WB, Dexter MW, Congswell RC. Vascular changes of skin in pregnancy. Surg Gynecol Obstet 1949;88:739–52.

151. Fabricant ND. Sexual functions and the nose. Am J Med Sci 1960;239:498–502.

152. Howard DJ. Life-threatening epistaxis in pregnancy. J Laryngol Otol 1985;99:95–9.

153. Pickles VR. Blood flow estimations as indices of mammary activity. J Obstet Gynaecol Br Emp 1953;60:301–11.

154. Mannell EW, Taylor HC Jr. Liver blood flow in pregnancy. Hepatic vein catheterization. J Clin Invest 1947;26:952–6.

155. McCall ML. Cerebral blood flow and metabolism in toxemias of pregnancy. Surg Gynecol Obstet 1949; 89:715–21.

156. Elkus R, Popovich J. Respiratory physiology in pregnancy. Clin Chest Med 1992;13:555–65.

157. Metcalfe J, Ueland K. The heart and pregnancy. In: Hurst JW, Logue RB, Schlant RC, et al, editors. The heart arteries and veins. New York: McGraw-Hill; 1978. p. 1721–34.

158. Rubler S, Damani P, Pinto E. Cardiac size and performance during pregnancy estimated with echocardiography. Am J Cardiol 1977;49:534–8.

159. Lard-Meeter K, van de Ley G, Bom T, et al. Cardiocirculatory adjustments during pregnancy: an echocardiographic study. Clin Cardiol 1979;49:560–5.

160. Kametas NA, McAuliffe F, Cook B, et al. Maternal left ventricular transverse and long axis systolic function during pregnancy. Ultrasound Obstet Gynecol 2001;18:467–74.

161. Henricks CH, Quilligan EJ. Cardiac output during labor. Am J Obstet Gynecol 1956;71:953–72.

162. Burch GE. Heart disease and pregnancy. Am Heart J 1977;93:104–16.

163. Adams JG, Alexander AM. Alterations in cardiovascular physiology during labor. Obstet Gynecol 1958;12:542–9.

164. Ueland K, Hansen JM. Maternal cardiovascular dynamics. III. Labor and delivery under local and caudal analgesia. Am J Obstet Gynecol 1969;103:8–18.

165. Robson C, Dunlop W, Boys RJ, et al. Cardiac output during labour. Br Med J (Clin Res Ed) 1987;295:1169–72.

166. Lee W, Rokey R, Cotton DB, et al. Maternal hemodynamics effects of uterine contractions by M-mode and pulsed-Doppler echocardiography. Am J Obstet Gynecol 1989;161:974–7.

167. Ueland K, Hansen JM. Maternal cardiovascular dynamics. II. Posture and uterine contractions. Am J Obstet Gynecol 1969;103:1–7.

168. Hamilton HF. Blood viscosity in pregnancy. J Obstet Gynaecol Br Emp 1950;57:530–8.

169. Rose DJ, Bader ME, Bader RA, et al. Catheterization studies of cardiac hemodynamics in normal and pregnant women with reference to left ventricular work. Am J Obstet Gynecol 1956;72:233–46.

170. Goeltner E, Quade C. Intrathorakaler Venendruck, Pulse und atmung während der Eröffnungswehen. Gynaecologia 1967;163:235–40 [in German].

171. Kjeldsen J. Hemodynamic investigations during labor and delivery. Acta Obstet Gynecol Scand 1979;89(Suppl):10–252.

172. Henricks CH. The hemodynamics of uterine contraction. Am J Obstet Gynecol 1958;76:969–81.

173. Cunningham I. Cardiovascular physiology of labor and delivery. J Obstet Gynaecol Br Commonw 1966;73:498–503.

174. Hansen JM, Ueland K. The influence of caudal analgesia on cardiovascular dynamics during normal labor and delivery. Acta Anaesthesiol Scand 1966;23(Suppl):449–52.

175. Wult KH, Kunzel W, Lehmann V. Clinical aspects of placental gas exchange. In: Longo LD, Bartels H, editors. Respiratory gas exchange and blood flow in the placenta. Bethesda (MD): US Department of Health, Education and Welfare; 1972. p. 505–21 US Dept of Health, Education and Welfare publication NIH 73-36.

176. Midwall J, Jaffin H, Herman MB, et al. Shunt flow and pulmonary hemodynamics during labor and delivery in Eisenmenger's syndrome. Am J Cardiol 1978;42:299–303.

177. Ueland K, Gills RE, Hansen JM. Maternal cardiovascular dynamics. I. Cesarean section under subarachnoid block anesthesia. Am J Obstet Gynecol 1968;100:42–54.

178. Ueland K, Hansen J, Eng M, et al. Maternal cardiovascular dynamics. V. Cesarean section under thiopental, nitrous oxide, and succinylcholine anesthesia. Am J Obstet Gynecol 1970;108: 615–22.

179. Ueland K, Akamatsu TJ, Eng M, et al. Maternal cardiovascular dynamics. VI. Cesarean section under epidural anesthesia without epinephrine. Am J Obstet Gynecol 1972;114:775–80.

180. Tihtonen K, Koobi T, Ylihankala A, et al. Maternal hemodynamics during cesarean delivery assessed by whole body impedance cardiography. Acta Obstet Gynecol Scand 2005;84:355–61.

181. Robson SC, Dunlop W. Hemodynamic changes during the early puerperium. Br Med J 1987;294: 1065.

182. Robson SC, Hunter S, Moore M, et al. Hemodynamic changes during the puerperium: a Doppler and M-mode echocardiographic study. Br J Obstet Gynaecol 1987;94:1028–35.

183. Robson SC, Boys RJ, Hunter S, et al. Maternal hemodynamics after normal delivery and delivery complicated by postpartum hemorrhage. Obstet Gynecol 1989;74:234–99.

184. Pouta AM, Raasanen JP, Airaksinen KEJ, et al. Changes in maternal heart dimensions and plasma atrial natriuretic peptide levels in the early puerperium of normal and preeclamptic pregnancies. BJOG 1996;103(10):988–92.

Cardiovascular Imaging and Diagnostic Procedures in Pregnancy

David L. Ain, MD, Jagat Narula, MD, PhD,
Partho P. Sengupta, MD*

KEYWORDS

- Cardiovascular imaging • Pregnancy • Echocardiography • CT • MRI • Ionizing radiation
- Coronary angiography

KEY POINTS

- Echocardiography is a useful initial imaging study in pregnant patients with signs or symptoms concerning for cardiac pathology. Transesophageal echocardiography can be used safely in pregnant women to diagnose aortic dissection.
- MRI studies with contrast can be considered for use in pregnancy only if determined to be essential and in specific situations, such as aortic syndromes, myocarditis, and cardiomyopathies.
- Imagining studies that involve exposure of pregnant women to ionizing radiation should be done only after informed consent is obtained.
- In selected situations, CT may be useful in pregnant patients with suspected pulmonary embolism or coronary artery disease, whereas direct coronary angiogram may be indicated in patients with acute coronary syndrome.

Cardiovascular disorders in the pregnant woman can pose challenges for diagnosis and management.[1] When the history or physical examination suggests a disease state, imaging studies are frequently considered. Diagnostic imaging procedures including echocardiography, chest radiography, angiography, computed tomography (CT), and cardiovascular magnetic resonance (MR) imaging may be indicated in the pregnant patient. Concerns related to the safety of these tests, specifically the possible effects of exposure to ionizing radiation and the use of intravenous contrast agents on fetal development and subsequent risk of malignancy, must be balanced against the importance of accurate diagnosis and assessment of a pathologic state. Such a calculus requires an understanding of the normal physiology of pregnancy, manifestations of preexisting cardiac disease in the pregnant woman, and signs and symptoms of nascent cardiovascular disease in pregnancy. Additionally the cardiologist must understand indications for and limitations of each diagnostic imaging test, potential harmful effects of various modalities, and precautions that must be taken to protect the fetus. Pregnancy among women with congenital heart disease is more common than in previous years,[2] and in this group the physiologic alterations can be significant. Cyanotic defects place mother and fetus at extremely high risk. In patients with these lesions, reliance on the history and clinical examination is most often not sufficient for assessment of cardiovascular status, and imaging studies—sometimes performed serially—become necessary throughout gestation. Other cardiovascular conditions are also high risk. These include pulmonary hypertension; dilated cardiomyopathy, especially with heart failure; Marfan syndrome, particularly with dilated

Disclosures: D.L. Ain, none; J. Narula, none; P.P. Sengupta, none.
The Zena and Michael A. Wiener Cardiovascular Institute, Mount Sinai School of Medicine, One Gustave L. Levy Place, Box 1030, New York, NY 10029, USA
* Corresponding author.
E-mail address: partho.sengupta@mssm.edu

Cardiol Clin 30 (2012) 331–341
doi:10.1016/j.ccl.2012.05.002
0733-8651/12/$ – see front matter © 2012 Elsevier Inc. All rights reserved.

aortic root; the presence of a prosthetic heart valve; coarctation of the aorta; and, obstructive valvular lesions. Assessment of the cardiovascular system in pregnant women with these conditions or with concerning symptoms or signs relies on the imaging techniques discussed in this article.

IONIZING RADIATION IN PREGNANCY

Perhaps the most anxiety-inducing aspect of diagnostic imaging in pregnant patients—for patients and clinicians—is the use of modalities that employ ionizing radiation. Major concerns involve potential increased risk of pregnancy loss, teratogenesis, growth retardation, cognitive and behavior abnormalities, and carcinogenesis after fetal exposure to radiation. Fortunately, the majority of diagnostic procedures that use radiation carry minimal risk to the fetus. The effects that radiation can have on the fetus depend on the gestational age and the dose of radiation.[3–5] Many of the data in this area have been extrapolated from studies of people who had a history of exposure in utero to radiation after detonation of the atomic bombs at Hiroshima and Nagasaki.[6–8] In general, exposure to doses less than 5 rad (50 mGy) is thought to have no untoward effects on a developing fetus, and doses less than 10 rad are thought to have risks so low that intervention is not warranted.[3] This dose level is higher than that caused by many common diagnostic studies. A 2-view series of chest radiographs, for example, exposes a fetus to 0.02 mrad to 0.07 mrad, whereas a single abdominal radiograph and CT scan of the abdomen and lumbar spine expose a fetus to 100 mrad and 3.5 rad, respectively.[3,9–11] The US Nuclear Regulatory Commission recommends that occupational radiation exposure of pregnant women not exceed 5 mGy (500 mrad) to the embryo/fetus during the entire pregnancy.[12]

Exposure in First 2 Weeks

During the first 2 weeks after conception, the developing embryo is most susceptible to ionizing radiation, and exposure to higher doses of radiation during this early period before implantation results in either destruction of the embryo or no detectable abnormalities.[5,13] Radiation-induced teratogenesis, growth restriction, or carcinogenesis is not observed during this stage of development,[14] presumably because of the pluripotent nature of each cell of the very early embryo.

For human exposure, a conservative estimate of the threshold for death at this stage is more than 0.1 Gy (10 rad).[15] A fetal dose of 1 Gy (100 rad) will likely kill 50% of embryos; the dose necessary to kill 100% of human embryos or fetuses before 18

weeks of gestation is approximately 5 Gy (500 rad) (Table 1).

Exposure After 2 Weeks

Major organogenesis occurs during weeks 3 to 8 after conception; during this period, exposure to radiation above a threshold level can potentially lead to malformations and growth restriction.[3] This threshold level is likely greater than 10 rad; one article, published in 2009, estimated that the risk of gross malformations is unchanged from baseline until the fetus is exposed to 20 rad.[16] The risk of mental retardation is greatest during weeks 8 to 15, with continued risk from weeks 15 to 25 and possibly thereafter[5,11]; however, the risks to the developing central nervous system beyond 15 weeks likely exist only at high doses (greater than 20 rad).[3]

Antenatal exposure to radiation, particularly in the last trimester, is associated with increased risk of cancer in childhood (Table 2).[17–19] Although the effect of radiation on risk of pregnancy loss, malformation, growth restriction, and cognitive impairment is thought deterministic—that is, related to doses above a threshold level, risk of carcinogenesis is thought stochiastic—related to random, mutagenic events.[19] One review concluded that risk of childhood cancer begins after exposure to doses as low as 1 rad and that each additional 100-rad exposure increases the risk by 6% above the baseline rate, which is 3.6 per 10,000.[13,19]

Current guidelines emphasize the low risk of untoward effects of radiation with doses less than 10 rad or 15 rad.[3] Fortunately, most cardiac imaging procedures expose fetuses to much less radiation. When in doubt, consultation with a medical physicist is appropriate. General recommendations regarding imaging studies that involve exposure of pregnant women to ionizing radiation include obtaining informed consent and minimizing the amount of exposure.

ECHOCARDIOGRAPHY

Ultrasonography is considered safe for the fetus at all gestational ages[20] and is, therefore, a reasonable initial imaging study in patients with signs or symptoms concerning for cardiac pathology. An understanding of both hemodynamic alterations and anatomic changes that occur during pregnancy is key to interpretation of echocardiograms in pregnant patients. The heart is displaced anteriorly and leftward, facilitating transthoracic parasternal and apical echocardiographic windows.[21] The heart enlarges throughout gestation; the right-sided chambers increase in size by 20% and the left atrium and left ventricle by 12% and

Table 1
Potential health effects (other than cancer) of prenatal radiation exposure

Acute Radiation Dose[a] to the Embryo/Fetus[b]	Time Postconception				
	Blastogenesis (up to 2 wk)	Organogenesis (2–7 wk)	Fetogenesis		
			(8–15 wk)	(16–25 wk)	(26–38 wk)
<0.05 Gy (5 rad)	Noncancer health effects NOT detectable				
0.05–0.50 Gy (5–50 rad)	Incidence of failure to implant may increase slightly, but surviving embryos probably have no significant (noncancer) health effects	• Incidence of major malformations may increase slightly • Growth retardation possible	• Growth retardation possible • Reduction in IQ possible (up to 15 points, depending on dose) • Incidence of severe mental retardation up to 20%, depending on dose	Noncancer health effects unlikely	
>0.50 Gy (50 rad); the expectant mother may be experiencing acute radiation syndrome in this range, depending on her whole-body dose.	Incidence of failure to implant likely is large,[c] depending on dose, but surviving embryos probably have no significant (noncancer) health effects	• Incidence of miscarriage may increase, depending on dose • Substantial risk of major malformations, such as neurologic and motor deficiencies • Growth retardation likely	• Incidence of miscarriage probably increases, depending on dose • Growth retardation likely • Reduction in IQ possible (>15 points, depending on dose) • Incidence of severe mental retardation >20%, depending on dose • Incidence of major malformations probably increases	• Incidence of miscarriage may increase, depending on dose • Growth retardation possible, depending on dose • Reduction in IQ possible, depending on dose • Severe mental retardation possible, depending on dose • Incidence of major malformations may increase	• Incidence of miscarriage and neonatal death probably increases depending on dose[d]

Note: This table is intended only as a guide. The indicated doses and times postconception are approximations.
[a] Acute dose: dose delivered in a short time (usually minutes). Fractionated or chronic doses: doses delivered over time. For fractionated or chronic doses the health effects to the fetus may differ from what is depicted here.
[b] Both the gray (Gy) and the rad are units of absorbed dose and reflect the amount of energy deposited into a mass of tissue (1 Gy = 100 rad). In this document, the absorbed dose is that dose received by the entire fetus (whole-body fetal dose). The referenced absorbed dose levels in this document are assumed to be from β-, γ-, or x-radiation. Neutron or proton radiation produces many of the health effects described herein at lower absorbed dose levels.
[c] A fetal dose of 1 Gy (100 rad) will likely kill 50% of the embryos. The dose necessary to kill 100% of human embryos or fetuses before 18 weeks' gestation is approximately 5 Gy (500 rad).
[d] For adults, the lethal dose (LD)50/60 (the dose necessary to kill 50% of the exposed population in 60 days) is approximately 3–5 Gy (300–500 rad) and the LD100 (the dose necessary to kill 100% of the exposed population) is approximately 10 Gy (1000 rad).
Centers for Disease Control and Prevention.

Table 2
Estimated risk for cancer from prenatal radiation exposure

Radiation Dose	Estimated Childhood Cancer Incidence[a,b]	Estimated Lifetime[c] Cancer Incidence[d] (Exposure at Age 10)
No radiation exposure above background	0.3%	38%
0.00–0.05 Gy (0–5 rad)	0.3%–1%	38%–40%
0.05–0.50 Gy (5–50 rad)	1%–6%	40%–55%
>0.50 Gy (50 rad)	>6%	>55%

[a] Data published by the International Commission on Radiation Protection.
[b] Childhood cancer mortality is approximately half of childhood cancer incidence.
[c] The lifetime cancer risks from prenatal radiation exposure are not yet known. The lifetime risk estimates given are for Japanese males exposed at age 10 years from models published by the United Nations Scientific Committee on the Effects of Atomic Radiation.
[d] Lifetime cancer mortality is approximately one-third of lifetime cancer incidence.

10%, respectively. In late pregnancy, the enlarged uterus can compress structures superior to it, leading to the appearance of posterior wall motion.[22] During gestation, a small pericardial effusion is not necessarily indicative of pathology; however, hemodynamically significant effusions should not be considered normal.

There is an early, progressive, and marked increase in left ventricular stroke volume throughout pregnancy.[23,24] This increase can appear as a high-output state, and one effect of the augmented stroke volume is increased velocity across valves, which may falsely increase systolic or diastolic gradients (**Fig. 1**).[25] As the heart enlarges, the mitral,

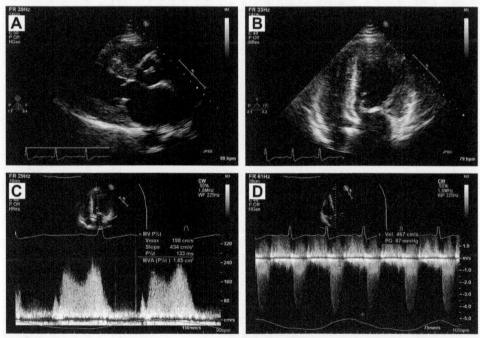

Fig. 1. Transthoracic echocardiogram of a 29-year-old pregnant woman at 36 weeks' gestation. The patient had known rheumatic valve disease, and she developed increased dyspnea with exertion during this pregnancy. This study showed rheumatic mitral valve disease (A, B) with moderate mitral valve stenosis (C). There was also mild aortic commisural fusion with severe valvular aortic stenosis (with a worsening gradient possibly due in part to increased cardiac output) (D). The study also revealed mild aortic regurgitation, concentric left ventricular hypertrophy, and hyperdynamic left ventricular function. She was treated with increased doses of a diutetic and labetalol. Forceps-assisted vaginal delivery was used to reduce Valsalva maneuvers. The patient and her child did well after delivery.

tricuspid, and pulmonary annuli dilate, and there is a concomitant increase in functional regurgitation through these valves.[26] As left ventricular volume increases and the position of the mitral valve leaflets change with respect to one another, pre-existing mitral regurgitation due to mitral valve prolapse may actually improve during pregnancy.[18]

Several conditions are diagnosed and can be followed by echocardiography throughout pregnancy (Table 3). Peripartum cardiomyopathy can develop during pregnancy or up to several months postpartum. Risk factors include twin pregnancy, high parity and gravity, and extremes of reproductive age.[27] Women commonly present with dyspnea, edema, and fatigue, with findings of biventricular failure on examination. The echocardiogram is fundamental to diagnosis, and it should be the initial test in women with history and examination concerning for heart failure. Echocardiography typically shows global cardiac dilation and reduced left ventricular function, consistent with—and often indistinguishable from—other forms of dilated cardiomyopathy. Left ventricular diastolic assessment often shows a restrictive pattern, and mitral and tricuspic regurgitation can be severe.[27]

Women with signs or symptoms of hypertrophic cardiomyopathy should also be evaluated with transthoracic echocardiography, because this condition is associated with complications in pregnancy.[28] Echocardiography can be used to confirm the diagnosis. In patients with hypertrophic obstructive cardiomyopathy there is typically an asymmetric, hypertrophic myocardium; the septum is disproportionally thick.[29] During rest or with Valsalva, Doppler echocardiography shows a high-velocity jet across the left ventricular outflow tract, consistent with obstruction.[29]

Mitral valve stenosis is the most common valve disease complicating pregnancy, and the normal hemodynamic changes associated with pregnancy can increase the pressure gradient across the valve (see Fig. 1).[30,31] Mitral valve prolapse is common in the general population[32] and, therefore, not infrequently discovered during physical examination of pregnant women. Because of the normal changes in the auscultatory examination (described previously), mitral valve prolapse should be confirmed by echocardiography.

Serial echocardiography is recommended for women with Marfan syndrome who elect to continue with a pregnancy.[33] If possible, these studies should be compared to a study done prior to conception to evaluate for progressive dilation of the aorta, with the caveat that dissection can occur in a nondilated aorta.[34,35] Although most cases of aortic dissection in pregnancy occur in women with Marfan syndrome,[34,35] women without connective tissue disease are also at risk, usually in the third trimester.[36] Transesophageal echocardiography can be used safely in pregnant women to diagnose aortic dissection and is a reasonable imaging study in the right clinical

Table 3
Use of echocardiography and MRI in pregnant patients

Modality	Appropriate	Inappropriate
Echocardiography	Suspected peripartum cardiomyopathy	Physiologic systolic murmur
	Suspected/known hypertrophic cardiomyopathy	Baseline assessment of cardiac function in the asymptomatic patient
	Evaluation of patient with Marfan syndrome	
	Known congenital heart disease	
	Suspected aortic dissection (transesophageal echocardiography)	
	Nonphysiologic systolic murmur	
	Diastolic murmur	
	Progressive or limiting dyspnea	
	Suspected heart failure	
	Suspected mechanical valve malfunction	
	Evaluation of pericadial effusion echocardiography)	
	Suspected coronary artery disease (stress echocardiography)	
Cardiac MRI	Suspected coronary artery disease	Acute coronary syndrome
	Evaluation of pericardial disease	
	Evaluation of aortic pathology	

context because it avoids exposure to ionizing radiation and iodinated contrast.[37]

CHEST RADIOGRAPHY

Chest radiography in pregnancy can be useful for assessment for cardiopulmonary disease. Case series from the middle of the twentieth century detail the changes that can be seen on chest radiographs in pregnancy. A slight prominence of the pulmonary conus is reported to be common, as is the appearance of both right and left atrial enlargement; the degree of atrial enlargement may be marked.[24,38,39] The heart may be rotated horizontally, the left cardiac border straightened, and increased lung markings present. These findings have all been reported in otherwise healthy women at varying stages of gestation.

Although these abnormalities suggest that pregnancy can lead to findings on chest radiographs similar to those seen in disease states, at least one study has findings that are at odds with this teaching. In 1975, Turner looked at 200 chest radiographs from pregnant women and analyzed lung parenchyma, cardiac contour, and vascular markings. He found no characteristic changes in pregnancy and concluded that abnormal findings should be investigated just as they are in nonpregnant patients.[40]

Indications for obtaining a chest radiograph in pregnancy are no different from those in nonpregnant patients. A chest radiograph should be considered in any pregnant patient who presents with new-onset dyspnea; in such a patient, it is a reasonable diagnostic study to evaluate for pulmonary edema, cardiomegaly, and atrial enlargement.[41] As discussed previously, radiation exposure from a chest radiograph is so low that it is likely not to pose any significant threat to the well-being of the fetus. Shielding of the pelvic area with a lead apron is nonetheless prudent.

STRESS TESTING WITH MYOCARDIAL PERFUSION IMAGING

Exercise stress testing can be used to aid in the diagnosis coronary disease in pregnant women. Low-level exercise is recommended when stress tests are performed on pregnant patients,[42] and stress echocardiography can be considered.[24] Fetal radiation exposure during stress testing with imaging with thallium 201 or technetium Tc 99m–labeled sestamibi is approximately 1 rad to 2 rad. This is due to the systemic distribution of the radioactive agents. Because of concerns about radiation exposure as well as lack of information about the safety profile of radiopharmaceutical agents

on the fetus, stress myocardial perfusion imaging is probably best avoided in pregnancy.[43]

CORONARY ANGIOGRAPHY

When an acute coronary syndrome is suspected, diagnostic coronary angiography may be undertaken in pregnancy patients with appropriate precautions. Owing to age and gender, symptomatic coronary artery disease is rare among pregnant women. Myocardial infarction complicates fewer than 1 in 10,000 pregnancies, and when it does occur during pregnancy, it is usually not a result of plaque rupture.[44] The most common cause of myocardial infarction in pregnancy is most likely spontaneous dissection of a coronary artery, but it may be caused by atherosclerosis or coronary embolism or occur as a result of thrombus due to a hypercoagulable state or as a complication of preeclampsia.[24] Vasculitis and anomalous origin of a coronary artery are other considerations in pregnant women with an acute coronary syndrome.

Calculations of fetal radiation exposure are more difficult with fluoroscopy than with other forms of ionizing radiation because fluoroscopy time and fetal exposure to the field of radiation vary widely.[9] With variations in fluoroscopy and fetal exposure times, calculations estimate that the radiation dose to the uterus during coronary angiography and percutaneous coronary intervention in the present era is approximately 0.6 mrad to 0.9 mrad.[9,45,46] The dose is most likely higher with percutaneous intervention involving placement of an intracoronary stent and potentially lower if a radial (as opposed to femoral) approach is used. As with any form of iodizing radiation during pregnancy, shielding the fetus with lead is appropriate (Fig. 2). The potential effects of iodinated contrast on neonatal thyroid function also must be considered (discussed later).

Percutaneous coronary intervention—with stenting as well as with balloon angioplasty alone—in pregnant women has been described in case reports.[47–53] The cardiovascular risks of angioplasty in pregnancy are similar to those in nonpregnant patients. According to European Society of Cardiology and American College of Cardiology/American Heart Association guidelines, coronary angioplasty is the preferred reperfusion therapy for ST-segment elevation acute myocardial infarction during pregnancy versus thrombolysis.[7,37]

CT

Pulmonary embolism is both more common and more complex to diagnose in pregnant compared

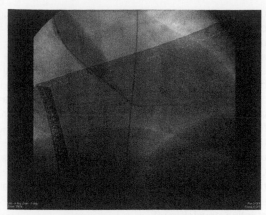

Fig. 2. Still frame from cineangiogram of a 39-year-old woman who presented with symptomatic aortic stenosis at 34 weeks' gestation. After balloon aortic valvuloplasty, peak and mean aortic valve gradients decreased from 50 mm Hg and 42 mm Hg, respectively, to 25 mm Hg and 20 mm Hg, respectively. Aortic valve area increased from 1 to 1.5 cm². The image shows balloon inflated in the aortic valve with shielding of the pelvis.

with non-pregnant patients. Pregnancy is known to be a risk factor for venous thromboembolic disease, with an increased risk 4-fold or 5-fold over baseline,[54,55] and thromboembolism remains a significant cause of maternal death.[56,57] Evaluation of pregnant patients with signs or symptoms of pulmonary embolism is made difficult because of the degree of overlap between these signs and symptoms and those present in healthy pregnant women. Dyspnea, tachypnea, tachycardia, leg edema, and elevated jugular venous pressure are often present in normal pregnancy. Scores that are commonly used to predict pretest probability of venous thromboembolism have not been validated in pregnant women. Additionally D-dimer is more likely elevated in pregnancy.

In pregnant women with symptoms of pulmonary embolism, compression ultrasonography of the lower extremities, after initiation of antithrombotic therapy, is the recommended first diagnostic study.[58] Faced with a negative study for deep vein thrombosis, the question of how to image the chest arises. CT pulmonary angiography and ventilation-perfusion lung scintigraphy are both used for diagnosis of pulmonary embolism. When deciding which study to select for a pregnant patient, factors to be considered include the diagnostic accuracy of each test, the amount of radiation exposure to the pregnant woman and the fetus, and the potential effects of fetal exposure to iodinated contrast material when CT pulmonary angiography is used.

The diagnostic accuracy of ventilation-perfusion scintigraphy and CT pulmonary angiography has

been examined in several, small-scale studies. A prospective study of 120 pregnant women who had clinical suspicion for pulmonary embolism and who underwent ventilation-perfusion scintigraphy found that 1.8% had high-probability scans, 73.5% had normal scans, and 24.8% had a nondiagnostic study.[59] Of the 104 women with nondiagnostic or normal studies who were not treated with anticoagulation, not one developed subsequent pulmonary embolism after a mean of 20 months' follow-up. Two recent retrospective studies compared CT pulmonary angiography and ventilation-perfusion scanning in pregnant women with clinical suspicion for pulmonary embolism. One found that both studies were comparable for diagnosis of pulmonary embolism with a similar proportion of indeterminate results (both 19%) between the 2 modalities.[60] The investigators speculate that the lower rate of nondiagnostic ventilation-perfusion studies compared with studies of nongravid patients may be due to a low average age (32 years ± 6) in their study. The rate of indeterminate CT studies may have been due to changes in the physiology of pregnant women, such as increased blood volume, that affects contrast dilution and delivery to the pulmonary arteries. The second study found that the likelihood of a diagnostic study for pulmonary embolism in pregnant patients is related to findings on the chest radiograph.[61] Women with a normal chest radiograph were more likely to have a diagnostic ventilation-perfusion scan.

Reports of the relative amount of radiation exposure between the 2 studies have varied. Fetal radiation exposure with ventilation-perfusion scintigraphy is approximately 4.5 mrad to 5.7 mrad.[9] CT pulmonary angiography was found in one retrospective series to deliver higher radiation dose than ventilation-perfusion scanning,[60] but several studies have created models to compare the effective-dose radiation from CT with ventilation-perfusion scintigraphy and found the exposure with CT equivalent or less than that of ventilation-perfusion nuclear studies.[62,63]

Exposure to iodinated contrast is likewise a concern with CT. There is a known risk of neonatal hypothyroidism after maternal ingestion of iodine during gestation,[64] which has led to investigation of the effect of intravenous iodinated contrast material on neonatal thyroid function. One retrospective study followed 115 consecutive patients with suspected pulmonary embolism admitted to a group of hospitals in the United Kingdom, 73 of whom underwent CT pulmonary angiography; the remaining 43 women had perfusion imaging.[65] After delivery, the neonates of all women in both groups underwent thyrotropin screening. The study found no significant difference in thyrotropin levels among the neonates when assessed based on antenatal exposure to iodinated contrast. This was a small study, and until the safety of iodinated contrast is firmly established, it is appropriate to use iodinated contrast material only when necessary and to evaluate neonates exposed to iodinated contrast material in utero with thyrotropin studies.

CARDIOVASCULAR MRI

Noninvasive imaging modalities can also be used for the diagnosis of coronary disease. Coronary CT angiography and cardiac MRI (discussed later) may be considered for evaluation of pregnant women with chest pain. A 2006 meta-analysis compared coronary CT angiography with MRI for the detection of significant coronary artery stenoses.[66] CT was found to have both sensitivity and specificity for coronary stenoses that were significantly higher than with MRI. The technologies have been evaluated in 2 subsequent trials. The first study compared CT and MRI studies done immediately prior to coronary angiography.[67] It found that although CT and MRI have similar specificities, CT has significantly better sensitivity than MR. The second trial also compared both modalities prior to invasive catheterization and found that both had similar diagnostic accuracy.[68] In pregnant patients with a chest pain syndrome, these results, as well as the risks of ionizing radiation and exposure to iodinated contrast and gadolinium (discussed later), must be weighed when selecting an imaging modality.

MRI has been used for fetal imaging with no evidence of negative impact on the fetus.[69] The lack of ionizing radiation with MRI is a clear advantage compared with modalities (discussed previously). Theoretic concerns with respect to the fetus include the possibility of teratogenesis and acoustic damage, but most studies have shown a good safety profile.[70–72] As with all studies, analysis of the potential benefit of the information derived and the possible risks, although small, should be performed and presented to patients when obtaining informed consent.

The decision to administer gadolinium-based intravenous contrast material for cardiovascular MRI must also be considered. Teratogenic effects of intravenous gadolinium have been demonstrated when used at high doses in animal studies.[73] After administration, gadolinium is known to cross the placenta, after which it is filtered by fetal kidneys and excreted into the amniotic fluid. To the authors' knowledge no studies or reports have described deleterious effects of gadolinium contrast, in

dosages commonly used for diagnostic imaging, on the human fetus.[74] Given the lack of data, however, MRI studies with contrast can be considered for use in pregnancy only if determined to be essential after a careful analysis of risk and potential benefits. This is reflected in current guidelines.[69]

In pregnant patients with suspected myocarditis or cardiomyopathy, MRI can evaluate ventricular function as well as the presence of tissue infiltration or scar. Cardiac MRI is also ideal for the evaluation of pericardial disease, and it is superior to CT for the characterization of effusions and potential neoplasms.[75,76] Cine acquisitions can also be used to distinguish between restrictive and constrictive physiology.[76]

MRI studies have a role in the diagnosis and evaluation of aortic pathology and have advantages over other modalities.[77] The quality of the images that can now be obtained allows for localization of the origin of aortic dissection and evaluation of branch vessels. MRI can also assess the intima as well as intramural pathology. 3-D magnetic resonance angiography can be constructed and—in the case of aortic dissection—magnetic resonance technology can be used to evaluate the true and false lumens within the aorta and its branches. In the diagnosis of an acute aortic process, the length of the MRI study and the need for timely diagnosis may favor CT or echocardiographic imaging (see **Table 3**). For vascular imaging, time-of-flight sequences can be used to selectively visualize arterial or venous signals without the administration

---

Box 1
Selected indications for imaging modalities in pregnancy

Chest radiography
> Dyspnea
> Abnormal lung examination

Coronary angiography
> Acute coronary syndrome
> Suspected coronary artery dissection

CT angiography
> Suspected pulmonary embolism (pulmonary angiography)
> Suspected aortic dissection

Ventilation-perfusion lung scintigraphy
> Suspected pulmonary embolism with normal chest radiograph

Coronary CT angiography
> Suspected coronary artery disease

of contrast. This technique adds time to the study, and results can be variable.[77]

SUMMARY

Evaluation of pregnant women with either pre-existing cardiovascular disease or evidence of undiagnosed cardiovascular pathology often relies on imaging techniques. The choice between the various imaging modalities should be informed by the diagnostic accuracy of each test—which is often different in a pregnant woman compared with a non-pregnant patient—and the risks posed to pregnant women and the fetus (**Box 1**). Any assessment of the cardiovascular system in pregnancy, whether by history, physical examination, or imaging, requires an understanding of the extraordinary capacity of the cardiovascular system to adapt to pregnancy. The changes in the heart and vascular system—and in blood volume, composition, and distribution—that occur in pregnancy alter the physical, radiographic, and echocardiographic examinations in both health and disease.

Complicating these decisions is that although the adverse events that can result from these diagnostic procedures are rare, the outcomes may be devastating. The decision for pregnant women to undergo a study that might have a negative impact on the health of the fetus can be traumatic in itself. Physicians who order or perform the study similarly have to balance concerns about doing harm with the diagnostic study, and the issue of liability exposure is one that frequently arises.[78,79] Cardiologists treating pregnant women should bear in mind the strengths and limitations of the imaging modalities (discussed previously) so that a thoughtful and informed approach to diagnostic imaging can be planned.

REFERENCES

1. Elkayam U. Pregnancy and cardiovascular disease. In: Zipes DP, Libby P, Bonow RO, et al, editors. Braunwald's Heart Disease. Philadelphia: Elsevier; 2005.
2. Siu SC, Coleman JM. Heart disease and pregnancy. Heart 2001;85:710.
3. American College of Radiology. ACR Guidelines and Technical Standards. Practice guidelines for imaging pregnant or potentially pregnant adolescents and women with ionizing radiation. 1st edition. Reston (Virginia): American College of Radiology; 2008. p. 1–15.
4. Osei EK, Faulker K. Fetal doses from radiological examinations. Br J Radiol 1999;72:773–80.
5. Groen RS, Bae JY, Lim KJ. Fear of the unknown: ionizing radiation exposure during pregnancy. Am J Obstet Gynecol 2012;206(6):456–62.
6. Yamazaki JN, Schull WJ. Perinatal loss and neurological abnormalities among children of the atomic bomb. JAMA 1990;264:605–9.
7. Blot WJ, Miller RW. Mental retardation following in utero exposure to the atomic bombs of Hiroshima and Nagasaki. Radiology 1973;106:617–9.
8. Otake M, Schull WJ. In utero exposure to A-bomb radiation and mental retardation; a reassessment. Br J Radiol 1984;57:409–14.
9. Cunningham FG, Gant NF, Leveno KJ, et al. General considerations and maternal evaluation. In: Cunningham FG, Leveno KJ, Bloom SL, editors. Williams obstetrics. 23rd edition. New York: McGraw-Hill; 2010.
10. Rosenstein M. Handbook of selected tissues doses for projections common in diagnostic radiology. Rockville (MD): Department of Health and Human Services, Food and Drug Administration; 1988. DHHS Pub No. (FDA) 89–8031.
11. Laws W, Rosenstein M. A somatic index for diagnostic radiology. Health Phys 1978;35:629.
12. Brent RL. The effect of embryonic and fetal exposure to x-ray, microwaves, and ultrasound: counseling the pregnant and nonpregnant patient about these risks. Semin Oncol 1989;16(5):347.
13. Klein JP, Hsu L. Neuroimaging during pregnancy. Semin Neurol 2011;31:361–73.
14. CDC guidelines on radiation exposure in pregnancy. Available at: www.bt.cdc.gov/radiation/prenatalphysician.asp. Accessed March 18, 2012.
15. Antman EM, Anbe DT, Armstrong PW, et al. ACC/AHA guidelines for the management of patients with ST-elevation myocardial infarction: executive summary. J Am Coll Cardiol 2004;44: 671–719.
16. Brent RL. Saving lives and changing family histories: appropriate counseling of pregnant women and men and women of reproductive age, concerning risk of diagnostic radiation exposure during and before pregnancy. Am J Obstet Gynecol 2009;200:4.
17. Stewart A, Kneale GW. Radiation dose effects in relation to obstetric x-rays and childhood cancers. Lancet 1970;1:1185–8.
18. Wakeford R, Little MP. Risk coefficients for childhood cancer after intrauterine irritation: a review. Int J Radiat Biol 2003;5:293–309.
19. Doll R, Wakeford R. Risk of childhood cancer from fetal irradiation. Br J Radiol 1997;70:130–9.
20. ACOG Committee on Obstetric Practice. ACOG Committee Opinion. Number 299, September 2004 (replaces No. 158, September 1995). Guidelines for diagnostic imaging during pregnancy. Obstet Gynecol 2004;104:647–51.

21. Dennis AT. Transthoracic echocardiography in obstetric anesthesia and obstetric critical illness. Int J Obstet Anesth 2011;21:160–8.

22. Armstrong WF, Ryan T. Feigenbaum's echocardiography. 7th edition. Philadelphia: Lipincott, Williams, and Wilkins; 2010.

23. Capeless EL, Clapp JF. Cardiovascular changes in early pregnancy. Am J Obstet Gynecol 1989;161: 1449–53.

24. Ueland K, Novy MJ, Peterson EN, et al. Maternal cardiovascular dynamics: IV. The influence of gestational age on the maternal cardiovascular response to posture and exercise. Am J Obstet Gynecol 1969; 104:856–64.

25. Oakley C, Warnes CA, editors. Heart disease in pregnancy. Chichester (England): Wiley; 2008.

26. Campos O, Andrade JL, Bocanegra J, et al. Physiologic multivalvular regurgitation during pregnancy: a longitudinal Doppler echocardiographic study. Int J Cardiol 1993;40:265–72.

27. Blauwet LA, Cooper LT. Diagnosis and management of peripartum cardiomyopathy. Heart 2011;97:1970–81.

28. Autore C, Conte MR, Piccinirino M, et al. Risk associated with pregnancy in hypertrophic cardiomyopathy. J Am Coll Cardiol 2002;40:1864–9.

29. Nishimura RA, Holmes DR. Hypertrophic obstructive cardiomyopathy. N Engl J Med 2004;350: 1320–7.

30. Avila WS, Rossi EF, Ramires JA, et al. Pregnancy in patients with heart disease: experience with 1,000 cases. Clin Cardiol 2003;26:135–42.

31. Elkayam U, Bitar F. Valvular heart disease and pregnancy part I. Native valves. J Am Coll Cardiol 2005; 46:223–30.

32. Freed LA, Levy D, Levine RA, et al. Prevalence and clinical outcome of mitral-valve prolapse. N Engl J Med 1999;341:1–7.

33. Uchida T, Ongino H, Ando M, et al. Aortic dissection in pregnant women with the Marfan syndrome. Jpn J Thorac Surg 2001;55:693–6.

34. Elkayam U, Ostrezega E, Shotan A, et al. Marfan syndrome in pregnancy. In: Elkayam U, Gleicher N, editors. Cardiac problems in pregnancy. 3rd edition. New York: Wiley-Liss; 1998.

35. Lind J, Wallenburg HC. The Marfan sydrome and pregnancy: a retrospective study in a Dutch population. Eur J Obstet Gynecol Reprod Biol 2001;98: 28–35.

36. Elkayam U, Hameed A. Vascular dissections and aneurysms during pregnancy. In: Elkayam U, Gleicher N, editors. Cardiac problems in pregnancy. 3rd edition. New York: Wiley-Liss; 1998.

37. European Society of Gynecology, Association for European Paediatric Cardiology, German Society for Gender Medicine, et al. ESC Guidelines on the management of cardiovascular diseases during pregnancy: the Task Force on the Management of Cardiovascular Diseases during Pregnancy of the European Society of Cardiology (ESC). Eur Heart J 2011;32(24):3147–97.

38. Hollander AG, Crawford J. Roentgenologic and electrocardiographic changes in the normal heart during pregnancy. Am Heart J 1943;26:364.

39. Keats TE, Martt JM. Selective dilation of the right atrium in pregnancy. Am J Roentgenol 1964;91:307.

40. Turner AF. The chest radiograph in pregnancy. Clin Obstet Gynecol 1975;18:65–74.

41. Morley CA, Lim BA. Lessson of the week: the risks of delay in diagnosis of breathlessness in pregnancy. BMJ 1995;311:183–4.

42. Elkayam U, Gleicher N. Cardiac evaluation during pregnancy. In: Elkayam U, Gleicher N, editors. Cardiac problems in pregnancy. 3rd edition. New York: Wiley-Liss; 1998. p. 23–32.

43. Baggish A, Boucher C. Radiopharmaceutical agents for myocardial perfusion imaging. Circulation 2008; 118:1668–74.

44. Hankins GD, Wendel GD, Leveno KL, et al. Myocardial infarction during pregnancy: a review. Obstet Gynecol 1985;65:139–46.

45. Finci L, Meier B, Steffenino G, et al. Radiation exposure during diagnostic catheterization and single- and double-vessel percutaneous transluminal coronary angioplasty. Am J Cardiol 1987;60:1401.

46. Gorson RO, Lassen M, Rosenstein M. Patient dosimetry in diagnostic radiology. In: Waggnener RG, Kereiakes JG, Shalek R, editors. Handbook of medical physics, vol. 2. Boca Raton (FL): CRC Press; 1984.

47. Klutstein MW, Tzivoni D, Bitran D, et al. Treatment of spontaneous coronary artery dissection: report of three cases. Cathet Cardiovasc Diagn 1997;40:372–6.

48. Craig S, Ilton M. Treatment of acute myocardial infarction in pregnancy with coronary artery balloon angioplasty and stenting. Aust N Z J Obstet Gynaecol 1999;39:194–6.

49. Sebastian C, Scherlag M, Kugelmass A, et al. Primary stent implementation for acute myocardial infarction during pregnancy. Cathet Cardiovasc Diagn 1998;45:275–9.

50. Glazier JJ, Eldin AM, Hirst JA, et al. Primary angioplasty using a urokinase coated hydrogel balloon in acute myocardial infarction during pregnancy. Cathet Cardiovasc Diagn 1995;36:216–9.

51. Sanchez-Ramos L, Chami YG, Bass TZ, et al. Myocardial infarction during pregnancy: management with transluminal coronary angioplasty and metallic intracoronary stents. Am J Obstet Gynecol 1994;171:1392–3.

52. Al-Aqeedi RF, Al-Nabti AD. Drug-eluting stent implantation for acute myocardial infarction during pregnancy with use of glycoprotein IIb/IIIa inhibitor. J Invasive Cardiol 2008;20:E146–9.

53. Ascarelli MH, Grider AR, Hsu HW. Acute myocardial infarction during pregnancy managed with

immediate percutaneous transluminal coronary angioplasty. Obstet Gynecol 1996;88:655–7.

54. Heit JA, Kobbervig CE, James AH, et al. Trends in the incidence of venous thromboembolism during pregnancy or postpartum: a 30-year population-based study. Ann Intern Med 2005;143:697–706.

55. Haemostatis, Thrombosis Task Force. Guidelines on the prevention, investigation and management of thrombosis associated with pregnancy: maternal and neonatal haemostasis working papers of the Haemostasis and Thrombosis Task Force. J Clin Pathol 1993; 26:489–96.

56. Horlander KT, Mannino DM, Leeper KV. Pulmonary embolism mortality in the United States, 1978-1998: an analysis using multiple-cause mortality data. Arch Intern Med 2003;163:1711–7.

57. The National Institute for Clinical Excellence. Why mothers die 2000-2002—report on confidential enquires into maternal deaths in the United Kingdom. London: Royal College of Obstetricians and Gynaecologists Press; 2003.

58. Marik PE, Plante LA. Venous thromboembolic disease and pregnancy. N Engl J Med 2008;359: 2025–33.

59. Chan WS, Ray JG, Murray S, et al. Suspected pulmonary embolism in pregnancy. Arch Int Med 2002;162:1170–5.

60. Revel MP, Cohen S, Sanchez, et al. Pulmonary embolism during pregnancy: diagnosis with lung scintigraphy or CT angiography? Radiology 2011;258: 590–8.

61. Cahill AG, Stout MJ, Macones GA, et al. Diagnosing pulmonary embolism in pregnancy using computed-tomographic angiography or ventilation-perfusion. Obstet Gynecol 2009;114:124–9.

62. Hurwtiz LM, Yoshizumi T, Reiman RE, et al. Radiation dose to the fetus from body MDCT during early gestation. Am J Roentgenol 2006;186:871.

63. Winer-Muram HT, Boone JM, Jennings SG, et al. Pulmonary embolism in pregnant patients: Fetal radiation dose with helical CT. Radiology 2002;224: 487–92.

64. Galina MP, Avnet ML, Einhorn A. Iodides during pregnancy: an apparent cause of neonatal death. N Engl J Med 1962;267:1124–7.

65. Rajaram S, Exley C, Fairlie F, et al. Effect of antenatal iodinated contrast agent on neonatal thyroid function. Br J Radiol 2011. [Epub ahead of print].

66. Schuijf JD, Bax JJ, Shaw LJ, et al. Meta-analysis of comparative diagnostic performance of magnetic resonance imaging and multislice computed tomography for noninvasive coronary angiography. Am Heart J 2006;151:404–11.

67. Dewey M, Teige F, Schnapauff D, et al. Noninvasive detectection of coronary artery stenoses with multislice computed tomography or magnetic resonance imaging. Ann Intern Med 2006;145:407–15.

68. Kefer J, Coche E, Legros G, et al. Head-to-head comparison of three-dimension navigator-gate magnetic resonance imaging an 16-slice computed tomography to detect coronary artery stenosis in patients. J Am Coll Cardiol 2005;46:92–100.

69. Kanal E, Barkovich AJ, Bell C, et al. ACR guidance document for safe MR practices: 2007. AJR Am J Roentgenol 2007;188:1447–74.

70. Mevissen M, Buntenkötter S, Löscher W. Effects of static and time-varying (50-Hz) magnetic fields on reproduction and fetal development in rats. Teratology 1994;50:229–37.

71. Clements H, Duncan KR, Fielding K, et al. Infants exposed to MRI in utero have a normal paediatric assessment at 9 m of age. Br J Radiol 2000;73: 190–4.

72. Kok RD, de Vries MM, Heerschap A, et al. Absence of harmful effects of magnetic resonance exposure at 1.5 T in utero during the third trimester of pregnancy: a follow-up study. Magn Reson Imaging 2004;22:851–4.

73. Okuda Y, Sagami F, Tirone P, et al. Reproductive and developmental toxicity study of gadobenate dimeglumine formulation (E7155) (3)—study of embryofetal toxicity in rabbits by intravenous administration. J Toxicol Sci 1999;24(Suppl 1):79–87 [in Japanese].

74. Webb JA, Thomsen HS, Morcos SK. The use of iodinated and gadolinium contrast media during pregnancy and lactation. Eur Radiol 2005;15: 1234–40.

75. Sechtem U, Tscholakoff D, Higgins CB. MRI of the normal pericardium. AJR 1986;147:239–44.

76. Breen J. Imaging of the pericardium. J Thorac Imag 2001;16:47–54.

77. Olin JW, Kaufman JA, Bluemke DA, et al. Atherosclerotic vascular disease conference: writing group IV: imaging. Circulation 2004;109:2626–933.

78. Berlin L. Radiation exposure and the pregnant patient. AJR Am J Roentgenol 1996;176:1377–9.

79. National Regulatory commission guidelines to radiation exposure. 2007. Available at: www.nrc.gov/reading-rm/doc-collections/cfr/part020/full-text.html. Accessed March 18, 2012.

Chest Pain Syndromes in Pregnancy

Gagan Sahni, MD

KEYWORDS

- Pregnancy • Acute myocardial infarction • Aortic dissection • Coronary dissection
- Pulmonary embolism • Venous thromboembolism • Amniotic fluid embolism

KEY POINTS

- Chest pain syndromes in pregnancy include acute myocardial infarction (AMI), aortic dissection and aortic syndromes, pulmonary embolism, and amniotic fluid embolism.
- The main risk factors associated with AMI in pregnancy are older maternal age(>35 years), hypertension, and diabetes mellitus.
- Most cases of aortic dissection and aortic syndromes occur in patients with Marfan syndrome, aneurysms associated with bicuspid valve, and other aortopathies that may get unmasked during pregnancy because of the accelerated aortic dilatation that occurs during pregnancy.
- The age-adjusted incidence of venous thromboembolism ranges from 4 to 50 times higher in pregnant compared with nonpregnant women, with most cases occurring postpartum versus peripartum.
- The basis of the management of amniotic fluid embolism, a rare but lethal condition, is support of the airway, tissue oxygenation, breathing, and circulation.

ACUTE MYOCARDIAL INFARCTION IN PREGNANCY

Introduction

Acute coronary syndromes and acute myocardial infarction (AMI) are rare in pregnancy (1–2 per 35,000 deliveries).[1] However, pregnancy has been shown to increase the risk of myocardial infarction (MI) 3- to 4-fold.[2] As the trend of child-bearing at older ages and advances in reproductive technology increase, so also does the incidence of AMI from atherosclerotic heart disease. The causes of acute coronary syndromes in pregnancy range from coronary dissection, to vasospasm, to acute plaque rupture. AMI can occur during any stage of pregnancy but is most common in the third trimester and in the 6-week period after delivery, occurring mostly in multigravidas (66%), most patients being older than 30 years (72%).[1,2]

Location of the AMI is mostly the anterior wall, largely because of the greater susceptibility of the territory of the left anterior descending artery (LAD) for coronary dissection.

Incidence

In the past decade in the United States there has been a higher incidence of detection of AMI in pregnancy, largely reflecting the changing epidemiology of increasing age of pregnancy as well as improvements in diagnostic capability. The average incidence varies from 1 in 24,000 according to Ladner and colleagues[2] to 1 in 16,129 deliveries as per James and colleagues.[3–5] The higher incidence reported by James and colleagues likely reflects improvements in diagnostic capability or a recent increase in the number of reported cases in several of these studies.[1–3]

Disclosures: None.
Mount Sinai Medical Center, Cardiovascular Institute, 1 Gustave L. Levy Place, Box 1030, New York, NY 10023, USA
E-mail address: gagan.sahni@mountsinai.org

Cardiol Clin 30 (2012) 343–367
doi:10.1016/j.ccl.2012.04.008

Risk Factors

The main risk factors associated with AMI in pregnancy are[1–3,6]:

- Maternal age greater than 35 years
- Hypertension
- Diabetes mellitus.

The magnitude of the increase in risk was evaluated in the series of 859 cases from the Nationwide Inpatient Sample.[3] In a multivariable regression model, the odds ratio was 21.7 for hypertension, 3.6 for diabetes, 6.7 for maternal age between 30 and 34 years, and 15 to 16 for maternal age 35 years and older.

Other independent risk factors in this report were smoking (odds ratio 8.4), thrombophilia, including a history of thrombosis and antiphospholipid syndrome (odds ratio 25.6), severe postpartum hemorrhage (odds ratio 5), migraine headaches (odds ratio 4.2) as a possible marker of vasospastic disease, and postpartum infection (odds ratio 2–3). The marked increase in risk with thrombophilia may reflect an interaction with the hypercoagulable state induced by pregnancy.[2,3]

It is not clear whether pregnancy itself is a risk factor for MI. In a report that had 3.6 million woman-years of observation, the incidence of a first-ever MI not related to pregnancy was 5.0 per 100,000 woman-years in women of childbearing age, with the risk increasing dramatically after age 35.[7] Because pregnancy lasts three-quarters of a year, this rate of MI is not different from the rates in the 2 large epidemiologic studies cited above (2.8–6.2 per 100,000 pregnancies).[2,3]

Mortality

Maternal mortality with AMI has significantly lowered in current reviews,[1–3] ranging from as low as 5.1% reported by James and colleagues[3] to 11% as reported by Roth and colleagues,[1] compared with the mortality of as high as 38% reported in studies from decades before the year 2000.[8] This improving mortality has been largely due to use of percutaneous coronary intervention (PCI) in acute coronary syndromes in pregnancy. The mortality rate is higher in the peripartum period (18%) than in the antepartum and postpartum periods (both 9%).[1] The incidence of fetal mortality was 9% (6 of 68), and most fetal deaths were associated with maternal mortality.[1]

Etiology

In a review of 103 pregnant patients presenting with acute coronary syndrome from 1995 to 2005, coronary artery morphology was evaluated in 96 by angiography or autopsy.[1] Coronary atherosclerosis with or without intracoronary thrombus was present in only 40% of patients. The remaining cases consisted of thrombus in a normal coronary artery (8%), coronary artery dissection (27%), spasm in (2%), emboli (2%), and normal coronary arteries (13%).

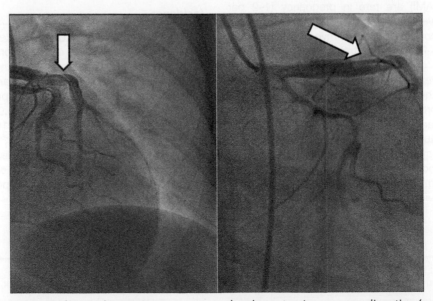

Fig. 1. Left coronary angiogram in a postpartum woman showing extensive coronary dissection (*arrows*). (*From* Alsleibi S, Dweik M, Afifi M, et al. Postpartum multivessel coronary artery dissection treated with coronary artery bypass grafting. J Cardiol Cases 2012;5(1):e23–7. doi: 10.1016/j.jccase.2011.11.003; with permission.)

Atherosclerotic disease was more prevalent in the pregnant women presenting with AMI in the antepartum period (54%) than in the peripartum (27%) or postpartum periods (29%).

Coronary dissection, which is a rare cause of AMI in the nonpregnant population, is the main cause of AMI in the peripartum period (50%) or postpartum period (34%), and rare in the antepartum period (11%).[7,9] The most commonly affected artery is the LAD,[1] followed by the right coronary artery (RCA), left circumflex artery (LCirc), and left main coronary artery (LM). The most common multivessel dissections involve the LM, LAD, and LCirc (**Fig. 1**).[1,8–11]

The timing of arterial dissection during or early after pregnancy is related to structural changes in the intima and media of the arterial wall produced by the effect of hormones such as progesterone, which produces loss of normal corrugation in elastic fibers, fragmentation of reticular fibers, and a decrease in the amount of acid mucopolysaccharides.[8,12,13] Other hypotheses include lytic action of proteases from eosinophils.[14–16] The hemodynamic changes of increase in blood volume and cardiac output magnify shear forces of blood in the large vessels, also resulting in a greater propensity for dissection.[17,18] The fact that coronary dissection occurs frequently in more than one vessel points toward generalized rather than localized pathogenesis.

The finding of spontaneous coronary artery dissection should also trigger the search for a previously undiagnosed connective tissue disease, such as Ehlers-Danlos syndrome or vasculitic syndromes such as Takayasu arteritis. Moreover, conventional risk factors such as hypertension also remain a risk factor for AMI related to spontaneous coronary artery dissection in the Nationwide Inpatient Sample.[3]

Normal coronaries were described in about 13% of recently reported cases, with almost equitable distribution throughout the 3 periods of pregnancy.[1] A transient coronary spasm is a possible explanation for these, caused by increased vascular reactivity to angiotensin II[19] or norepinephrine,[20] endothelial dysfunction,[21] increased renin-angiotensin production due to decreased uterine perfusion in supine position,[17] ergot derivatives used to control postpartum hemorrhage or to suppress lactation,[22–26] pheochromocytoma,[27] or cocaine abuse.[28,29]

Coronary thrombosis without atherosclerotic coronary artery disease, seen in approximately 8% of cases,[1] are likely due to a hypercoagulable state of pregnancy caused by alterations in the coagulation and fibrinolytic systems, which include decreased levels of tissue plasminogen activator (tPA),[16,30] increased levels of tPA inhibitor,[31,32] increases in levels of coagulation factors,[33] and decreased levels of functional protein S.[34–36] Smoking in pregnant women further increases platelet aggregability.[37]

Diagnosis

AMI in pregnant women is diagnosed in the same way as in nonpregnant patients, including the constellation of symptoms, electrocardiographic changes, and cardiac markers.[38] At the same time, however, the diagnostic approach is also influenced by fetal safety and normal changes during pregnancy.

Electrocardiograms (ECGs) done during normal pregnancy frequently show a left or right axis deviation, a small Q in lead III, nonspecific T-wave inversions, or an increased R/S ratio in leads V1 and V2, which can make the ECG diagnosis of ischemia in acute coronary syndromes more challenging. ECGs showing ST-segment depression mimicking myocardial ischemia have been observed in healthy women after the induction of anesthesia for cesarean section, and this result can be misleading.[1,39–41] One such study[40] reported significant ST-segment changes by Holter monitoring in 42% of 26 patients undergoing elective cesarean sections and in 38.5% of patients postoperatively.

Echocardiography is safe during pregnancy, and can be used to evaluate the presence of wall-motion abnormalities.

Interpretation of biochemical markers is somewhat complicated by changes that may occur during normal labor and delivery.[42] An increase in the concentration of creatine kinase and its MB fraction by nearly 2-fold within 30 minutes after delivery was reported by Shivvers and colleagues,[42] and is probably related to the uterus and placenta, which embody substantial amounts of these enzymes. Mean creatine kinase-MB levels continued to increase and reached a maximum at 24 hours after delivery. By contrast, use of troponin I levels has been validated for the diagnosis of AMI in pregnancy.[43] Troponin levels may show a small increase after normal delivery and remain below the upper limit of normal,[42–45] except in women with preeclampsia and gestational hypertension, in whom it may show a mild elevation.[44,45]

Exercise testing can be performed during pregnancy for the diagnosis of myocardial ischemia or risk stratification following AMI. Fetal bradycardia, reduction of fetal heart rate variation, and absence of body movement have been described during moderate to heavy maternal exercise.[46,47] Because of these findings, the use of a submaximal protocol (70% of maximal predicted heart rate) with fetal monitoring, if possible, is preferred.[48,49] The use of stress echocardiography may increase the sensitivity of the test for detection of myocardial ischemia and viability.[48] The use of radiation during pregnancy should be kept to a minimum, and nuclear imaging should be avoided because radionuclide imaging using [99m]technetium-labeled sestamibi or [201]thallium is expected to yield 1 rad of radiation to the conceptus,[48] which is teratogenic in the first trimester and if used in the second and third trimesters still poses a risk of intrauterine growth retardation, central nervous system abnormalities, and perhaps even malignancy.

Cardiac catheterization and interventional procedures also result in an approximate fetal exposure of 1 rad despite abdominal shielding, because of intra-abdominal scatter, and the more difficult and lengthier procedures could easily result in fetal exposure of 5 to 10 rad. Termination of pregnancy is not recommended for fetal doses of less than 5 rad because most researchers agree that it represents no measurable noncancer risk to the embryo or fetus at any stage of gestation.[50] However, congenital defects in the fetus and death of the human embryo are possible on exposure to greater than 10 rad, and termination of pregnancy is recommended for such exposure.[50,51] Using the radial or brachial approaches, appropriate abdominal shielding, minimizing fluoroscopy time, and so forth are important in reducing fetal risk.

Cardiac catheterization was reported in 386 (45%) of 859 patients with AMI in pregnancy postpartum by James and colleagues.[3] Of these, 81% needed angioplasty, stent placement, or coronary bypass. The procedure resulted in fatal coronary dissection in one patient and coronary dissection leading to bypass surgery in another. Because of the possible increased risk of coronary dissection, noninvasive risk stratification may be preferred during pregnancy or the early postpartum period in stable and low-risk patients.[38]

The technology of coronary computed tomographic angiography (CCTA) is also being applied to noninvasive imaging of acute coronary syndromes in pregnancy as a viable alternative to invasive catheterization, although it does preclude any intervention if a coronary abnormality is found. Besides being noninvasive, CCTA has the added advantage of identifying abnormalities such as intramural hematomas associated with coronary dissections in the tunica media (**Fig. 2**), aortic dissection, or pulmonary embolism (PE).

Treatment

The treatment of pregnant women with AMI and its complications should in general follow the usual standard of care,[52,53] although both maternal and fetal considerations should affect the choice of therapy. Therefore the treatment plan should be carefully concerted by both the cardiologist and obstetrician. If possible, the patient should be treated in an intensive care unit that can also provide maternal monitoring and a comprehensive obstetric service. A plan should be established for urgent delivery of a potentially viable fetus in the case of clinical deterioration of the mother (**Table 1**).

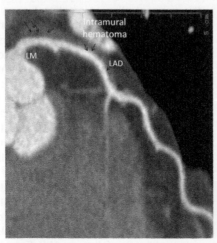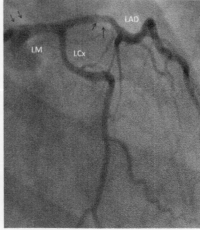

Fig. 2. Cardiac computed tomographic angiogram (CTA) (*left*) showing coronary intramural hematoma (*arrows*) in the left main (LM) and left anterior descending (LAD) artery resulting from a coronary dissection in the tunica media in a woman 2 weeks postpartum. The relatively unremarkable angiogram (*right*) done a few days before the CTA missed the diagnosis of coronary dissection. LCx, left circumflex artery. (*Courtesy of* Harvey Hecht, MD, Mount Sinai Medical Center, New York.)

Table 1
Recommendations for the management of coronary artery disease in pregnancy (European Society of Cardiology)

Recommendations	Class[a]	Level[b]
ECG and troponin levels should be performed in the case of chest pain in a pregnant woman	I	C
Coronary angioplasty is the preferred reperfusion therapy for STEMI during pregnancy	I	C
A conservative management should be considered for non–ST-elevation ACS without risk criteria	IIa	C
An invasive management should be considered for non–ST-elevation ACS with risk criteria (including NSTEMI)	IIa	C

Abbreviations: ACS, acute coronary syndrome; ECG, electrocardiogram; NSTEMI, non–ST-elevation myocardial infarction; STEMI, ST-elevation myocardial infarction.
[a] Class of recommendation.
[b] Level of evidence.
Data from The Task Force on the Management of Cardiovascular Diseases during Pregnancy of the European Society of Cardiology (FSC). Eur Heart J 2011;32:3147–97.

Revascularization

Percutaneous coronary intervention PCI has been well documented during pregnancy, and is considered safe for maternal and fetal survival.[1,3,54–57] In most cases PCI is preferred over thrombolysis because of the decreased risk of hemorrhage in pregnancy and because coronary dissection is a significant cause of AMI in pregnancy. The cardiovascular risks of angioplasty in pregnancy are similar to those in the nonpregnant patient. As in coronary angiography, the bleeding and radiation risks can be minimized by use of a radial approach,[58] appropriate abdominal shielding, and reducing fluoroscopy time. The use of an intra-aortic balloon pump to improve left ventricular output and coronary perfusion is also considered safe,[59,60] although the patient should be positioned in the left lateral recumbent position to reduce compression of the inferior vena cava.

James and colleagues[3] reported PCI in 135 patients with stenting in 127 of these. Roth and colleagues[1] reported PCI in 38 of 92 patients (41%) in their series with 23 antepartum, 6 peripartum, and 9 postpartum. All reported stenting during the acute phase of MI during pregnancy was performed with bare-metal stents; the safety of drug-eluting stents in pregnant women is currently still unknown. Because drug-eluting stents require prolonged antiplatelet therapy with clopidogrel and the incidence of cesarean deliveries in patients with heart disease is relatively high, the use of a drug-eluting stent during pregnancy may be problematic and should be avoided if possible.[38]

Coronary artery bypass graft surgery Hundreds of cases of cardiopulmonary bypass have been reported in literature since it was first used in pregnancy in 1959. Over time there have been significant improvements in maternal and fetal outcomes. At present, maternal mortality in coronary artery bypass grafting (CABG) is the same as that in the general population, at 1.7% to 3%, with a fetal mortality rate of 9.5% to 19%.[61–64] In a systematic review of cardiovascular surgery cases published between 1984 and 1996, Weiss and colleagues[65] reported a higher mortality of 6% in pregnant compared with nonpregnant patients. However, most these deaths occurred in patients with aortic dissection or PE, and there were no deaths in women undergoing CABG.

Surgical revascularization was reported in 61 women of 859 with AMI during pregnancy by James and colleagues.[3] No information, however, was provided on the outcome of these surgeries. The review by Roth and colleagues[1] reported 10 women of 92 patients who underwent CABG, 7 of which were to treat coronary dissection. Surgery was completed in the antepartum period in 5 patients (usually after the second week of pregnancy), of whom 1 had Turner syndrome and underwent the operation for aortic dissection with occlusion of the ostium of the RCA. One intrauterine fetal death was reported in a patient undergoing CABG surgery for dissection of the LM subsequent to PCI.

Surgery in the first trimester is associated with more fetal congenital malformations but does not affect fetal mortality.[62,63] The timing of the CABG does affect fetal mortality, and if the fetus is of more than 28 weeks' gestation, consideration must be given to deliver the child immediately before or during the same cardiac surgery.[63] A first consideration that can improve fetal outcomes is to position the patient in the left lateral recumbent position during surgery to prevent aortic and caval compression. Second, high-flow extracorporeal circuits (2.5–2.7 L/m^2/min) and normothermic or mildly hypothermic conditions should be used because these techniques have been shown to improve fetoplacental perfusion.[61,62] Third, continuous fetal monitoring should be used throughout surgery as an indirect means of assessing fetoplacental perfusion. Fetal bradycardia and loss of beat-to-beat variability suggest poor fetoplacental perfusion, and can be corrected by increasing the flow rate (5 L/min or greater) and maternal temperature. Fourth, an adequate mean arterial pressure must be maintained throughout surgery, as placental perfusion is dependent on mean arterial pressures of 70 mm Hg or greater in the relaxed uterus, and higher pressures in the contracting uterus.[63] Uterine activity should also be monitored because cardiopulmonary bypass and rewarming can place the patient at risk for early contractions.[61] Controlling contractions is crucial in avoiding placental insufficiency and secondary fetal hypoxia. Finally, hemodilution must be kept to a minimum to maximize oxygen-carrying capacity to the fetus, and the time necessary for cardiopulmonary bypass should be kept to a minimum.

Thrombolytic therapy Thrombolytic therapy (TT) is considered to be relatively contraindicated in pregnancy,[52] and because pregnant patients have been traditionally excluded from clinical trials, the available information is anecdotal.[66–68] Recent clinical experience with the use of TT in pregnancy has been mostly with tissue plasminogen activator (tPA) and primarily in patients with stroke, prosthetic heart valve thrombosis, PE, or deep vein thrombosis (DVT).[69,70] Several studies have demonstrated that placental transfer of streptokinase[71] and tPA[72] is too low to cause fibrinolytic effects in the fetus. Both urokinase and tPA were not found to be teratogenic in rats or mice,[70,73] and available reports do not support such an effect in humans. Although maternal and fetal outcomes were favorable in most cases,[70] some reports have documented complications such as maternal hemorrhage, preterm delivery, fetal loss, spontaneous abortion, minor vaginal bleeding, massive subchorionic hematomas, abruptio placenta, uterine bleeding requiring emergency cesarean section, and postpartum hemorrhage requiring transfusion.[69–74] Occasional fetal loss did not seem to be related to this therapy, although such a relation could not always be ruled out.[69,70]

Drug Therapy

Drugs that can be used with relative safety in pregnancy are discussed in detail in *Cardiovascular Drugs in Pregnancy* by William H. Frishman and colleagues. The most appropriate medication regimen for pregnant patients with ischemic heart disease or AMI is unknown. There is a significant amount of anecdotal evidence supporting the use of salicylates, β-blockers, nitroglycerin, calcium antagonists, and heparin during pregnancy, but little is known about the optimal combination of these medications.

Aspirin: risk category C
The safety of aspirin during the first trimester of pregnancy is questionable, because animal studies have shown birth defects, including fissure of the spine and skull; facial and eye defects; and malformations of the central nervous system, viscera, and skeleton.[75] The safety of high-dose aspirin during pregnancy is also debatable, and its chronic use should be avoided because it may lead to increased maternal and fetal hemorrhage, increased perinatal mortality, intrauterine growth retardation, and premature closure of the ductus arteriosus.[76,77] On the other hand, the safety of low-dose aspirin (<150 mg/d) has been suggested by a meta-analysis[77] and a large randomized trial[78] that enrolled more than 9000 patients during both the second and third trimesters. Although aspirin is secreted in breast milk in low concentrations, no adverse effects have been reported.[75] The American Academy of Pediatrics suggests cautious use of aspirin during lactation.[79]

Thienopyridine derivatives: risk category B
Information on the use of clopidogrel, prasugrel, or ticlopidine in pregnancy is very limited. Clopidogrel was administered in 6 patients[80–84] for a period of several weeks during weeks 6 to 37 of pregnancy. One case of intrauterine mortality was reported[81]; this patient's clinical condition was complicated by CABG, and thus no conclusion could be reached regarding the effects of the drug on the fetus. One report[83] described a patient with essential thrombocytopenia and a history of AMI treated with clopidogrel throughout pregnancy without complications. At least 1 week is needed for the elimination of clopidogrel for safe application of regional anesthesia. It is not known whether these drugs are excreted in human milk, and breastfeeding is therefore not recommended in women taking ticlopidine or clopidogrel.[79] It is noteworthy that the newer antiplatelet drugs such as ticagrelor have been given a risk category of C.

Morphine sulfate: risk category C
One report of 448 exposures during pregnancy showed no evidence of teratogenic effects. Placental transfer of morphine is very rapid and may cause neonatal respiratory depression when it is given shortly before delivery. Morphine enters breast milk only in trace amounts unless it is given

in high and repeated doses, and the drug is considered compatible with breastfeeding.[79]

Nitrates: nitroglycerin (risk category B) and isosorbide dinitrate (risk category C)

Intravenous, transdermal, and oral nitrates have been used as antianginals in MI and acute coronary syndromes, to treat hypertension,[85] for acute tocolysis to avoid preterm labor,[86] and for relaxation of uterus in postpartum patients with retained placenta.[87] However, careful titration is required to avoid maternal hypotension and reduced uterine perfusion.[88] No data are available on breastfeeding, and nitrates are not recommended for use in nursing mothers.[76]

β-Blockers: risk category C

β-Blocking agents have been extensively used in pregnancy for the management of hypertension, arrhythmias, mitral stenosis, Marfan syndrome (MFS), and myocardial ischemia.[89] There have been no reports of teratogenic effects, but side effects such as bradycardia, hypoglycemia, hyperbilirubinemia, and apnea at birth have been anecdotally reported. In addition, a possible increase in the rate of fetal growth retardation was linked to the use of atenolol,[90] especially when it is used in the first trimester. Because nonselective β-blockers may facilitate increases in uterine activity, use of β1 selective agents may be preferred.[90] Nursing infants should be monitored for adverse effects because all β-blockers accumulate in greater concentrations in breast milk than in plasma, with the least transmission being that of metoprolol tartrate, the most widely studied β-blocker in pregnancy.

Calcium-channel blockers: risk category C

At present only nifedipine, a dihydropyridine calcium-channel blocker (CCB), which has been commonly used for the treatment of hypertension, preeclampsia, and tocolysis, has been shown to be safe during gestation.[91] Information regarding the use of verapamil and diltiazem during pregnancy is limited, and a surveillance study has suggested that diltiazem may have teratogenic effects and that verapamil in the third trimester may cause dysfunctional uterine bleeding.[75] Concurrent use of CCB and magnesium sulfate should be done cautiously because of the potential for synergistic effects.[92] Nifedipine, verapamil, and diltiazem are all excreted in human milk; therefore, breastfeeding has been recommended with caution in women taking these drugs, although the American Academy of Pediatrics considers their use to be compatible with breastfeeding.[79]

Angiotensin-converting enzyme inhibitors and angiotensin receptor blockers: risk category C in first trimester and risk category D in second, third trimesters

The use of angiotensin-converting enzyme (ACE) inhibitors is contraindicated in pregnant patients[76] because of the fetotoxic effect predominately affecting the developing fetal kidneys. Other adverse events include oligohydramnios, intrauterine growth retardation, prematurity, bony malformations, limb contractures, patent ductus arteriosus, pulmonary hypoplasia, respiratory distress syndrome, hypotension, anuria, and neonatal death.[93] In 1992 the US Food and Drug Administration (FDA) warned against the use of ACE inhibitors in the second and third trimesters of pregnancy. Shotan and colleagues[93] in 1994 and, later, Cooper and colleagues[94] reported evidence for teratogenic effects and recommended avoiding these drugs during the first trimester as well. The effect of angiotensin receptor blockers (ARBs) is similar to that of ACE inhibitors, and the use of both groups of drugs should be avoided in all patients who develop AMI during pregnancy.[95,96] ACE inhibitors are detected in breast milk (the least 1% with captopril); the use of the drug, however, is considered compatible with breastfeeding[75] after 4 weeks, once the neonatal kidney is less susceptible to the drug's nephrotoxic effects. It is not known whether ARBs are excreted in human milk, but significant levels of losartan and its active metabolite were shown to be present in rat milk.[97]

Eplerenone: risk category B

Eplerenone is an aldosterone blocker indicated to improve survival in patients with AMI and left ventricular systolic dysfunction (left ventricular ejection fraction <40%) with clinical evidence of congestive heart failure or diabetes. Because of the lack of safety information in humans, eplerenone should be used in pregnancy only if the potential benefit justifies potential risks. No information is available regarding the concentration in human breast milk. Breastfeeding is therefore not recommended in women taking eplerenone.

HMG-CoA reductase inhibitors (statins): risk category X

Available information on the use of these drugs during pregnancy in humans is very limited. Animal studies have demonstrated increased incidence of skeletal abnormalities with lovastatin as well as maternal, fetal, and neonatal mortality with fluvastatin.[75,96] Information obtained from a worldwide postmarketing surveillance based on 137 reports to the manufacturer of inadvertent exposure to simvastatin or lovastatin during pregnancy did not show an adverse pregnancy outcome.[98] However, because these drugs inhibit the synthesis of mevalonic acid, which plays an important role in DNA replication and is essential for the synthesis of steroids and cell membranes in fetal development, and because information on the use of these drugs in pregnancy is limited, the use of HMG-CoA inhibitors is not recommended in pregnancy.

Unfractionated heparin (risk category C) and low molecular weight heparin (risk category B)

Both unfractionated heparin (UFH) and low molecular weight heparin (LMWH) do not cross the placenta, and several reports have indicated a lack of fetal adverse effects.[99] LMWH has advantages over UFH because it has a longer half-life, greater bioavailability, decreased affinity for heparin-binding proteins,[100] and thus more predictable therapeutic effect. Numerous studies have shown its safety during pregnancy[101]; its use for long-term management is therefore convenient and feasible. Discontinuation of treatment with either form of heparin (6 hours with UFH and 24 hours with LMWH) is desirable before delivery. If indicated, treatment can be resumed after delivery as soon as hemostasis appears to be adequate.

Glycoprotein IIb/IIIa inhibitors: eptifibatide and tirofiban (risk category B), abciximab (risk category C)

Because pregnant patients have been excluded from randomized trials, available information is limited to a few isolated reports.[56,102,103] Until more information on fetal safety becomes available, a cesarean section should be considered as the method of delivery to avoid the risk of fetal intracranial hemorrhage if delivery occurs while the antiplatelet effects of these agents are present.

Management of Labor and Delivery

- Because of the increased hemodynamic stress associated with labor, it has been recommended that induction of labor or scheduled cesarean delivery should be delayed, if possible, for at least 2 to 3 weeks after an AMI[1] if there is no obstetric indication or evidence of any fetal compromise.
- Mode of delivery in gestational MI should be decided by obstetric indications and the clinical status of the mother. In most cases it is advisable to proceed with vaginal delivery over elective cesarean section, because this eliminates the potential risks associated with anesthesia and a major surgical procedure that includes hemodynamic fluctuations, greater blood loss, pain, infection, respiratory complications, damage to pelvic organs, and potential unfavorable effects on future reproductive health (risks of miscarriage, ectopic gestation, placenta previa, and placenta accreta).[104] An elective cesarean section, on the other hand, is useful for avoiding long or stressful labor, and allows better control of the time of delivery to allow the planned presence of a multidisciplinary team including an experienced obstetrician, obstetric anesthesiologist, cardiologist, and pediatrician. In the study by Roth and colleagues,[1] only 10 of the 103 reviewed patients with pregnancy-related AMI delivered by cesarean section, a rate lower than the contemporary rate of 30% in the general population. These data therefore suggest that vaginal delivery can be accomplished relatively safely in the stable patient with pregnancy-associated AMI as long as measures aimed to reduce cardiac workload and oxygen demands are taken.

- Instrumental vaginal delivery and other methods to shorten the second stage of labor are recommended to avoid excessive maternal effort and the catecholamine surges and increased shear forces associated with it.
- The patient should be positioned in the left lateral position to improve cardiac output during labor and delivery.
- In addition, the patient's pain, fear, and apprehension, which may lead to tachycardia and hypertension and thus to an increase in myocardial oxygen demand, should be prevented and treated with early epidural anesthesia.
- Vital signs as well as oxygen saturation, ECG, and fetal heart rate should be monitored continuously. For prevention or treatment of myocardial ischemia during labor, intravenous nitroglycerin, β-blockers, and calcium antagonists can be used with caution regarding the tocolytic effects of nitroglycerin and the CCBs.
- Tachycardia and hypotension should be promptly corrected to prevent placental hypoperfusion. Ephedrine is usually the vasopressor agent of choice for hypotension associated with regional anesthesia, because it helps maintain placental perfusion.[105]
- Ergot alkaloids immediately after delivery should be avoided because of the risk of coronary artery spasm. After initial recovery, the patient should be monitored for 48 hours postpartum in a coronary intensive care or general intensive care unit, because of the significant hemodynamic changes that occur during this time.

AORTIC DISSECTION AND AORTIC SYNDROMES

Incidence

The overall incidence of aortic dissection is 0.4 case per 100,000 person-years within the female population aged between 15 and 45 years. The incidence in the general population of aortic dissection is 2.6 to 3.5 cases per 100,000 person-years across all ages.[106] The majority of the dissections and/or ruptures occur in the third trimester (50%) and the peripartum period (30%). Most of the cases occur in patients with MFS, aneurysms associated with bicuspid valve, and other aortopathies that may be unmasked during pregnancy because of the accelerated aortic dilatation that occurs during pregnancy.

Mortality

Type A aortic dissection is a life-threatening event to both mother and baby, and accounted for 14% of maternal cardiac deaths in the 2006-2008 UK Confidential Enquiries into Maternal Deaths.[107] Prehospital mortality rates could be as high as 53% in some studies.[108] The mortality from untreated proximal aortic dissections increases by 1% to 3% per hour after presentation and is approximately 25% during the first 24 hours, 70% at 1 week, and 80% at 2 weeks[109,110]; the early recognition of this entity during pregnancy is therefore of prime importance. A study over a 27-year period found that misdiagnosis occurred in 85% of patients presenting with acute aortic dissection.[109] Several case reports describe how the diagnosis was initially missed in the peripartum period.

Pathophysiology and Risk Factors

The physiologic changes in pregnancy include increased maternal blood volume, stroke volume, and cardiac output.[18,111] Moreover, the effect of maternal hormones on remodeling the tunica media and intima of the arterial wall[12,112] cause increased shear forces on the aortic wall. These combined changes begin in the first and second trimesters but are most notable in the third trimester and peripartum.

However, these hemodynamic stressors in pregnancy alone cannot account for the high incidence of aortic dissection and are likely secondary contributors. Several observational studies have identified preexisting risk factors such as premature atherosclerosis and arterial hypertension, hereditary connective tissue disease such as MFS and Ehlers-Danlos syndrome, previous aortic surgery, bicuspid aortic valve disease, coarctation, aortitis, surgical manipulation, cardiac catheterization, and cocaine exposure as the most common risk factors in aortic dissection occurring in women younger than 45 years.[106–108,111,113–117]

In one of the few prospective studies of pregnant patients with MFS, 4.4% of carefully monitored patients developed aortic dissection.[118,119] In unmonitored patients, the risk is likely higher, with 10% of patients with aortic root diameter greater than 40 mm presenting with aortic dissection during pregnancy. In fact about half of pregnant women with MFS and aortic root dilatation greater than 40 mm will have a dissection, rupture, prophylactic surgery, or life-threatening growth, although a normal dimension does not exclude the possibility of dissection.[111,114,115] Most of the dissections that occur are proximal or type A dissections.

Clinical Presentation

Arterial hypertension (93%), sudden onset of severe chest pain (73%), and neurologic symptoms, such as syncope (40%), are the leading symptoms of acute aortic dissection[106] in pregnancy. The presence of severe chest or interscapular pain requiring opioid analgesia, especially in the presence of systolic hypertension, should be investigated. However, 10% of dissections are painless at presentation, more often in chronic dissections or preexisting connective tissue diseases.[109,110,120] There could be differential peripheral pulses in both arms with a difference in blood pressure greater than 20 mm Hg taken in both arms. Congestive cardiac failure is a less common but well-described presentation of thoracic aortic dissection.[110,120,121] Hypotension in the presence of aortic dissection is an ominous sign indicating cardiac tamponade or hypovolemia from aortic rupture.

Diagnosis

As per the American College of Cardiology/American Heart Association/American Thoracic Society (ATS) guidelines[122] for imaging in pregnant patients suspected of having aortic dissection or aneurysm, magnetic resonance imaging (MRI) without gadolinium is recommended over computer tomographic (CT) imaging to avoid exposing both mother and fetus to ionizing radiation. Barring the risks of ionizing radiation, the sensitivity of CT in diagnosis of aortic dissection is equivalent to that of MRI and may be used if the patient is unstable, intolerant of MRI because of claustrophobia, or if MRI is not available (Fig. 3). Transesophageal echocardiogram is an

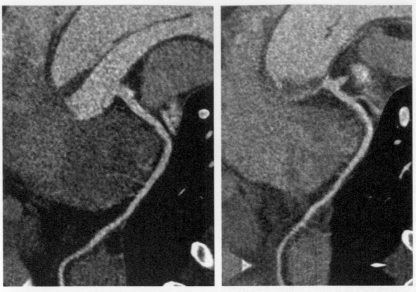

Fig. 3. Cardiac computed tomography in a patient in third trimester of pregnancy, showing a type A dissection involving aortic root and ascending aorta, with images in end diastole (*left*) and end systole (*right*) showing the dissection flap compressing the left main coronary ostium during systole. (*Courtesy of* Harvey Hecht MD, Mount Sinai Hospital, New York.)

alternative option (Class IC indication) if the patient is clinically unstable.

The yield of a chest radiograph is low, as a widened mediastinum is not seen in 40% of cases and in 12% no abnormalities can be seen at all.[106]

Management

Medical therapy

β-Blockers should be started to minimize aortic dilatation, lower blood pressure, and limit shear forces of aortic dissection during pregnancy. Labetolol or metoprolol is the preferred β-blocker in pregnant women because atenolol may impair fetal growth. Propranolol blocks the inhibitory effects of epinephrine on myometrial activity and the nonselective β-blocking effect of propranolol may, therefore, facilitate an increase in uterine activity. Intravenous labetolol could be used for urgent lowering of blood pressure and heart rate, in addition to adequate opioid analgesia to reduce shear forces. It is recommended that in the nonpregnant patient, β-blockers be titrated up to a resting heart rate of less than 60 beats/ min. Because heart rate is increased during gestation, the dose should be titrated to reduce resting heart rate by at least 20%.[111] Because of increased sympathetic output during

pregnancy the heart rate is increased, and a higher dose of β-blockers may be needed to achieve adequate control of heart rate. β-Blocking agents are excreted in breast milk, and nursing infants should therefore be monitored for adverse effects.

In addition to β-blockade, vasodilators may be required to control blood pressure. Intravenous sodium nitroprusside is the most established agent and offers the advantage of being rapidly titratable. Intravenous hydralazine, nitroglycerine, or sodium nitroprusside have all been studied in pregnancy. Vasodilator therapy without prior β-blockade may cause reflex tachycardia and increased force of ventricular contraction, leading to greater aortic wall stress and potentially causing false-lumen propagation. ACE inhibitors and ARBs are teratogens and are thus contraindicated during pregnancy.

Surgical treatment

For type A proximal aortic dissections during the first or second trimester, urgent surgical repair with aggressive fetal monitoring is preferred. Fetal loss during hypothermia and cardiopulmonary bypass is common. Death rates during surgery decreased from 30% in 1990-1994 to 0% in 2002-2004 in one study and a similar 1.5% to 3% mortality rate in other series, while fetal death rates decreased from 50% to 10% for the same periods.[123] Because cardiac surgery continues to be associated with increased fetal loss,[65,123,124] cesarean section should be performed before or concomitantly with thoracic surgery if fetal maturity can be confirmed.[125,126]

Measures to reduce fetal mortality during surgery if done before 30 weeks of gestation include the use of intraoperative cardiotocography (CTG) for monitoring the fetal heart, use of high-flow, high-pressure normothermic perfusion and a perfusion index of 3.0 during cardiopulmonary bypass, which is probably safest for the fetus, and measures to prevent hypothermia (which causes fetal bradycardia).[65,123,124]

For acute arch or type B dissection, medical therapy is preferred unless percutaneous stent grafting or open surgery is mandated by malperfusion, aortic rupture, or subacute aortic leaking.[121]

Prophylactic aortic root and ascending aorta repair is also indicated in pregnant patients with MFS if the size exceeds 50 mm or if there is rapidly progressive dilatation of more than 10 mm during surveillance in pregnancy or greater than 50 mm with bicuspid aortic valve, because of the high risk of rupture and dissection.[38] Successful surgeries during gestation or shortly after delivery[108,116,124,127] have been reported in several women with MFS.

Mode of delivery

Cesarean delivery is preferred in patients with an aortic diameter greater than 45 mm, or greater than 40 mm in MFS, aortic dissection, severe aortic regurgitation, or heart failure. Vaginal delivery is safe in patients with MFS with aortic diameter of less than 40 mm.[111,114–117] To minimize the stress of labor in vaginal delivery, epidural anesthesia should be used to reduce pain, and forceps or vacuum should be used to shorten the second stage of labor.

Because around 70% to 90% of patients with MFS present with lumbosacral dural ectasia, an anesthetist should be consulted before delivery.[128] Although dural ectasia is not an absolute contraindication for epidural anesthesia, the increased risk of dural puncture or inadequate anesthesia should be discussed with the patient.

Both systolic and diastolic blood pressures increase markedly during uterine contractions and with labor pains. These changes should be anticipated and prevented with epidural anesthesia, β-blockers, and vasodilatory agents. Postpartum hemorrhage of the uterine vasculature 3 days after

cesarean section secondary to MFS has been reported, and should be anticipated.

Prevention and preconception counseling

It is difficult to identify aortic aneurysms associated with bicuspid aortic valve, coarctation, and other aortopathies that are usually asymptomatic until they manifest with acute aortic syndromes in pregnancy.

However, women with MFS should be counseled before conception about the risk for potential pregnancy-related cardiovascular and obstetric complications as well as the 50% probability of transmitting the syndrome to their offspring. The woman and her family should also be informed of the need for close follow-up during pregnancy as well as the use of β-blockers and possibly other cardiac medications, and the potential side effects to the fetus. The possibility and limitations of prenatal diagnosis with the use of both genetic linkage and fetal echocardiography[129] should be explained.

In addition, the patient should be informed about the likelihood of morbidity and possibly reduced longevity[114] even after successful pregnancy. Based on most series, aortic dissection occurred in MFS women in their third decade of life; therefore, it is advisable to plan a pregnancy at a younger age.[114,123]

MFS patients and those with bicuspid aortic valve who are considering pregnancy should be evaluated using echocardiography, MRI, CT, and/or abdominal ultrasonography to comprehensively assess the heart and the aorta, with particular attention paid to the aortic root. It has thus been recommended that transthoracic echocardiography be performed every 4 to 8 weeks in the antenatal monitoring of the MFS patient and be continued until 6 months postpartum.[38] Progressive aortic dilatation and/or an aortic root dimension of 40 mm or greater suggest increased gestational risk for aortic dissection, such that pregnancy should be discouraged or prepregnancy aortic repair should be undertaken. If such a patient is already pregnant, therapeutic abortion should be considered. For bicuspid aortic valve, prophylactic prepregnancy repair should be considered for aortic diameter greater than 50 mm.

All patients with MFS or bicuspid aortic valve with dilated aorta should be administered β-blockers with close fetal monitoring, and this should continue until 3 months postpartum, as dissection (type A or B) can occur during this period.

PULMONARY EMBOLISM
Epidemiology

PE is a leading cause of pregnancy-related mortality in the developed world, accounting for 20% of maternal deaths in the United States.[130]

Pregnancy and the puerperium are associated with an increased incidence of venous thromboembolism (VTE), occurring in 1 in 500 to 1 in 2000 pregnancies (0.05%–0.20%).[131–136] The age-adjusted incidence of VTE ranges from 4 to 50 times higher in pregnant women than in nonpregnant women, with most cases occurring postpartum versus peripartum.

The incidence of pregnancy-associated DVT is about 3 times higher than that of pregnancy-associated PE.[131]

Risk Factors

Pregnancy and the postpartum period may be marked by the presence of all 3 components of Virchow's triad: venous stasis, endothelial injury, and a hypercoagulable state. Inherited or acquired thrombophilias such as factors unrelated to pregnancy further increase thromboembolic risk.[137,138] For example, the thrombotic risk for a woman with factor V Leiden mutation during pregnancy or the puerperium has been estimated at approximately 1 in 400 to 1 in 500, compared with 1 in 1400 in the general population.[139]

The most significant risk factors for VTE in pregnancy are a prior history of unprovoked DVT or PE (Box 1) and thrombophilias. Fifteen percent to 25% of VTEs are recurrent events, and 50% of the women who develop a thrombotic event during pregnancy have either a thrombophilic disorder or a previous idiopathic VTE.[140]

Diagnosis

Clinical examination

The clinical diagnosis of both DVT and PE is notoriously insensitive and nonspecific, especially during pregnancy when women often present with lower extremity swelling and discomfort, and dyspnea may occur in up to 70% of normal pregnancies. In a study of 38 pregnant women with confirmed PE, dyspnea (62%), pleuritic chest pain (55%), cough (24%), and perspiration (18%) were the 4 most common features at presentation[141]; Powrie and colleagues[142] reported an abnormal alveolar-arterial gradient (>15 mm Hg) in 8 of 17 (58%) pregnant women with confirmed PE. However, in most studies of pregnant women with clinical suspicion of PE, there was no significant risk association between any of these features and the presence of PE. Although there

are some specific risk factors (see Box 1) that help to predict the pretest probability of VTE, at present VTE is ultimately confirmed in fewer than 10% of pregnant women who present with clinical features.[134] Although an array of diagnostic tests are currently available, clinicians are often uncertain as to the best diagnostic algorithm, which has now been suggested by the ATS Guidelines (Fig. 4) using the Grades of Recommendation, Assessment, Development, and Evaluation (GRADE) System.

Ultrasound scanning

Direct evidence for the use of bilateral compression ultrasonography (CUS) of the lower extremities for diagnosis of PE in pregnancy currently does not exist. The benefit of using ultrasonography early in the diagnostic algorithm is potential avoidance of radiation-associated tests in the setting of a positive study (see Fig. 4). Selection of women with signs and symptoms of DVT could increase the positive yield of CUS. Chan and colleagues[143] have reported 3 objective variables ("LEFt": symptoms in the left leg [L]; calf circumference difference >2 cm [E]; and first-trimester presentation [Ft]) to be highly predictive of DVT in pregnancy; in their study of 194 pregnant women, the presence of 2 or 3 of these variables was associated with DVT in 58.3% of cases.

Chest radiography

In pregnant women with suspected PE, chest radiography (CXR) is the first radiation-associated procedure suggested by the ATS.[144] If the CXR is normal, ventilation/perfusion (V/Q) scan is the next imaging test recommended. If the CXR is abnormal, chest CT pulmonary angiogram (CTPA) is suggested. Use of chest radiographs to selectively triage only patients with normal CXR findings to undergo V/Q scan can increase the prevalence of definitive V/Q results.[145,146] Two studies (n = 105 and n = 24) performed in pregnant women with suspected PE have reported definitive V/Q results (normal and high probability) in 94% and 96% of cases when the presenting CXR is normal.[146,147]

Ventilation/perfusion scanning

Direct evidence for the use of lung scintigraphy for diagnosis of PE in pregnancy is derived from 4 retrospective management studies performed in the pregnant population that reported the prevalence of diagnostic V/Q scan results (high probability, very low probability, and normal) to range from 75% to 94%, with the upper value observed in a group selected by normal CXR and no prior history of asthma or chronic obstructive pulmonary disease.[146,148–150]

Box 1
Risk factors for venous thromboembolism in pregnancy

Hypercoagulable Risk Factors in Pregnancy

- Increase in coagulation factors, particularly factors I, II, VII, VIII, IX, and X
- Fibrinogen levels double in pregnancy
- Factors V, VII, and X increase in the first few days after delivery
- Decrease in levels of the endogenous anticoagulant Protein S
- Increase in resistance to the anticoagulant Protein C in second and third trimesters
- Fibrinolysis is suppressed through increases in plasminogen activator inhibitor type 2 produced from the placenta, and plasminogen activator inhibitor type 1 produced from the endothelium

Venous Stasis

- Compression of iliac veins by gravid uterus
- Hormonally mediated vein dilatation
- Immobilization

Obstetric Risk Factors

- Preeclampsia
- Dehydration/hyperemesis/ovarian hyperstimulation syndrome
- Multiple pregnancy or assisted reproductive therapy
- Emergency and elective cesarean section
- Midcavity or rotational forceps
- Prolonged labor longer than 24 hours
- Peripartum hemorrhage

Preexisting Risk Factors

- Previous VTE
- Family history of VTE
- Known thrombophilias such as factor V Leiden mutation, antithrombin III deficiency
- Antiphospholipid antibody syndrome
- Medical comorbidities such as heart, lung disease, systemic lupus erythematosus, cancer, sickle cell disease
- Age older than 35 years
- Parity greater than 3
- Body mass index greater than 30 kg/m^2
- Smoker
- Gross varicose veins

Transient Risk Factors

- Concomitant systemic infection (eg, pyelonephritis)
- Immobility
- Surgical procedure in pregnancy or less than 6 weeks postpartum

---

Dose-reduction techniques for lung scintigraphy include using one-half the usual administered activity of technetium-99m (Tc-99m) macroaggregated albumin for the perfusion scan and increasing the scan time to achieve adequate counts. When possible, a xenon-133 ventilation scan should be performed instead of a Tc-99m aerosol ventilation study, because the effective dose to the mother is lower. Although some experts recommend omitting the ventilation scan,

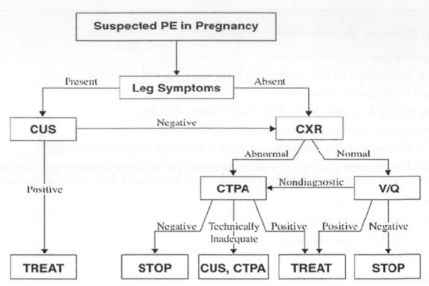

Fig. 4. Diagnostic algorithm for suspected pulmonary embolism in a pregnancy. CTPA, computed tomographic pulmonary angiography; CUS, compression ultrasonography; CXR, chest radiography; V/Q, ventilation/perfusion. (*Adapted from* Leung AN, Bull TM, Jaeschke R, et al. An official American Thoracic Society/Society of Thoracic Radiology clinical practice guideline: evaluation of suspected pulmonary embolism in pregnancy. ATS/STR Committee on Pulmonary Embolism in Pregnancy. Am J Respir Crit Care Med 2011;184(10):1200–8; with permission.)

this may decrease the diagnostic accuracy of the study. Further dose-reduction techniques include hydration to encourage frequent urinary voiding and reduction of fetal exposure.[144]

D-dimer
A degradation product of cross-linked thrombus, D-dimer levels have a high negative predictive value in the normal population. However, in pregnancy D-dimer levels become elevated as a result of physiologic changes in the coagulation system, and there is a 39% relative increase in D-dimer concentration for each trimester compared with the previous[151] and even more if there is a concomitant problem (eg, preeclampsia, threatened miscarriage, or antepartum hemorrhage). Direct data come from a retrospective study of 37 pregnant women[152] with suspected PE who had both V/Q scans and D -dimer testing. Sensitivity and specificity for suspected PE was calculated to be 73% and 15%, respectively, and the negative likelihood ratio was 1.8, suggesting that a negative D-dimer is inadequate to rule out PE in pregnancy. In addition, 2 case reports have documented negative D-dimer levels in the setting of acute PE in pregnancy.[153,154]

Computed tomographic pulmonary angiography
The main risk of iodinated contrast agents given during CTPA to rule out PE is related to the

presence of free iodine with possible induction of neonatal hypothyroidism. A retrospective study of 344 pregnant women who underwent a CTPA examination for suspected PE found normal thyroxine levels in all neonates at time of birth.[155] No animal studies have demonstrated teratogenicity to the developing fetus from iodinated contrast. Iodinated contrast agents are classified as category B by the US FDA.[156] A recent retrospective management study comparing CTPA (n = 106) with V/Q scan (n = 99) in the diagnosis of PE in pregnancy has reported negative predictive values of 99% and 100%, respectively.[149] **Fig. 5** however, there is the consideration that CTPA exposes the fetus to lower radiation doses but has a higher maternal exposure in comparison with V/Q scanning (**Table 2**), keeping in mind that the mortality associated with untreated PE far outweighs the potential oncogenic and teratogenic risk incurred by fetal exposure to diagnostic imaging for PE. The European Society of Cardiology recommends CTPA over VQ scanning for the diagnosis of PE in pregnancy,[38] whereas the ATS is equivocal with the choice of imaging, depending on the initial CXR being normal or not.[144]

Magnetic resonance imaging
The main risk to the fetus from gadolinium administration for MRI is exposure to potentially free unchelated gadolinium in the amniotic fluid. Animal studies have demonstrated teratogenic effects,

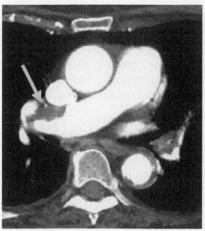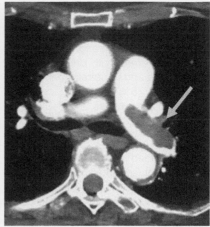

Fig. 5. Computed tomography scan showing massive bilateral pulmonary embolism (seen as filling defect denoted with *arrows*) in a patient presenting with sudden shortness of breath 2 days postpartum. (*Courtesy of Partho Sengupta, MD, Mount Sinai Medical Center, New York.*)

but only at markedly increased doses and/or for extensive periods of exposure,[157] and limited human observational studies have not documented any adverse fetal effects.[158] Gadolinium-based contrast agents are classified as category C by the FDA[156] and MRI with gadolinium is relatively contraindicated in pregnancy because of the uncertain long-term effects of gadolinium on the fetus.[159] Moreover, no accuracy or management studies that evaluate the performance of MRI for PE in pregnancy have been performed in the pregnant population. There are unenhanced MR techniques that have been described for the diagnosis of PE that require no use of gadolinium and with no risk of ionizing radiation to the fetus or mother, which could be a promising imaging modality for the future.[160]

Management

Detailed discussion of use of various anticoagulants and thrombolytics in pregnancy is outlined in a another article by Sorel Goland elsewhere in this issue, but here these are briefly discussed in the context of PE.

Low molecular weight heparins

LMWH has also become the drug of choice for the treatment of VTE in pregnancy and puerperium. LMWHs have been used in pregnancy since 1992, and the efficacy and safety of several LMWH preparations was shown in a review of 2777 pregnant women, treated for DVT or PE.[161] The risk of recurrent VTE with treatment doses of LMWH was 1.15%. The observed rate of major bleeding was 1.98%. Protamine sulfate reverses up to 60% of factor Xa inhibition versus 100% for UFH. Heparin-induced thrombocytopenia is markedly lower with LMWH than with UFH, as is heparin-induced osteoporosis (0.04%). LMWHs are not teratogenic or fetotoxic and do not cross the placenta, and are classified by the FDA as pregnancy category B, whereas UFH[156] is category C (**Table 3**). In clinically suspected DVT or PE, treatment with LMWH should be given until the diagnosis is excluded by objective testing.

Table 2
Fetal and maternal radiation doses associated with diagnostic tests for PE

Diagnostic Test	Fetal Dose (mGy)	Maternal Dose (Whole-Body Effective Dose in mSv)
CXR	0.002	0.1
V/Q scan	0.32–0.74	1–2.5
CTPA	0.03–0.66	4–18

Table 3
FDA pregnancy categories of anticoagulants and thrombolytics

Drug	FDA Category
Unfractionated heparin	C
Enoxaparin	B
Dalteparin	B
Danaparoid	B
Recombinant alteplase	C
Streptokinase	C
Urokinase	C
Warfarin	X

LMWH has also been shown to be effective in preventing pregnancy-related complications in women with thrombophilia and/or antiphospholipid antibody syndrome. Administration of enoxaparin, 20 mg daily, to women with primary early recurrent pregnancy loss and impaired fibrinolytic capacity produced up to 75% to 80% successful live births in different case series.[162,163] Similar results have been seen in patients with factor V Leiden mutation.[164]

Dosage The recommended therapeutic dose is calculated on body weight (eg, enoxaparin 1 mg/kg body weight twice daily; dalteparin 100 IU/kg body weight twice daily) aiming for 4- to 6-hour peak anti-Xa values of 0.6 to 1.2 IU/mL.[165]

Monitoring The necessity to monitor anti-Xa values regularly in patients with VTE is still controversial. Whereas it is considered necessary in patients with mechanical valves in whom LMWH is used (see section Anticoagulation in Pregnancy), this is not so clear in patients with VTE. Given the need for dose increase as pregnancy progresses to maintain a certain therapeutic anti-Xa level, it seems reasonable to also determine anti-Xa levels during pregnancy in patients with VTE.

Unfractionated heparin
UFH also does not cross the placenta, but is associated with more thrombocytopenia, osteoporosis, and more frequent dosing when given subcutaneously in comparison with LMWH. UFH is favored in patients with renal failure and when urgent reversal of anticoagulation by protamine is needed, as well as in the acute treatment of massive pulmonary emboli.

Dosage In patients with acute PE with hemodynamic compromise, intravenous administration of UFH is recommended (loading dose of 80 U/kg, followed by a continuous intravenous infusion of 18 U/kg/h).[165]

Monitoring The activated partial thromboplastin time (aPTT) has to be determined 4 to 6 hours after the loading dose, 6 hours after any dose change, and then at least daily when in the therapeutic range. The therapeutic target aPTT ratio is usually 1.5 to 2.5 times the average laboratory control value. The dose is then titrated to achieve a therapeutic aPTT, defined as the aPTT that corresponds to an anti-Xa level of 0.3 to 0.7 IU/mL. When hemodynamics are improved and the patient is stabilized, UFH can be switched to LMWH in therapeutic doses and maintained during pregnancy. LMWH should be switched to intravenous UFH at least 36 hours before the

induction of labor or cesarean delivery. UFH should be discontinued 4 to 6 hours before anticipated delivery, and restarted 6 hours after delivery if there are no bleeding complications. Neither UFH nor LMWH is found in breast milk in any significant amount, and neither represents a contraindication to breastfeeding.

Thrombolytics
Thrombolytics are considered to be relatively contraindicated during pregnancy and peripartum, and should only be used in high-risk patients with severe hypotension or shock.[166] The risk of hemorrhage, mostly from the genital tract, is around 8%.[167] In 200 reported patients, streptokinase was mostly used and, more recently, recombinant tissue plasminogen activator. Neither of these thrombolytics crosses the placenta in significant amounts. Fetal loss of 6% and 6% preterm delivery were reported.[168] When thrombolysis has been given, the loading dose of UFH should be omitted and an infusion started at a rate of 18 U/kg/h. After stabilization of the patient, UFH can be switched to LMWH for the residual duration of pregnancy.

Bechtel and colleagues[169] reported the successful use of catheter-directed mechanical fragmentation and local thrombolytic infusion, with the theoretical advantage of rapid clot lysis and avoidance of hemorrhagic complications. Disadvantages are the need of sophisticated material, pulmonary artery catheterization, and radiation exposure. No conclusions can be made regarding the superiority of this method.

Embolectomy
Embolectomy, another treatment option when conservative treatment fails, is indicated to prevent death in patients who are hemodynamically unstable despite anticoagulation and treatment with vasopressors. Early experience with embolectomy was associated with a high incidence of mortality and neurologic sequelae, but technologic advances and extracorporeal bypass have significantly reduced the mortality associated with this procedure.[168] Pregnant women may be good candidates for surgery, as they tend to be younger and healthier than the average patient with VTE. Embolectomy has been associated with a 20% to 40% incidence of fetal loss,[168] however, so this treatment must be restricted to cases whereby woman's life is endangered.

Inferior vena cava filters
Inferior vena cava (IVC) filters have been used in pregnancy, and their indications are the same as for the nonpregnant population. Patients with such indications include: (1) patients with acute

VTE and contraindications to anticoagulation, (2) patients who have an episode of acute VTE while appropriately anticoagulated, and (3) patients who are critically ill and at risk for recurrent embolism whereby recurrent embolism is likely to be fatal.[168] In patients with hemodynamic compromise from PE, a repeat embolic event may be catastrophic. High risk for fatal recurrent embolism is an indication for the placement of an IVC filter, and retrievable filters are a valuable option in pregnancy.[170]

Management of delivery

Because of reports of spinal hematomas and cord compression during epidural anesthesia in nonpregnant women treated with LMWH, it is prudent to take measures to minimize the risk of hemorrhage when administering epidural anesthesia to women previously on LMWH. These measures include delaying epidural insertion until 10 to 12 hours after the last dose of LMWH and not restarting it until at least 6 to 8 hours after the epidural catheter has been removed.[101,161]

Prevention

Early mobilization and graduated compression stockings are mildly effective, safe, and noninvasive methods for prevention of VTE; they are probably all that is needed to prevent VTE in low-risk groups. Prospective, nonrandomized studies showed that in women with risk factors not receiving anticoagulation, the recurrence rate of VTE ranged from 2.4% to 12.2%, in comparison with 0% to 2.4% in patients who did receive anticoagulation.[171] LMWH has become the drug of choice for the prophylaxis and treatment of VTE in pregnant patients.[161] The dose of LMWH for thromboprophylaxis is based on the booking weight. There are no data to guide appropriate doses of LMWH for pregnant women who are obese or puerperal. It is agreed that women of higher weights should receive higher doses, but there are no studies available on the optimal dose and weight ranges. Patients at high risk for VTE (see **Table 2**) should receive the usual prophylactic dose of enoxaparin, 0.5 mg/kg body weight or dalteparin, 50 IU/kg body weight twice daily.

AMNIOTIC FLUID EMBOLISM
Introduction

Amniotic fluid embolism (AFE) is a rare but lethal condition also known as anaphylactoid syndrome of pregnancy. It usually occurs during or soon after delivery but can occur at any time during pregnancy.[172–175] AFE has also been described with the following procedures: vacuum aspiration of the uterus in the first trimester, second-

trimester termination of pregnancy, amniocentesis, amnioinfusion, and as late as 48 hours after a cesarean delivery.[172,173]

AFE was first described in a report by Meyer in 1926, who suggested that there was an occlusion of the pulmonary blood vessels by amniotic fluid or fetal cells,[174] but it was not widely recognized until 1941 when an autopsy series of 8 women who had died of sudden shock during labor reported squamous cells and mucin of fetal origin in the maternal pulmonary vasculature.[176,177] The modern concept of an anaphylactoid syndrome of pregnancy was suggested by Clark and colleagues.[178]

Outcomes

AFE has a high mortality rate of 61% to 85%,[172,179,180] although some recent reports found it to be as low as 16% to 37%[181,182] in United States and United Kingdom registries. Apart from the high mortality associated with AFE, the incidence of neurologic handicap is also significant, with reports quoting figures between 7%[172] and 85%.[180]

Incidence

The incidence of AFE is reported to be between 1 in 8000 and 1 in 80,000 live births.[172–174,179–181,183]

Risk Factors

AFE was associated with maternal age greater than 35 (odds ratio [OR] 2.2, 95% confidence interval [CI] 1.5–2.1), grand multiparity of more than 5 pregnancies (adjusted OR 10.9, 95% CI 2.81–42.7), placenta previa and abruptio placenta (OR 30.4, 95% CI 15.4–60.1), cesarean delivery (OR 5.7, 95% CI 3.7–8.7), medical induction of labor (OR 1.5, 95% CI 0.9–2.3), eclampsia and preeclampsia, and forceps and vacuum delivery.[181,184] Despite the associations, our current understanding of the pathogenesis suggests that these factors are probably not the cause of AFE syndrome, which at best is considered unpredictable and unpreventable.

Pathophysiology

Amniotic fluid probably enters the maternal circulation through the endocervical veins, the placental insertion site, or a site of uterine trauma. Once it reaches the maternal circulation it can precipitate cardiogenic shock, respiratory failure, and, possibly, an inflammatory response. Invasive hemodynamic measurements from women with AFE show a biphasic pattern of cardiogenic shock, with an initial phase of acute pulmonary hypertension due to diffuse vasospasm of the pulmonary vasculature lasting 15 to 30 minutes followed by left ventricular dysfunction. The mechanism of left ventricular failure during the later phase is unclear. Animal data suggest that it may be due to hypoxic injury to the left ventricle, release of maternal inflammatory mediators, or a direct depressant effect of amniotic fluid on the myocardium.[185–188]

Clinical Presentation

80% of patients with AFE present with[172,173,179,180]:

- Hypotension due to cardiogenic shock
- Coagulopathy due to disseminated intra-vascular coagulation (DIC)
- Acute respiratory failure or adult respiratory distress syndrome.

Most patients present with rapid cardiorespiratory collapse caused by these symptoms. Nonspecific symptoms (eg, chills, nausea, vomiting, agitation, mental confusion) may precede the onset of dyspnea and hypotension. Tonic-clonic seizure activity may also occur. There also appears to be a less severe presentation of AFE whereby only some of the major symptoms and signs occur. Such patients generally present with the sudden onset of milder dyspnea and hypotension. The clinical course tends to be abbreviated and the prognosis is much better than in women who have the full syndrome.[189,190]

Differential Diagnosis

The aforementioned signs and symptoms may also be seen in the following conditions:

- Obstetric-related hemorrhage and hypo-volemia
- Cardiogenic shock
- Massive thromboembolism
- Septic shock
- Eclampsia
- Incorrect drug administration
- Allergic reaction to a drug
- Transfusion reaction
- Peripartum cardiomyopathy
- Aspiration.

Diagnosis

- AFE is a clinical diagnosis that is based on the constellation of clinical findings, rather than isolated symptoms and signs. Clinicians should suspect AFE whenever shock and/or respiratory compromise develops during labor or immediately postpartum. Other causes of sudden intrapartum or postpartum cardiorespiratory failure must be excluded (see the differential diagnosis above).
- Amniotic fluid debris (squamous cells, trophoblastic cells, mucin, and lanugo) can sometimes be identified in blood samples drawn from the distal port of a pulmonary artery catheter. However, finding amniotic fluid debris should not be considered diagnostic of AFE because such debris is common in the maternal circulation of women without AFE.[191]
- Serologic assays of monoclonal antibodies to the mucin-like glycoprotein sialyl Tn and immunohistochemical staining that uses a monoclonal antibody (TKH-2) to detect a common fetal antigen in the mother's blood appear to have a high sensitivity for AFE.[192–194] However, these methods have not been fully validated and cannot be recommended for routine clinical practice.
- Other important tests to evaluate AFE should include a chest radiograph, ECG, full blood count and platelet count, coagulation profile, and arterial blood gas.
- Transesophageal echocardiography has been used to evaluate patients with suspected AFE, and shows the acute right ventricular overload with a D-shaped left ventricle on short-axis views, due to septal flattening from increased pulmonary pressures. Pulmonary trunks are dilated, with no other clinical conditions to explain the findings. During the later phase the left ventricular function is also globally depressed.[175,180,183]

Management

The basis of the management of AFE is support of the airway, tissue oxygenation, breathing, and circulation.[179]

- To maintain tissue oxygenation, 100% supplemental oxygen is indicated with intubation and ventilation to maintain positive end-respiratory pressure and to attempt to achieve a level of arterial oxygen partial pressure greater than 60 mm Hg with the saturation above 90%. The administration of diuretics is recommended.
- For circulatory support the Advanced Cardiac Life Support (ACLS) protocol should be initiated with the mother in the left lateral decubitus position. Colloids and crystalloids should be administered with inotropes such as dopamine, dobutamine, or phenylephrine. The aim is to improve the circulation and maintain a urine output of more than

25 mL/h with the mean arterial pressure higher than 65 mm Hg. Other treatment modalities include nitric oxide (a selective pulmonary vasodilator), cardiopulmonary bypass, extracorporeal membrane oxygenation, and intra-aortic balloon counterpulsation. Delivery of the fetus improves the survival of the fetus and helps with the maternal cardiopulmonary resuscitation. Intact fetal survival is possible if the fetus is delivered within 5 minutes. Improvement in maternal outcome is possible if the fetus is delivered within 4 minutes of developing malignant arrhythmia via a perimortem cesarean section.

- In cases where the mother develops convulsions or an altered level of consciousness, her hypoxia needs to be corrected and antiepileptic drugs may be used. Central venous pressure and pulmonary arterial lines are recommended in the fluid management of these patients.
- An important step in management is to correct the coagulopathy, which can be done using fresh-frozen plasma, packed red blood cells, and platelets. Cryoprecipitate is not the first-line therapy but has a role in volume-overloaded patients and also contains fibronectin, which assists the reticuloendothelial system with the filtration of antigenic and toxic substances. Recombinant factor VIIa may be useful to treat the DIC caused by AFE. Obstetric hemorrhage should be aggressively prevented by balloon tamponade of the uterus, and uterine artery embolization may be of help.
- Other treatment modalities such as high-dose steroids (500 mg hydrocortisone sodium succinate every 6 hours until improvement), antithrombin III infusion, leukotriene inhibitors, inhaled prostacyclines, hemofiltration, or exchange transfusion have been described anecdotally, and are unlikely to be tested scientifically.

REFERENCES

1. Roth A, Elkayam U. Acute myocardial infarction associated with pregnancy. J Am Coll Cardiol 2008;52:171–80.
2. Ladner HE, Danielson B, Gilbert WM. Acute myocardial infarction in pregnancy and puerperium: a population based study. Obstet Gynecol 2005;105:480–4.
3. James AH, Jamison MG, Biswas MS, et al. Acute myocardial infarction in pregnancy: a United States population-based study. Circulation 2006;113: 1564–71.
4. The Task Force on the Management of Cardiovascular Disease during Pregnancy of the European Society of Cardiology. Expert consensus document on management of cardiovascular disease during pregnancy. Eur Heart J 2003;24:761–81.
5. Badui E, Enciso R. Acute myocardial infarction during pregnancy and puerperium: a review. Angiology 1996;47:739–56.
6. Roos-Hesselink JW, Duvekot JJ, Thorne SA. Pregnancy in high risk cardiac conditions. Heart 2009; 95(8):680.
7. Petitti DB, Sidney S, Quesenberry CP Jr, et al. Incidence of stroke and myocardial infarction in women of reproductive age. Stroke 1997;28(2):280.
8. Koul AK, Hollander G, Moskovits N, et al. Coronary artery dissection during pregnancy and the postpartum period: two case reports and review of literature. Catheter Cardiovasc Interv 2001;52: 88–94.
9. Mather PJ, Hansen CL, Goldman B, et al. Postpartum multivessel coronary dissection. J Heart Lung Transplant 1994;13(3):533.
10. Appleby CE, Barolet A, Ing D, et al. Contemporary management of pregnancy-related coronary artery dissection: a single-centre experience and literature review. Exp Clin Cardiol 2009;14(1): e8–16.
11. Maeder M, Ammann P, Drack G, et al. Pregnancy-associated spontaneous coronary artery dissection: impact of medical treatment case report and systematic review. Z Kardiol 2005;94:829–35.
12. Manalo-Estrella P, Barker AE. Histopathologic findings in human aortic media associated with pregnancy. Arch Pathol 1967;83:336–41.
13. Bonnet J, Aumailley M, Thomas D. Spontaneous coronary artery dissection: case report and evidence for a defect in collagen metabolism. Eur Heart J 1986;7:904–9.
14. Borczuk AC, van Hoeven KH, Factor SM. Review and hypothesis: the eosinophils and peripartum heart disease: coincidence of pathogenetic significance? Cardiovasc Res 1997;33:527–32.
15. Rabinowitz M, Virmani R, McAllister HA. Spontaneous coronary artery dissection and eosinophilic inflammation: a cause and effect relationship? Am J Med 1982;72:923–8.
16. Basso C, Morgagni GL, Thiene G. Spontaneous coronary artery dissection: a neglected cause of acute myocardial ischemia and sudden death. Heart 1996;75(5):451.
17. Sasse L, Wagner R, Murray FE. Transmural myocardial infarction during pregnancy. Am J Cardiol 1975;35:448–52.
18. Elkayam U, Gleicher N. Hemodynamics and cardiac function during normal pregnancy and

the puerperium. In: Elkayam U, Gleicher N, editors. Cardiac problems in pregnancy. 3rd edition. New York: Wiley-Liss; 1998. p. 3–20.

19. Gant NF, Daley GL, Chand S. A study of angiotensin II pressor response throughout primigravid pregnancy. J Clin Invest 1973;52:2682–9.

20. Nisell H, Hjemdahl P, Linde B. Cardiovascular responses to circulating catecholamines in normal pregnancy and in pregnancy induced hypertension. Clin Physiol 1985;5:479–93.

21. Roberts JM, Taylor RN, Musci TJ. Preeclampsia: an endothelial cell disorder. Am J Obstet Gynecol 1989;161:1200–4.

22. Lin YH, Seow KM, Hwang JL. Myocardial infarction and mortality caused by methylergonovine. Acta Obstet Gynecol Scand 2005;84:1022.

23. Taylor GJ, Cohen B. Ergonovine-induced coronary artery spasm and myocardial infarction after normal delivery. Obstet Gynecol 1985;66: 821–2.

24. Mousa HA, McKinley CA, Thong J. Acute postpartum myocardial infarction after ergometrine administration in a woman with familial hypercholesterolemia. BJOG 2000;107:939–40.

25. Sutaria N, O'Toole L, Northridge D. Postpartum acute MI following routine ergometrine administration treated successfully by primary PTCA. Heart 2000;83:97–8.

26. Tsui BC, Stewart B, Fitzmaurice A, et al. Cardiac arrest and myocardial infarction induced by postpartum intravenous ergonovine administration. Anesthesiology 2001;94:363–4.

27. Jessurun CR, Adam K, Moise KJ, et al. Pheochromocytoma induced myocardial infarction in pregnancy. Tex Heart Inst J 1993;20:120–2.

28. Iadanza A, Del Pasqua A, Barbati R, et al. Acute ST elevation myocardial infarction in pregnancy due to coronary vasospasm: a case report and review of the literature. Int J Cardiol 2007;115:81–5.

29. Livingston JC, Mabie BC, Ramanathan J. Crack cocaine, myocardial infarction, and troponin I levels at the time of cesarean delivery. Anesth Analg 2000;91:913–5.

30. Koh CL, Viegas OA, Yuen R, et al. Plasminogen activators and inhibitors in normal late pregnancy, postpartum and postnatal period. Int J Gynaecol Obstet 1992;38:9–18.

31. Fletcher AP, Alkjaersig NK, Burstein R. The influence of pregnancy upon blood coagulation and plasma fibrinolytic enzyme function. Am J Obstet Gynecol 1979;134:743–51.

32. Gore M, Eldon S, Trofatter KF. Pregnancy induced changes in the fibrinolytic balance: evidence for defective release of tissue plasminogen activator and increased levels of fast acting tissue plasminogen activator inhibitor. Am J Obstet Gynecol 1987;156:674–80.

33. MacKinnon S, Walker ID, Davidson JF. Plasma fibrinolysis during and after normal childbirth. Br J Haematol 1987;65:339–42.

34. Yoshimura T, Ito M, Nakamura T. The influence of labor on thrombotic and fibrinolytic system. Eur J Obstet Gynecol Reprod Biol 1992;44:195–9.

35. Comp PC, Thurnau GR, Welsh J. Functional and immunologic protein S levels are decreased during pregnancy. Blood 1986;68:881–5.

36. Taylor GW, Moliterno DJ, Hillis LD. Peripartum myocardial infarction. Am Heart J 1993;126:1462–3.

37. Davis RB, Leuschen MP, Boyd D. Evaluation of platelet function in pregnancy. Comparative studies in non smoker and smokers. Thromb Res 1987;46: 175–86.

38. Regitz-Zagrosek V, Blomstrom Lundqvist C, Borghi C, et al; European Society of Gynecology; Association for European Paediatric Cardiology; German Society for Gender Medicine; Authors/ Task Force Members. The Task Force on the Management of Cardiovascular Diseases during Pregnancy of the European Society of Cardiology (ESC). Eur Heart J 2011;32:3147–97

39. Mathew JP, Fleisher LA, Rinehouse JA, et al. ST segment depression during labor and delivery. Anesthesiology 1993;78:997–8.

40. Moran C, Ni Bhuinnedin M, Geary M, et al. Myocardial ischemia in normal patients undergoing elective cesarean section: a peripartum assessment. Anaesthesia 2001;56:1051–8.

41. McLintic A, Pringle SD, Lilley S, et al. Electrocardiographic changes during cesarean section under regional anesthesia. Anesth Analg 1992;74:51–6.

42. Shivvers SA, Wians FH, Keffer JH, et al. Maternal cardiac troponin I levels during normal labor and delivery. Am J Obstet Gynecol 1999;180:122–7.

43. Shade GH Jr, Ross G, Bever FN, et al. Troponin I in the diagnosis of acute myocardial infarction in pregnancy, labor, and post partum. Am J Obstet Gynecol 2002;187(6):1719.

44. Fleming SM, O'Gorman T, Finn J, et al. Cardiac troponin I in pre-eclampsia and gestational hypertension. Br J Obstet Gynaecol 2000;107:1417–20.

45. Atalay C, Erden G, Turhan T, et al. The effect of magnesium sulfate treatment on serum cardiac troponin I levels in preeclamptic women. Acta Obstet Gynecol Scand 2005;84:617–21.

46. Manders MA, Sonder GJ, Mulder EF, et al. The effect of maternal exercise on fetal heart rate and movement pattern. Early Hum Dev 1997;48: 237–47.

47. Avery ND, Stocking KD, Tranmer JE, et al. Fetal responses to maternal strength conditioning exercises in late gestation. Can J Appl Physiol 1999; 24:362–76.

48. Schinkel AF, Bax JJ, Geleijnse ML, et al. Noninvasive evaluation of ischemic heart disease: myocardial

perfusion imaging or stress echocardiography? Eur Heart J 2003;24:789–800.

49. Collins JS, Bossone E, Eagle KA, et al. Asymptomatic coronary artery disease in a pregnant patient. Herz 2002;27:548–54.

50. International Commission on Radiological Protection, Annals of the ICRP. Tarrytown (NY): Pergamon, Elsevier Science, Inc; 2000. Publication 84: Pregnancy and Medical Radiation 30(1).

51. Colletti PM, Lee K. Cardiovascular imaging in the pregnant patient. In: Elkayam U, Gleicher N, editors. Cardiac problems in pregnancy. 3rd edition. New York: Wiley-Liss; 1998. p. 33–6.

52. Antman EM, Anbe DT, Armstrong PW, et al. ACC/AHA Guidelines for the management of patients with ST-elevation myocardial infarction: executive summary. J Am Coll Cardiol 2004;44:671–719.

53. Wright RS, Anderson J, Zidar JP. 2011 ACCF/AHA Focused Update Incorporated Into the ACC/AHA 2007 Guidelines for the management of patients with unstable angina/non ST elevation MI. J Am Coll Cardiol 2011;57:e215–367.

54. Bredy PL, Singh P, Frishman WH. Acute inferior wall myocardial infarction and percutaneous coronary intervention of the right coronary during active labor. Cardiol Rev 2008;16:260–8.

55. Reizig K, Diar N, Walcker JL. Myocardial infarction, pregnancy and anesthesia. Ann Fr Anesth Reanim 2000;19:544–8.

56. Sebastian C, Scherlag M, Kugelmass A, et al. Primary stent implantation for acute myocardial infarction during pregnancy: use of abciximab, ticlopidine, and aspirin. Cathet Cardiovasc Diagn 1998;45:275–9.

57. Eickman FM. Acute coronary artery angioplasty during pregnancy. Cathet Cardiovasc Diagn 1996;38:369–72.

58. Sharma GL, Loubeyre C, Morice C. Safety and feasibility of the radial approach for primary angioplasty in acute myocardial infarction during pregnancy. J Invasive Cardiol 2002;14:359–62.

59. Ko WJ, Ho HN, Chu SH. Postpartum myocardial infarction rescued with an intraaortic balloon pump and extracorporeal membrane oxygenator. Int J Cardiol 1998;63:81–4.

60. Garry D, Leikin E, Fleisher AG, et al. Acute myocardial infarction in pregnancy with subsequent medical and surgical management. Obstet Gynecol 1996;87:802–4.

61. Chambers CE, Clark SL. Cardiac surgery during pregnancy. Clin Obstet Gynecol 1994;37:316–23.

62. Bernal JM, Miralles PJ. Cardiac surgery with cardiopulmonary bypass during pregnancy. Obstet Gynecol Surv 1986;41:1–6.

63. Parry AJ, Westaby S. Cardiopulmonary bypass during pregnancy. Ann Thorac Surg 1996;61:1865–9.

64. Pomini F, Mercogliano D, Cavalletti C, et al. Cardiopulmonary bypass in pregnancy. Ann Thorac Surg 1996;61:259–68.

65. Weiss BM, von Segesser LK, Alon E, et al. Outcome of cardiovascular surgery and pregnancy: a systemic review of the period 1984-1996. Am J Obstet Gynecol 1998;179:1643–53.

66. Klutstein MW, Tzivoni D, Bitran D, et al. Treatment of spontaneous coronary artery dissection. Cathet Cardiovasc Diagn 1997;40:372–6.

67. Schumacher B, Belfort MA, Card RJ. Successful treatment of acute myocardial infarction during pregnancy with tissue plasminogen activator. Am J Obstet Gynecol 1997;176:716–9.

68. Bac DJ, Lotgering FK, Verkaalk AP, et al. Spontaneous coronary artery dissection during pregnancy and post-partum. Eur Heart J 1995;16:136–8.

69. Murugappan A, Coplin WM, Al-Sadat AN, et al. Thrombolytic therapy of acute ischemic stroke during pregnancy. Neurology 2006;66:768–70.

70. Leonhardt G, Gaul C, Nietsch HH, et al. Thromobolytic therapy in pregnancy. J Thromb Thrombolysis 2006;21:271–6.

71. Pfeifer GW. Distribution studies on placental transfer of 131Istreptokinase during labor. Ann Med 1970;19:17–8.

72. Lecander I, Nilsson M, Astedt B. Depression of plasminogen activator activity during pregnancy by the placental inhibitor PAI 2. Fibrinolysis 1988;2:165–7.

73. Shepard TH. Catalog of teratogenic agents. 6th edition. Baltimore (MD): Johns Hopkins University Press; 1989. p. 655.

74. Usta IM, Abdallah M, El-Hajj M. Massive subchorionic hematomas following thrombolytic therapy in pregnancy. Obstet Gynecol 2004;103:1079–82.

75. Briggs GG, Freeman RK, Yaffe SJ. Drugs in pregnancy and lactation. 7th edition. Philadelphia: Lippincott Williams &Wilkins; 2005.

76. Qasgas SA, Mc Pherson C, Frishman WH, et al. Cardiovascular pharmacotherapeutic considerations during pregnancy and lactation. Cardiol Rev 2004;12:240–61.

77. Imperiale TF, Petrulis AS. A meta-analysis of low-dose aspirin for the prevention of pregnancy-induced hypertensive disease. JAMA 1991;266:260–4.

78. CLASP (Collaborative Low-dose Aspirin Study in Pregnancy) Collaborative Group. CLASP: a randomized trial of low-dose aspirin for the prevention and treatment of pre-eclampsia among 9364 pregnant women. Lancet 1994;343:619–29.

79. American Academy of Pediatrics Committee on Drugs. The transfer of drugs and other chemicals into human milk. Pediatrics 1994;93:137–50.

80. Sullebarger JT, Fontanet HL, Matar FA, et al. Percutaneous coronary intervention for myocardial

infarction during pregnancy: a new trend? J Invasive Cardiol 2003;15:725–8.

81. Shah P, Dzavik V, Cusimano RJ, et al. Spontaneous dissection of the left main coronary artery. Can J Cardiol 2004;20:815–8.

82. Martin M, Romero E, Moris C. Acute myocardial infarction during pregnancy. Treatment with clopidogrel. Med Clin (Barc) 2003;121:278–9 [in Spanish].

83. Klinzing P, Markert UR, Liesaus K, et al. Case report: successful pregnancy and delivery after myocardial infarction and essential thrombocythemia treated with clopidogrel. Clin Exp Obstet Gynecol 2001;28:215–6.

84. Nallamothu BK, Saint M, Saint S, et al. Double jeopardy. N Engl J Med 2005;353:75–80.

85. Cetin A, Yurtcu N, Guvenal T, et al. The effect of glyceryl trinitrate on hypertension in women with severe preeclampsia, HELLP syndrome and eclampsia. Hypertens Pregnancy 2004;23:37–46.

86. Chandraharan E, Arulkumaran S. Acute tocolysis. Curr Opin Obstet Gynecol 2005;17:151–6.

87. Bullarbo M, Tjumum J, Ekerhovd E. Sublingual nitroglycerin for management of retained placenta. Int J Gynaecol Obstet 2005;91:228–32.

88. Kahler C, Schleussmer E, Moller A, et al. Nitric oxide donors: effects on fetoplacental blood flow. Eur J Obstet Gynecol Reprod Biol 2004;115:10–4.

89. Hurst AK, Hoffman R, Frishman WH, et al. The use of beta-adrenergic blocking agents in pregnancy and lactation. In: Elkayam U, Gleicher N, editors. Cardiac problems in pregnancy. 3rd edition. New York: Wiley-Liss; 1998. p. 357–72.

90. Magee LA, Elran EI, Bull SB, et al. Risks and benefits of beta receptor blockers for pregnant hypertension: overview of the randomized trials. Eur J Obstet Gynecol Reprod Biol 2000;88:15–26.

91. Childress CH, Katz VL. Nifedipine and its indications in obstetrics and gynecology. Obstet Gynecol 1994;83:616–24.

92. Waisman GD, Mayorga LM, Cámera MI, et al. Magnesium plus nifedipine: potentiation of hypotensive effect in preeclampsia. Am J Obstet Gynecol 1988;159:308–9.

93. Shotan A, Widerhorn J, Hurst A, et al. Risks of angiotensin converting enzyme inhibition during pregnancy: experimental and clinical evidence, potential mechanisms and recommendations for use. Am J Med 1994;96:451–6.

94. Cooper WO, Hernandez-Diaz S, Arbogast PG, et al. Major congenital malformations after first trimester exposure to ACE inhibitors. N Engl J Med 2006;354:2443–51.

95. Lambot MA, Vermeylen D, Vermeylen JC. Angiotensin II receptor inhibitors in pregnancy. Lancet 2001;357:1619–20.

96. Quan A. Fetopathy associated with exposure to angiotensin-converting enzyme. 16th edition. Drug information for the health care professional, vol. 1. Rockville (MD): United States Pharmacopeial Convention; 1996.

97. Quan A. Fetopathy associated with exposure to angiotensin converting enzyme inhibitors and angiotensin receptor antagonists. Early Hum Dev 2006;82:23–8.

98. Manson JM, Freyssinges C, Ducrocq MB, et al. Postmarketing surveillance of lovastatin and simvastatin exposure during pregnancy. Reprod Toxicol 1996;10:439–46.

99. Bates SM, Greer IA, Hirsh J, et al. Use of antithrombotic agents during pregnancy: the Seventh ACCP Conference on Antithrombotic and Thrombolytic Therapy. Chest 2004;126:627s–44s.

100. Oran B, Lee-Parritz A, Ansell J. Low molecular weight heparin for the prophylaxis of thromboembolism in women with prosthetic mechanical heart valves during pregnancy. Thromb Haemost 2004; 92:747–51.

101. Sanson BJ, Lensing AW, Prins MH, et al. Safety of low-molecular weight heparin in pregnancy: a systematic review. Thromb Haemost 1999;81:668–72.

102. Miller RK, Mace K, Polliotti B, et al. Marginal transfer of ReoPro (abciximab) compared with immunoglobulin G (F105), insulin and water in the perfused human placenta in vitro. Placenta 2003;24:727–38.

103. Boztosun B, Olcay A, Avci A, et al. Treatment of acute myocardial infarction in pregnancy with coronary artery balloon angioplasty and stenting: use of tirofiban and clopidogrel. Int J Cardiol 2008;127: 413–6.

104. Ecker J, Frigoletto F. Cesarean delivery and the risk-benefit calculus. N Engl J Med 2007;356: 885–8.

105. Hands ME, Johnson MD, Salzman DH, et al. The cardiac, obstetric and anesthetic management of pregnancy complicated by acute myocardial infarction. J Clin Anesth 1990;2:258–68.

106. Hagan PG, Nienaber CA, Isselbacher EM, et al. The International Registry of Acute Aortic Dissection (IRAD): new insights into an old disease. JAMA 2000;283:897–903.

107. Centre for Maternal and Child Enquiries (CMACE). Saving mothers' Lives: reviewing maternal deaths to make motherhood safer: 2006-2008. The Eighth Report on Confidential Enquiries into Maternal Deaths in the United Kingdom. BJOG 2011; 118(Suppl 1):1–203.

108. Thalmann M, Sodeck GH, Domanovits H, et al. Acute type A aortic dissection and pregnancy: a population-based study. Eur J Cardiothorac Surg 2011;39:e159–63.

109. Mészáros I, Mórocz J, Szlávi J, et al. Epidemiology and clinicopathology of aortic dissection. A population-based longitudinal study over 27 years. Chest 2000;117:1271–8.

110. Khan AK, Nair CK. Clinical, diagnostic and management perspectives of aortic dissection. Chest 2002;122:311–28.

111. Elkayam U, Ostrzega E, Shotan A, et al. Cardiovascular problems in pregnant woman with the Marfan syndrome. Ann Intern Med 1995;123:117–22.

112. Campisi D, Bivona A, Paterna S, et al. Oestrogen binding sites in fresh human aortic tissue. Int J Tissue React 1987;9:393–8.

113. Nolte JE, Rutherford RB, Nawaz S, et al. Arterial dissections associated with pregnancy. J Vasc Surg 1995;21:515–20.

114. Rossiter JP, Repke JT, Morales AJ, et al. A prospective longitudinal evaluation of pregnancy in the Marfan syndrome. Am J Obstet Gynecol 1995;173:1599–606.

115. Lipscomb KJ, Smith JC, Clarke B, et al. Outcome of pregnancy in women with Marfan's syndrome. Br J Obstet Gynaecol 1997;104:201–6.

116. Zeebregts CJ, Schepens MA, Hameeteman TM, et al. Acute aortic dissection complicating pregnancy. Ann Thorac Surg 1997;64:1345–8.

117. Lind J, Wallenburg HC. The Marfan syndrome and pregnancy: a retrospective study in a Dutch population. Eur J Obstet Gynecol Reprod Biol 2001;98:28–35.

118. Pacini L, Digne F, Boumendil A, et al. Maternal complication of pregnancy in Marfan syndrome. Int J Cardiol 2009;136:156–61.

119. Strickland RA, Oliver WC Jr, Chantigian RC, et al. Anesthesia, cardiopulmonary bypass, and the pregnant patient. Mayo Clin Proc 1991;66(4):411–29.

120. Spittell PC, Spittell JA Jr, Joyce JW, et al. Clinical features and differential diagnosis of aortic dissection: experience with 236 cases (1980 through 1990). Mayo Clin Proc 1993;68:642–51.

121. Erbel R, Alfonso F, Boileau C, et al. Diagnosis and management of aortic dissection—Recommendations of the Task Force on Aortic Dissection, European Society of Cardiology. Eur Heart J 2001;22:1642–81.

122. Hiratzka LF, Bakris GL, Beckman JA, et al. 2010 ACCF/AHA/AATS/ACR/ASA/SCA/SCAI/SIR/STS/SVM guidelines for the diagnosis and management of patients with Thoracic Aortic Disease: a report of the American College of Cardiology Foundation/American Heart Association Task Force on Practice Guidelines, American Association for Thoracic Surgery, American College of Radiology, American Stroke Association, Society of Cardiovascular Anesthesiologists, Society for Cardiovascular Angiography and Interventions, Society of Interventional Radiology, Society of Thoracic Surgeons, and Society for Vascular Medicine. Circulation 2010;121(13):e266.

123. Immer FF, Bansi AG, Immer-Bansi AS, et al. Aortic dissection in pregnancy: analysis of risk factors and outcome. Ann Thorac Surg 2003;76:309–14.

124. Gott VL, Cameron DE, Alejo DE, et al. Aortic root replacement in 271 Marfan patients: a 24-year experience. Ann Thorac Surg 2002;73:438–43.

125. Akashi H, Tayama K, Fujino T, et al. Surgical treatment for acute type A aortic dissection in pregnancy: a case of aortic root replacement just after cesarean section. Jpn Circ J 2000;64:729–30.

126. Jondeau G, Nataf P, Belarbi A, et al. Aortic dissection at 6 months gestation in women with Marfan's syndrome: simultaneous Bentall intervention and cesarean section. Arch Mal Coeur Vaiss 2000;93:185–7 [in French].

127. Naito H, Naito H, Tada K. Open heart operation for a pregnant patient with Marfan syndrome. Masui 2005;54:525–9 [in Japanese].

128. Lacassie HJ, Millar S, Leithe LG, et al. Dural ectasia: a likely cause of inadequate spinal anaesthesia in two parturients with Marfan's syndrome. Br J Anaesth 2005;94(4):500.

129. Ramaswamy P, Lytrivi ID, Nguyen K, et al. Neonatal Marfan syndrome: in utero presentation with aortic and pulmonary artery dilatation and successful repair of an acute flail mitral valve leaflet in infancy. Pediatr Cardiol 2006;27:763–5.

130. Centers for Disease Control and Prevention. Pregnancy-related mortality surveillance—United States, 1991-1999. MMWR Morb Mortal Wkly Rep 2003;52:1–8.

131. Heit JA, Kobbervig CE, James AH, et al. Trends in the incidence of venous thromboembolism during pregnancy or postpartum: a 30-year population-based study. Ann Intern Med 2005;143:697–706.

132. O'Connor DJ, Scher LA, Gargiulo NJ 3rd, et al. Incidence and characteristics of venous thromboembolic disease during pregnancy and the postnatal period: a contemporary series. Ann Vasc Surg 2011;25:9–14.

133. Sullivan EA, Ford JB, Chambers G, et al. Maternal mortality in Australia, 1973-1996. Aust N Z J Obstet Gynaecol 2004;44:452–7 [discussion: 377].

134. Marik PE, Plante LA. Venous thromboembolic disease and pregnancy. N Engl J Med 2008;359:2025.

135. Greer IA. Thrombosis in pregnancy: maternal and fetal issues. Lancet 1999;353:1258.

136. Prevention of venous thrombosis and pulmonary embolism. NIH Consensus Development. JAMA 1986;256:744.

137. Kujovich JL. Hormones and pregnancy: thromboembolic risks for women. Br J Haematol 2004;126:443.

138. Morris JM, Algert CS, Roberts CL. Incidence and risk factors for pulmonary embolism in the postpartum period. J Thromb Haemost 2010;8:998.

139. McColl MD, Ramsay JE, Tait RC, et al. Risk factors for pregnancy associated venous thromboembolism. Thromb Haemost 1997;78:1183.

140. Brill-Edwards P, Ginsberg JS, Gent M, et al. Safety of withholding heparin in pregnant women with a history of venous thromboembolism. Recurrence of Clot in This Pregnancy Study Group. N Engl J Med 2000;343:1439–44.

141. Gherman RB, Goodwin TM, Leung B, et al. Incidence, clinical characteristics, and timing of objectively diagnosed venous thromboembolism during pregnancy. Obstet Gynecol 1999;94:730–4.

142. Powrie RO, Larson L, Rosene-Montella K, et al. Alveolar-arterial oxygen gradient in acute pulmonary embolism in pregnancy. Am J Obstet Gynecol 1998;178:394–6.

143. Chan WS, Lee A, Spencer FA, et al. Predicting deep venous thrombosis in pregnancy: out in "LEFt" field? Ann Intern Med 2009;151:85–92.

144. Leung AN, Bull TM, Jaeschke R, et al. An official American Thoracic Society/Society of Thoracic Radiology clinical practice guideline: evaluation of suspected pulmonary embolism in pregnancy. ATS/STR Committee on Pulmonary Embolism in Pregnancy. Am J Respir Crit Care Med 2011; 184(10):1200–8.

145. Forbes KP, Reid JH, Murchison JT. Do preliminary chest X-ray findings define the optimum role of pulmonary scintigraphy in suspected pulmonary embolism? Clin Radiol 2001;56:397–400.

146. Scarsbrook AF, Bradley KM, Gleeson FV. Perfusion scintigraphy: diagnostic utility in pregnant women with suspected pulmonary embolic disease. Eur Radiol 2007;17:2554–60.

147. Ridge CA, McDermott S, Freyne BJ, et al. Pulmonary embolism in pregnancy: comparison of pulmonary CT angiography and lung scintigraphy. AJR Am J Roentgenol 2009;193:1223–7.

148. Chan WS, Ray JG, Murray S, et al. Suspected pulmonary embolism in pregnancy: clinical presentation, results of lung scanning, and subsequent maternal and pediatric outcomes. Arch Intern Med 2002;162:1170–5.

149. Shahir K, Goodman LR, Tali A, et al. Pulmonary embolism in pregnancy: CT pulmonary angiography versus perfusion scanning. AJR Am J Roentgenol 2010;195:W214–20.

150. Revel MP, Cohen S, Sanchez O, et al. Pulmonary embolism during pregnancy: diagnosis with lung scintigraphy or CT angiography? Radiology 2011; 258:590–8.

151. Kline JA, Williams GW, Hernandez-Nino J. D-dimer concentrations in normal pregnancy: new diagnostic thresholds are needed. Clin Chem 2005; 51:825–9.

152. Damodaram M, Kaladindi M, Luckit J, et al. D-dimers as a screening test for venous thromboembolism in pregnancy: is it of any use? J Obstet Gynaecol 2009;29:101–3.

153. Levy MS, Spencer F, Ginsberg JS, et al. Reading between the (Guidelines). Management of submassive pulmonary embolism in the first trimester of pregnancy. Thromb Res 2008;121:705–7.

154. To MS, Hunt BJ, Nelson-Piercy C. A negative D-dimer does not exclude venous thromboembolism (VTE) in pregnancy. J Obstet Gynaecol 2008;28: 222–3.

155. Bourjeily G, Chalhoub M, Phornphutkul C, et al. Neonatal thyroid function: effect of a single exposure to iodinated contrast medium in utero. Radiology 2010;256:744–50.

156. Food and Drug Administration. Content and format of labeling for human prescription drug and biological products; requirements for pregnancy and lactation labeling. Fed Regist 2008;29: 30831–68.

157. Lin SP, Brown JJ. MR contrast agents: physical and pharmacologic basics. J Magn Reson Imaging 2007;25:884–99.

158. Webb JA, Thomsen HS, Morcos SK. The use of iodinated and gadolinium contrast media during pregnancy and lactation. Eur Radiol 2005;15: 1234–40.

159. Chen MM, Coakley FV, Kaimal A, et al. Guidelines for computed tomography and magnetic resonance imaging use during pregnancy and lactation. Obstet Gynecol 2008;112:333–40.

160. Kluge A, Müller C, Hansel J, et al. Real-time MR with TrueFISP for the detection of acute pulmonary embolism: initial clinical experience. Eur Radiol 2004;14(4):709–18.

161. Greer IA, Nelson-Piercy C. Low-molecular-weight heparins for thromboprophylaxis and treatment of venous thromboembolism in pregnancy: a systematic review of safety and efficacy. Blood 2005;106: 401–7.

162. Gris JC, Neveu S, Tailland ML, et al. Use of enoxaparin in primary early recurrent aborters with an impaired fibrinolytic capacity. Thromb Haemost 1995;73:362–7.

163. Brenner B, Hoffman R, Blumenfeld Z, et al. Gestational outcome in thrombophilic women with recurrent pregnancy loss treated with enoxaparin. Thromb Haemost 2000;83:693–7.

164. Younis JS, Ohel G, Brenner B, et al. The effect of thrombophylaxis on pregnancy outcome in patients with recurrent pregnancy loss associated with Factor V Leiden mutation. BJOG 2000;107:415–9.

165. Bates SM, Greer IA, Pabinger I, et al. Venous thromboembolism, thrombophilia, antithrombotic therapy, and pregnancy: American College of Chest Physicians evidence-based clinical practice guidelines (8th edition). Chest 2008;133(Suppl 6): 844S–86S.

166. Torbicki A, Perrier A, Konstantinides S, et al. Guidelines on the diagnosis and management of acute pulmonary embolism: the Task Force for the Diagnosis and Management of Acute Pulmonary Embolism of the European Society of Cardiology (ESC). Eur Heart J 2008;29:2276–315.

167. Turrentine MA, Braems G, Ramirez MM. Use of thrombolytics for the treatment of thromboembolic disease during pregnancy. Obstet Gynecol Surv 1995;50:534–41.

168. Ahearn GS, Hadjiliadis D, Govert JA, et al. Massive pulmonary embolism during pregnancy successfully treated with recombinant tissue plasminogen activator: a case report and review of treatment options. Arch Intern Med 2002;162:1221–7.

169. Bechtel JJ, Mountford MC, Ellinwood WE. Massive pulmonary embolism in pregnancy treated with catheter fragmentation and local thrombolysis. Obstet Gynecol 2005;106(5 Pt 2):1158–60.

170. Kawamata K, Chiba Y, Tanaka R, et al. Experience of temporary inferior vena cava filters inserted in the perinatal period to prevent pulmonary embolism in pregnant women with deep vein thrombosis. J Vasc Surg 2005;41:652–6.

171. Bauersachs RM, Dudenhausen J, Faridi A, et al. Risk stratification and heparin prophylaxis to prevent venous thromboembolism in pregnant women. Thromb Haemost 2007;98:1237–45.

172. Stafford I, Sheffield J. Amniotic fluid embolism. Obstet Gynecol Clin North Am 2007;34:545–53.

173. Swayze CR, Barton JR, Skerman JH. Amniotic fluid embolism. Semin Anesth Perioperat Med Pain 2000;19:181–7.

174. Schoening AM. Amniotic fluid embolism: historical perspectives and new possibilities. MCN Am J Matern Child Nurs 2006;31:78–83.

175. O'Shea A, Eappen S. Amniotic fluid embolism. Int Anesthesiol Clin 2007;45:17–28.

176. Meyer JR. Embolia pulmonar amnio caseosa. Brasil Medico 1926;2:301 [in Portuguese].

177. Steiner PE, Lushbaugh CC. Landmark article, Oct. 1941: maternal pulmonary embolism by amniotic fluid as a cause of obstetric shock and unexpected deaths in obstetrics. JAMA 1986;255(16):2187.

178. Clark SL, Hankins GD, Dudley DA, et al. Amniotic fluid embolism: analysis of the national registry. Am J Obstet Gynecol 1995;172:1159–67.

179. Banks A, Levy D. Life-threatening complications of pregnancy: key issues for anaesthetists. Curr Anaesth Crit Care 2006;17:163–70.

180. James CF, Feinglass NG, Menke DM, et al. Massive amniotic fluid embolism: diagnosis aided by emergency transesophageal echocardiography. Int J Obstet Anesth 2004;13:279–83.

181. Abenhaim HA, Azoulay L, Kramer MS, et al. Incidence and risk factors of amniotic fluid embolisms: a population-based study on 3 million births in the United State. Am J Obstet Gynecol 2008;199(1):49.e1.

182. Tuffnell DJ. United Kingdom amniotic fluid embolism register. BJOG 2005;112(12):1625.

183. McDonnel NJ, Chan BO, Frenley RW. Rapid reversal of critical haemodynamic compromise with nitric oxide in a parturient with amniotic fluid embolism. Int J Obstet Anesth 2007;16:269–73.

184. Knight M, Tuffnell D, Brocklehurst P, et al, UK Obstetric Surveillance System. Incidence and risk factors for amniotic-fluid embolism. Obstet Gynecol 2010;115(5):910.

185. Clark SL, Cotton DB, Gonik B, et al. Central hemodynamic alterations in amniotic fluid embolism. Am J Obstet Gynecol 1988;158(5):1124.

186. Clark SL, Montz FJ, Phelan JP. Hemodynamic alterations associated with amniotic fluid embolism: a reappraisal. Am J Obstet Gynecol 1985;151(5):617.

187. Shechtman M, Ziser A, Markovits R, et al. Amniotic fluid embolism: early findings of transesophageal echocardiography. Anesth Analg 1999;89(6):1456.

188. Stanten RD, Iverson LI, Daugharty TM, et al. Amniotic fluid embolism causing catastrophic pulmonary vasoconstriction: diagnosis by transesophageal echocardiogram and treatment by cardiopulmonary bypass. Obstet Gynecol 2003;102(3):496.

189. Masson RG, Ruggieri J, Siddiqui MM. Amniotic fluid embolism: definitive diagnosis in a survivor. Am Rev Respir Dis 1979;120(1):187.

190. Wasser WG, Tessler S, Kamath CP. Nonfatal amniotic fluid embolism: a case report of post-partum respiratory distress with histopathologic studies. Mt Sinai J Med 1979;46(4):388.

191. Lee W, Ginsburg KA, Cotton DB, et al. Squamous and trophoblastic cells in the maternal pulmonary circulation identified by invasive hemodynamic monitoring during the peripartum period. Am J Obstet Gynecol 1986;155(5):999.

192. Aguilera LG, Fernandez C, Laza AP, et al. Fatal amniotic fluid embolism diagnosed histologically. Acta Aneasthesiol Scand 2002;46:334–7.

193. Oi H, Kobayashi H, Hirashima Y, et al. Serological and immunohistochemical diagnosis of amniotic fluid embolism. Semin Thromb Hemost 1998;24(5):479.

194. Kobayashi H, Ooi H, Hayakawa H, et al. Histological diagnosis of amniotic fluid embolism by monoclonal antibody TKH-2 that recognizes NeuAc alpha 2-6GalNAc epitope. Hum Pathol 1997;28(4):428.

Valvular Heart Disease and Pregnancy

Thomas A. Traill, BM, FRCP

KEYWORDS

- Pregnancy • Mitral stenosis • Bicuspid aortic valve • Marfan syndrome
- Hypertrophic cardiomyopathy • Prosthetic heart valves

KEY POINTS

- Among women with valvular heart disease, those with mitral stenosis carry the greatest potential for problems during pregnancy. Balloon commissurotomy may be needed before, or even during, pregnancy.
- Asymptomatic women with aortic stenosis and only mild or moderate left ventricular outflow obstruction generally tolerate pregnancy well, as do those with regurgitant lesions.
- In Marfan syndrome, pregnancy should not be undertaken if the aortic root dimension exceeds 4 cm. Even if the aortic root is normal, a small increased risk of dissection is present.
- Women with well-functioning bioprosthetic valves and normal hemodynamics may safely undertake a pregnancy. However, bioprostheses deteriorate rapidly in young people, and therefore preconception counseling should be kept under frequent review.

INTRODUCTION

How heart valve disease may complicate pregnancy is a topic of considerable historical significance. In approximately 1880 a young Scottish physician, James Mackenzie, had his "attention brought to the subject of heart disease and pregnancy by a tragic experience…" in which a young woman with mitral stenosis developed pulmonary congestion in the middle trimester and eventually succumbed during labor. Inspired by her loss, and by the recognition that the clinical evaluation of heart disease lacked a physiologic understanding of its effect on the circulation, Mackenzie became one of the first of a new kind of 20th century bedside medical physiologist, and he has been claimed to be the first to specialize in what would now be recognized as clinical hemodynamically based cardiology. His monograph "Heart Disease and Pregnancy,"[1] published in 1921, was the first modern text on this topic, and remains a classic of clinical study.[2] Although heart valve lesions retain their potential to complicate the physiologic effects of pregnancy, and mitral stenosis in particular remains a clinical challenge, over the past 100 years these threats have been mitigated by improved public health, clinical and echocardiographic assessment of patients, cardiac surgery, and interventional cardiology.

MITRAL STENOSIS
Epidemiology

With the virtual disappearance of rheumatic heart disease in the United States and Western Europe, the most valuable contemporary experience with pregnant women who have mitral stenosis tends to lie in regions of the world where first-rate medicine, and its accompanying technology, are available to poor overcrowded populations and public health resources are still overstretched. These regions, the sources of significant case series, include southern Africa, Brazil, Poland, India, and Southeast Asia.[3–7]

Division of Cardiology, Johns Hopkins University School of Medicine, 601 North Caroline Street, JHOC 7262, Baltimore, MD 21287-0960, USA
E-mail address: ttraill@jhmi.edu

Cardiol Clin 30 (2012) 369–381
doi:10.1016/j.ccl.2012.04.004
0733-8651/12/$ – see front matter © 2012 Elsevier Inc. All rights reserved

cardiology.theclinics.com

Pathophysiology

In mitral stenosis, the adverse effects of pregnancy stem from three physiologic changes: the inevitable increase in ventricular filling pressures that stem from increased blood and extracellular fluid volume; the increase in cardiac output, typically by as much as 50%; and an increase in heart rate that further compromises left ventricular filling.

Increased blood volume and cardiac output present a problem in any obstructive valvular lesion. The Gorlin formula predicts that the gradient across a stenosis is proportional to the square of the flow. Hence, in pregnancy, as in any high-flow state, a 50% increase in cardiac output entails that the valve gradient more than doubles, even assuming that blood flow remains laminar. This mechanism is true in aortic stenosis just as in mitral stenosis, but in aortic stenosis the left atrial pressure is not directly affected. In mitral stenosis, the increase in blood volume and gradient are additive to the left atrial and pulmonary venous pressure.

The third hemodynamic mechanism at work applies especially to mitral stenosis, namely the effect of an increase in heart rate. As much as it is a disease of a narrowed mitral orifice, with an elevated atrioventricular filling pressure gradient, mitral stenosis is a disease characterized by slow left ventricular filling. The normal process of active rapid filling, in which the first 200 ms of diastole are all that are required for completion of the rapid filling phase, allows heart rate to increase during physiologic stress and diastole to shorten, without curtailing filling. In mitral stenosis, filling is monophasic and slow, so that any increase in heart rate, through reducing filling time, leads to a decrease in left ventricular diastolic volume and stroke output and a corresponding increase in left atrial pressure that is in addition to the increases imposed by changes in blood volume and cardiac output.

Preconception Evaluation

Women with mitral stenosis referred for preconception evaluation may seem disarmingly well, yet they remain, as they were in Mackenzie's day, a group with a high potential to surprise the clinician when these complex hemodynamic factors come into play during the second and third trimesters.[8–10] Guidelines typically advise against pregnancy for a woman with valve area less than 1.1 cm^2, or who has significant pulmonary hypertension. Women with symptomatic mitral stenosis (New York Heart Association [NYHA] class II to IV symptoms) or severe pulmonary hypertension (defined as pulmonary artery pressure >75% of systemic pressure) should be referred for prophylactic percutaneous mitral balloon valvotomy (PMBV) or open commissurotomy before becoming pregnant, as per the 2006 American College of Cardiology/American Heart Association (ACC/AHA) guidelines.[11]

Clinical Presentation

Preconception screening can only achieve so much, however, and this is especially true in mitral stenosis; patients with the condition may have no inkling that they have heart disease until they develop pulmonary congestion or acute pulmonary edema during their pregnancy.[12] When patients with mitral stenosis begin to run into trouble during a pregnancy, usually toward the end of the second or beginning of the third trimester, the earliest symptoms, which include fatigue, dyspnea, and edema, may be difficult to distinguish from the normal effects of pregnancy. Experience is needed to determine what is pathologic, and may be usefully supplemented by investigations, such as an echocardiogram and a chest radiograph.

The incidence of maternal cardiac complications related to pregnancy is directly related to the severity of the mitral stenosis, as was illustrated in a report of 80 pregnancies in 74 women with rheumatic mitral stenosis.[10] The rate of cardiac complications (pulmonary edema or less frequently arrhythmias) ranged from 26% with mild mitral stenosis (valve area >1.5 cm^2) to 38% with moderate mitral stenosis to 67% in the 9 women with severe mitral stenosis.

Management

When symptoms prove to be caused by the valvular lesion, then the available options include diuretics, β-blockers, and a mitral valve procedure, either surgical or, in the most common situation of a pliable mitral valve with pure stenosis, with a catheter-based balloon. Conservative measures should also include bedrest and correction of anemia. Termination of pregnancy should be considered when symptoms supervene early in a pregnancy and if balloon commissurotomy is deemed contraindicated or proves unsuccessful.

Medical therapy

Treating pulmonary congestion with diuretics is second nature to cardiologists but must be coordinated with the obstetrics team, who will monitor the patient carefully for signs of placental insufficiency. Loop diuretics are preferred to thiazides. If a diuretic requirement develops before approximately 24 weeks, then chances are high that the patient will require additional measures, either commissurotomy or early delivery, and she should be followed very closely.

β-Blocking therapy is sometimes perceived as counterintuitive in a patient with progressive left heart failure, but in mitral stenosis, through slowing the heart rate and thereby devoting more of any given minute to diastole, β-blockers increase cardiac output and lower left atrial pressure.[13] Generally, in an ill patient, short-acting β1 selective members of the class are preferred, typically metoprolol given twice daily. Mixed β selectivity is to be avoided lest β2 blockade aggravate bronchospasm. Researchers have suggested that β-blockade may have adverse effects in patients with severe pulmonary hypertension through depressing right ventricular function,[14] but this has not been reported in the obstetrics literature, nor has it been the authors' experience. The potential benefit β-blockers when administered in addition to diuretics has been illustrated in a study of 25 pregnant women with mitral stenosis; 92% improved to or remained in NYHA functional class I or II, and all safely delivered healthy infants at term.[13] These results reflect a significant benefit, because the mortality rate for pregnant women with MS increases from 1 to 5% when class III or IV symptoms develop.

Deciding to anticoagulate patients during pregnancy is difficult, because warfarin is associated with a well-documented, albeit sometimes overemphasized, risk. However, patients with significant mitral stenosis are at risk of embolism even when they are in sinus rhythm, and this becomes especially a concern during the hypercoagulable state of pregnancy.[15] Generally, women who are encouraged to conceive have only mild disease and it is reasonable not to advise anticoagulation, but when disease is more than mild, the risk/benefit quotient swings more toward recommending warfarin.

Surgical mitral valvuloplasty

In 1952, three reports were published on closed surgical mitral valvotomy performed on pregnant women, all with good outcomes,[16–18] and since that time there has been a burgeoning literature on surgical management of valvular disease complicating pregnancy.[19–25] Although published accounts would be expected to have a generally optimistic tone, especially considering that the patients are young with generally little in the way of comorbidity, the results of valve replacement surgery in pregnancy are only fair, with maternal mortality rates in the region of 9%, ranging from 3% to 20%.[24] The seemingly high rate of 9% was reported in a comprehensive review that culled a large number of studies from a broad sweep of the literature, including several procedures performed as emergencies. Well-timed surgery in a woman who has received good obstetric and cardiologic care should have a mortality rate comparable to that for nonpregnant women at the same center. Fetal mortality rates are higher than the maternal mortality rate, reportedly 30%.[24] Scant current information is available on long-term outcome of babies born after maternal heart surgery in pregnancy, but at least a suspicion exists that these babies may be prone to developmental delay.

Percutaneous mitral balloon valvotomy

In the case of mitral stenosis, fortunately, cardiac surgery during pregnancy has largely given way to balloon valvotomy.[26–29] This trend has been true not only in countries with high health care expenditure but also in regions where resources are more limited. In certain regions, the trend has moved from closed surgical commissurotomy, without the heart-lung machine, to balloon catheter, almost bypassing the open surgical procedure, with its attendant complexity and risk. In either setting the results have been good, so much so that patients who might previously have been adequately managed with conservative measures and prolonged bedrest are referred for procedures. Pregnant women for whom medical management fails should undergo PMBV at experienced centers for relief of the stenosis.[11,30] Results have been excellent and, provided the usual precautions are taken, the risk posed to the fetus from radiation exposure is slight, certainly less than the risk associated with cardiopulmonary bypass. Thus, whereas in past years, one might often have tried to delay mitral valve surgery until it was plain that termination was the only alternative, today balloon valvotomy is often advised before a patient becomes severely in jeopardy.

Labor and Delivery

Generally the choice of how to deliver women with mitral valve disease should be made on obstetric grounds, as is the case for most of the cardiac conditions discussed in this issue, including the other valvular lesions to be considered. The risk of cesarean section is amplified by the presence of heart disease, and, if the patient's hemodynamic situation has been appropriately managed up to her confinement, then labor should be well-tolerated. Exceptions exist, however; in particular the occasional patient who needs to be delivered before term because of worsening hemodynamic stress, yet, for the same reasons, cannot safely receive oxytocin. Under these circumstances, when induction seems impossible or unsafe, cesarean section may be the only safe approach.

That vaginal delivery should usually be preferred to cesarean section, unless obstetric considerations determine otherwise, is not to say that normal labor is free of hemodynamic stress or risk.[31] During the first two stages, successive uterine contractions lead to a stepwise increase in atrial pressures, as blood volume is squeezed out from the endometrium and placenta. In mitral stenosis, this can lead to striking increase in pulmonary wedge pressure, and may mandate using diuretics during the first and second stage. The most vulnerable time, however, is immediately after delivery. When the inferior vena cava is released from the pressure of the gravid uterus, an abrupt increase in venous return, and therefore left atrial pressure, may occur. Hence, acute pulmonary edema may occur immediately after delivery, even when the conduct of labor seems to have been successful. For women with severe mitral stenosis or symptoms of heart failure at the time of labor, invasive hemodynamic monitoring with a right heart catheter is appropriate.[31,32] Fluid management to achieve a goal pulmonary capillary wedge pressure of approximately 14 mm Hg is generally recommended, although this may need to be adjusted on an individual basis. Invasive hemodynamic monitoring should be continued in the immediate postpartum period because of large intravascular volume shifts.

Routine endocarditis prophylaxis is not necessary for either cesarean or vaginal delivery.[11] However, continuation of antibiotics for secondary prophylaxis of rheumatic fever is recommended.

AORTIC STENOSIS
Introduction

For several years, the combination of aortic stenosis and pregnancy was believed to be particularly risky.[33–35] Several reports described maternal sudden deaths during or immediately after pregnancy. However, the more recent literature is consistent with wide clinical and anecdotal experience that women with moderate degrees of symptomless left ventricular outflow narrowing can generally be guided through pregnancy safely.[36,37] If cardiac function is normal and the patient is free of symptoms, sudden cardiac death and life-threatening cardiac failure are vanishingly uncommon. Some patients with high gradients may develop a degree of fluid retention and dyspnea in the weeks before term, but they can generally be managed with cautious diuretic therapy and, in some cases, bedrest.

Most cases of aortic stenosis are from a bicuspid aortic valve, which is discussed separately.

Pathophysiology

This generally favorable view of aortic stenosis stems from the fact that the hemodynamic problem is more straightforward than that of mitral stenosis. Increased cardiac output entails an increase in left ventricular outflow gradient, but the rise in pressure is borne by the hypertrophied left ventricle, in systole, not by the pulmonary veins. Increase in extracellular fluid volume and plasma volume may increase left ventricular diastolic cavity size, but at the expense of only a modest rise in left atrial pressure. In most patients with aortic stenosis, the hypertrophied ventricle is preload-sensitive, and pregnancy is unlikely to lead to a catastrophic decrease in filling pressure; if things do not go well, change tends to be gradual. Most important, the effect of reducing filling time is much less pronounced than in mitral stenosis, so that the inevitable rise in heart rate during pregnancy presents less of a problem.

Because the hemodynamic picture in women with aortic stenosis is more straightforward than that of patients with mitral stenosis, how things will go during a pregnancy is easy to predict and, as a percentage, women with aortic stenosis offer fewer surprises than women with mitral stenosis. However, in the developed world, women with aortic stenosis are much more numerous than those with mitral disease, and hence still represent a significant concern.

Clinical Presentation

If a woman with aortic stenosis has an outflow velocity of less than 4 m/s, hence an estimated valve area of more than 1 cm^2, and if she is free of symptoms and has normal cardiac function, the likelihood of significant difficulty during pregnancy is very low. A small number of patients with velocities in the region of 4 m/s do develop dyspnea and breathlessness as they near term, and some may even require diuretics, but the likelihood of catastrophe is minimal. The authors' own experience and reports in the literature include patients with very high gradients, as high as 150 mm Hg, who tolerate pregnancy without real difficulty.[38] Among 29 Canadian patients with severe aortic stenosis, whose peak gradients averaged 67 mm Hg, 3 developed hemodynamic distress during pregnancy and 1 required valvuloplasty.[39] The other 2 were managed successfully with medical regimens.

However, when patients are or have been symptomatic before pregnancy, or have impaired cardiac function, then aortic stenosis presents much more of a concern. Sudden cardiac death is seldom the first symptom, but may occur in patients with left ventricular failure or after a history of presyncope. Therefore, a substantial number of aortic valve procedures have been performed during pregnancy in women with severe aortic stenosis who became seriously symptomatic. Valvuloplasty using a balloon catheter may be preferred for obvious reasons over surgical valve replacement,[40,41] at least as a temporizing measure.[42] It does not have as high a long-term success rate as does mitral balloon valvuloplasty, but it may tide patients over long enough for them to reach term. Alternatively, some patients may require surgical valve replacement, with good and fairly good results for mother and fetus, respectively.[24]

BICUSPID AORTIC VALVE
Incidence

In practically all pregnant women with aortic stenosis, the lesion is congenital, with bicuspid aortic valve (also called *bicommissural valve*) by far the most common form. Bicuspid valve is detected in approximately 1 per 100 live births. The prevalence is 2% in the general population, with a 4:1 male predominance.

Along with the valve lesion, patients with bicuspid valve frequently have an aortopathy that is pathologically and histologically similar to that of Marfan syndrome, and that leads to fusiform aneurysm of the ascending aorta. The degree of ectasia does not correlate with the hemodynamic severity of the valve lesion; some patients with aneurysms have no physiologic disturbance at all. Therefore the expression "poststenotic dilatation" is inappropriate and has fallen largely out of use.

Preconception Counseling

Women with a bicuspid aortic valve should receive counseling regarding potential risks and treatments before and during pregnancy. Potential risks that should be discussed include heritable congenital heart disease, aortic enlargement or dissection, and complications of aortic stenosis and/or aortic regurgitation.

Bicuspid aortic valve is heritable in some families.[43,44] The frequency of bicuspid aortic valve in first-degree relatives was assessed in a study of 30 consecutive patients with bicuspid aortic valve and 190 (91%) of 210 first-degree relatives who underwent echocardiography.[43] Bicuspid aortic valve was found in 9% of first-degree relatives, and 11 of the 30 families had at least one

additional member with this lesion. In a literature review, fetal congenital heart disease occurred in 5 of 121 pregnancies (4.1%) in women with congenital aortic stenosis.[45] The authors suggest fetal ultrasound when the mother has bicuspid aortic valve.

Aneurysms accompanying bicuspid aortic valve can dissect,[46] and pregnancy itself carries a well-documented risk of aortic dissection.[3,47,48] Therefore, reports of dissection complicating pregnancy include several in which bicuspid aortic valve was present. The numbers of these events and reports do not represent a large numerator, and the denominator of all women with bicuspid valves is extensive, so the absolute risk of pregnancy in a woman with a bicuspid valve is too small for any accurate or useful estimate.

The 2008 ACC/AHA adult congenital heart disease guidelines[49–51] recommend that women with bicuspid aortic valve and ascending aortic diameter greater than 45 mm should be counseled about the high risks of pregnancy. Some enlargement of the aorta to levels below 45 mm is very common, and should probably not be seen as a contraindication to pregnancy, having a risk similar to that in the general population of pregnant women. A single, retrospective study of fewer than 100 patients offered a generally optimistic view consistent with this recommendation.[52]

Patients with severe aortic stenosis, symptoms, or left ventricular ejection fraction less than 40% are advised to delay conception until the aortic stenosis has been addressed.[49]

Preconception Management

Some young women with congenital aortic stenosis can be treated with percutaneous aortic balloon valvotomy (PABV), which reduces the transvalvular gradient but does not affect the risk of ascending aorta complications.

For asymptomatic women who want to become pregnant, PABV was considered reasonable if they have minimally calcified valves and are younger than 30 years. Selected patients older than 30 years who have minimally calcified valves may also benefit from PABV. This treatment consideration is a potentially important issue in women planning pregnancy, because PABV has limited efficacy and an appreciable complication rate in older adults.

Management During Pregnancy

If a woman with bicuspid aortic stenosis presents early in pregnancy with severe aortic stenosis and/or a left ventricular ejection fraction below 40%, some experts suggest termination of pregnancy followed by reparative surgery before another attempt at pregnancy. The magnitude of risk should be explained to the patient, although data are limited.

Alternatively, pregnant women with severe aortic stenosis who have no or only mild symptoms can often be managed conservatively with bedrest, β-blockers, and oxygen, if needed.[49] Intervention during pregnancy is recommended only for refractory NYHA class III or IV symptoms. Case reports suggest that balloon valvotomy can reduce the risks of gestation, labor, and delivery and avoid the risks of valve replacement.[35,40,41] However, even in experienced hands, balloon valvotomy can induce aortic regurgitation, recurrent stenosis is common within 6 to 12 months, and the ascending aorta still harbors an abnormal media.

Surgical aortic valve replacement is often required in symptomatic women with valve calcification or unfavorable anatomy. The choices are a usually a homograft valve, a pulmonary autograft (Ross procedure), and a mechanical valve. The Ross procedure, which replaces the aortic valve with the patient's own pulmonary valve and replaces the pulmonary valve with a homograft, has the advantage of avoiding the fetal risks of anticoagulation. However, cardiovascular complications are common after the Ross procedure, and reoperation is often required, involving one or both valves. The efficacy of the Ross procedure was evaluated in eight nonanticoagulated women who had 14 pregnancies.[53] No maternal deaths and no thromboembolic or hemorrhagic events occurred, and no evidence was seen of deterioration of valve function.

Labor and Delivery

Cesarean delivery is recommended in the presence of aortic aneurysm, dissection, or critical aortic stenosis, because intrapartum increases in cardiac output related to contractions may significantly increase the risk of a cardiac event. Delivery at a center experienced with high-risk heart disease is recommended for patients with greater than mild aortic stenosis or dilated aortic diameter (>40 mm).

Endocarditis prophylaxis is not indicated during an uncomplicated vaginal or cesarian delivery unless the bicuspid aortic valve has been treated with a valve replacement.[49]

MARFAN SYNDROME

In the United States, the estimated prevalence of Marfan syndrome is 4 to 6 cases per 10,000 persons, affecting both genders equally. Eighty percent of patients have some cardiovascular involvement, which includes aortic dilatation (mainly of the ascending part), aortic regurgitation, and mitral and tricuspid valve prolapse with or without regurgitation. Pregnancy in women with Marfan syndrome is associated with the potential for a catastrophic and even fatal acute aortic dissection, and the risk of having a child who will inherit the syndrome. The approach to pregnancy in patients with Marfan syndrome is therefore challenging and deserves special considerations.

Epidemiology and Maternal Risk

At least some useful though uncontrolled data and individual case reports attest to the risk of dissection during pregnancy in women with Marfan syndrome, and to the relative safety of pregnancy after successful prophylactic replacement of the aortic root, but even in that setting the potential exists for catastrophe.[54–57] The solid data include four series collected at centers with extensive experience in management of patients with Marfan syndrome.[58–61] Interpretation of the data must take into account the likelihood of ascertainment effects; for example, some of the patients were diagnosed with Marfan syndrome and seen in those centers only because they had sustained aortic dissection. Nevertheless, the four series describe outcomes of 374 pregnancies in 180 patients. Many of the pregnancies were sanctioned by detailed preconception evaluations, and these had good outcomes. Altogether, among the 180 women, 18 aortic dissections occurred. Of these, most occurred in women who had not been evaluated before conception, or who had been advised against pregnancy, but not all. Of 12 type A dissections (3.2% of pregnancies), 5 occurred in women known to have the syndrome and whose aortas had been measured before conception; three measurements were 40 mm and the other two were 42 and 45 mm. The remaining 6 dissections (1.6%) were type B, and therefore preconception echocardiography can hardly have been expected to predict risk.

A more recent prospective series of 23 women followed through 33 pregnancies, in whom the aorta was mildly if at all enlarged, with an average dimension of 37 mm (25–45 mm), was complicated by a single type B dissection.[62] This developed in a woman who had previously undergone aortic root replacement after a type A dissection. The overall data are not sufficiently detailed to allow a percent estimate of risk in women known to have Marfan syndrome but with mild or minimal vascular involvement, nor how these risks will prove to be influenced by β-blocker treatment or angiotensin receptor blockers.

Preconception Counseling

The consensus, such as there is, has been to permit pregnancy in women whose aortic roots measure less than 40 mm, and the data support this up to a point. However, even with normal or near-normal aortic dimensions, the rate of dissection in patients with Marfan syndrome exceeds that in women who do not have connective tissue disorders, and pregnancy should be undertaken only after a detailed discussion about its potential risk of death.

This discussion inevitably also includes a discussion of the genetic implications; Marfan syndrome has autosomal dominant inheritance. Penetrance is high, and families have a tendency to "breed true," in the sense that some kindreds may have mostly ophthalmologic disease, some skeletal, and others cardiovascular. Anticipation is not a feature of Marfan syndrome. Recently, the discovery of an increasing number of disease-causing mutations in the fibrillin 1 gene allowed the possibility of preimplantation genetic diagnosis, and it has been used successfully by several couples.[63]

Management during pregnancy

Among women with Marfan syndrome who become pregnant, a multidisciplinary approach to prenatal care is recommended, preferably at a center with experience in the management of this disease.

Monitoring Serial clinical assessment should include echocardiographic monitoring in all pregnant women with Marfan syndrome, even among women with baseline aortic root diameter of 40 mm or less.[58–60] The 2010 American College of Cardiology/American Heart Association/American Association for Thoracic Surgery (ACC/AHA/AATS) guidelines[49] recommend monthly or bimonthly echocardiographic measurement of the ascending aortic dimensions throughout pregnancy for all pregnant women with known aortic root or ascending aortic dilatation . For pregnant women with aortic arch or descending or abdominal aortic dilatation, MRI is recommended over CT to avoid exposing the mother and fetus to ionizing radiation. MRI without gadolinium contrast is preferred and generally sufficient for monitoring aortic size. Transesophageal echocardiography is an alternative for imaging the thoracic aorta.

Medical therapy B-Blockers should be given to all patients with Marfan syndrome in an attempt to minimize aortic dilatation and risk of aortic dissection during pregnancy.

Antibiotic prophylaxis is optional at delivery (unless bacteremia is suspected) for patients with prior valve replacement surgery or prior endocarditis.

Delivery Women with Marfan syndrome with aortic root aneurysm (aortic root >40 mm) should be delivered at an institution where cardiothoracic surgery is available.

Obstetric complications seem to be increased in women with Marfan syndrome. This finding was illustrated in a retrospective multicenter study of 111 completed pregnancies among 63 women with Marfan syndrome,[45] in which a high rate of premature deliveries (15%), mainly from preterm premature rupture of membranes and cervical insufficiency, and a markedly increased combined rate of fetal and neonatal mortality (7%) were seen. For comparison, in the US general population, the preterm birth rate is approximately 12%, neonatal mortality is approximately 0.4%, and fetal mortality is approximately 0.7%.

Patients who have an aortic root diameter that remains 40 mm or less and have no heart failure resulting from valvular regurgitation may proceed with a vaginal delivery if no other obstetric indications for cesarean delivery are present. With vaginal delivery, epidural anesthesia to minimize pain; forceps or vacuum delivery without maternal pushing; and continued use of a β-blocker during labor are appropriate ancillary measures to minimize surges in blood pressure and cardiac output. Cesarean delivery is preferred in patients with an aortic diameter greater than 40 mm, aortic dissection, severe aortic regurgitation, or heart failure.

Before attempting epidural anesthesia, the possible presence of dural ectasia should be considered.[64] Dural sac dilation can be present in up to 90% of patients with Marfan syndrome and may be associated with low back pain, headache, or proximal leg pain, weakness, or numbness. Although dural ectasia is not an absolute contraindication for epidural anesthesia, if suspected, it should be evaluated with lumbosacral MRI or CT, and the increased risk of dural puncture or inadequate anesthesia should be discussed with the patient.

REGURGITANT LESIONS

The natural history of chronic nonrheumatic mitral regurgitation in young women is very favorable, and therefore unless mitral regurgitation is acute, from chordal rupture or endocarditis, it is exceptional that this lesion should cause concern, either at preconception counseling or during pregnancy. Because systemic vascular resistance is reduced in pregnancy, both from widespread vasodilatation and by virtue of the low-resistance placental circulation, forward stroke output is favored at the expense of the regurgitant fraction and left ventricular volume loading is somewhat mitigated. By the same token, the increase in blood volume is likely only to cause a modest increase in pressure of an already dilated left atrium. In practice, patients with nonrheumatic mitral regurgitation have done well, with no reported cases of emergency repair performed during pregnancy. Acute mitral regurgitation can be more complicated to manage, but again, a pregnancy in itself does not aggravate the hemodynamic changes, and management is comparable to that of acute mitral regurgitation in other settings.

Rheumatic mitral regurgitation may present a more complex clinical problem. The hemodynamic load that it imposes may not be severe on its own, but a significant leak, contributing to increased left atrial pressure, when left ventricular filling rate is reduced, raises the likelihood of early pulmonary congestion and the potential for emergent surgical intervention.

Aortic regurgitation has seldom proved to be a clinical concern in obstetric practice. The hemodynamic factors at play are similar to those in chronic mitral regurgitation; the unloading effect of the decrease in systemic vascular resistance outweighs the effect of increased blood volume. The most important thing when aortic regurgitation is detected during pregnancy is to consider what may be its cause. Although bicuspid aortic valve is the most common cause of aortic regurgitation in a pregnant patient, connective tissue disorder, endocarditis, aortitis (Takayasu syndrome), and even aortic dissection are important to consider.

RIGHT-SIDED VALVE DISEASE

Congenital pulmonic stenosis has seldom led to hemodynamic embarrassment during pregnancy, and today, in the United States, more than mild disease is most unusual in young adults, because the lesion is so readily treated with balloon valvotomy in childhood. However, as an obstructive lesion, it carries at least the potential to cause right heart failure when severe and untreated. In practice this has seldom proved the case; in a small series of women with severe pulmonic stenosis, whose gradients were as high as 80 mm Hg, hemodynamic and clinical outcomes were very favorable.[65] However, one study reported that obstetric,

noncardiac problems were increased in a group of patients with congenital pulmonary valve disease.[66]

The authors' own small experience with tricuspid stenosis (in patients with degenerating bioprostheses) has been similar. An inevitable rise in right atrial pressure has been well tolerated, and has not led to problems for mother or fetus.

HYPERTROPHIC CARDIOMYOPATHY

Hypertrophic cardiomyopathy (HCM) is included in this contribution, rather than in the discussion of peripartum and other forms of dilated cardiomyopathy, because of its former name, the murmur, and the hemodynamics. HCM is well tolerated in pregnancy, because the reduction in systemic vascular resistance from vasodilation seems to be adequately offset by the increase in blood volume; preload volume is maintained; and in many patients the hemodynamics are disturbed very little.[67–70]

Outcomes in Pregnancy

The data supporting usually favorable outcomes of HCM in pregnancy conclusions were provided in a report of 100 women with HCM who had a total of 199 births.[70] Among 40 patients who were followed closely, only 1 of 28 previously asymptomatic patients progressed to NYHA class III or IV during pregnancy. In comparison, this progression occurred in 5 of 12 previously symptomatic patients. One patient had atrial fibrillation and one had syncope.

Nevertheless, a very broad range of severity is seen among young people with HCM, from those who may be genotype-positive yet with minimal disturbance of left ventricular architecture to those with severe disability, with high-risk family history, and who may have been subjected to myectomy or are awaiting transplantation. Among the last, pregnancy clearly would be hazardous. In the series mentioned earlier[70] two deaths occurred, both sudden and in patients at particularly high risk. One patient had massive left ventricular hypertrophy and a resting outflow gradient of 115 mm Hg. The other patient had a family history of eight deaths in young patients, five of which were sudden.

Even among the large middle-ground of women with murmurs, palpitations, and subtle if any hemodynamic disturbance, in whom common sense would mandate permitting or continuing a pregnancy, catastrophic outcomes occasionally occur.[71–75] Predicting them is as difficult as is prognostication in general in this condition, for the same reasons, and is based on an assessment of severity and risk that comes from the patient's history, family history, and extent of architectural distortion of the left ventricle and septum. For the most part, women in the middle ground do well.

Preconception genetic counseling is also recommended if either the mother or the father has diagnosed HCM.

Management During Pregnancy

Many patients with HCM are on treatment with ß-blockers, either for arrhythmia prophylaxis or for symptom relief. Today wide experience shows that this treatment is well tolerated by the developing fetus, and stopping therapy because of pregnancy would seldom be advised. Specific antiarrhythmic medication is more of a concern.[76] Amiodarone has been given to pregnant women, but the accumulated evidence implies that it should be avoided, because besides causing neonatal hypothyroidism almost automatically, it may also lead to clinically important growth retardation and teratogenic effects. Disopyramide and verapamil are less problematic but less likely to be considered important for the mother. Of course, experience is increasing with implanted defibrillators in pregnant women,[77,78] even with placing them during pregnancy in patients whose arrhythmic risk is only detected after conception.

Delivery

The mode of delivery of women with HCM should be determined based on obstetric considerations, just as in patients with valvular disease discussed in the preceding paragraphs. Because these patients are so sensitive to a decrease in left ventricular filling volume, spinal and epidural anesthesia carry the risk of causing intractable hypotension. Although they should be used,[79,80] because adequate pain relief is important to avoid intense catecholamine stimulation, their use requires careful clinical or invasive hemodynamic monitoring. Careful monitoring is advisable in the first 24 hours after delivery, when large fluid shifts can lead to acute pulmonary edema in the setting of a non-compliant and hypertrophied left ventricle.

PROSTHETIC HEART VALVES AND PREGNANCY

The main issue concerning management of pregnant women with mechanical prostheses is their anticoagulation, and this is the subject of another article in this issue. For many who have experience in this area, the presence of a mechanical prosthesis is itself a contraindication to pregnancy, owing largely to the need for anticoagulation with warfarin, and ideal management of the patient entails that this situation be avoided. Rather than place a mechanical prosthesis in a woman who wishes to be a mother, the cardiologist and cardiac surgeon should strive to manage her with a biologic prothesis, a valve repair, or a homograft, or should defer surgery if that is feasible.

Risks with Bioprosthetic Valves

However, women of childbearing age generally experience deterioration of bioprostheses at a considerably faster rate than middle-aged or elderly patients, with significant deterioration by the time of maximum hemodynamic stress in the later months of pregnancy. However, this is mostly reported in anecdotal reports[81] and has not been borne out by studies.[82–86]

Risks with Mechanical Valves

Mechanical heart valves are associated with an increased incidence of thromboembolic events during pregnancy. Therapeutic anticoagulation throughout pregnancy is essential to reduce the risk of thromboembolic complications, with the risk of valve thrombosis increased with the use unfractionated heparin and, to a lesser degree, low-molecular-weight heparin compared with warfarin. Each of these choices of anticoagulation is discussed separately elsewhere in this issue. The risk of valve thrombosis and thromboembolic events depends on the type and location of the prosthetic valve, and other factors that increase thromboembolic risk, including

- History of a prior thromboembolic event,
- Atrial fibrillation,
- Prosthesis in the mitral position, and
- Multiple prosthetic valves.

Risk of Infection

The 2008 ACC/AHA guidelines for management of adults with congenital heart disease and valvular disease[11,49] include antibiotic prophylaxis recommendations stating that antibiotic prophylaxis against infective endocarditis is reasonable to consider at membrane rupture and before vaginal delivery in select patients with the highest risk of adverse outcomes. This group includes patients with prosthetic cardiac valve or prosthetic material used for cardiac valve repair, and patients with unrepaired or palliated cyanotic heart disease, including surgically constructed palliative shunts and conduits. However, sufficient proof of efficacy of prophylaxis in this setting is not available.

Management of Valve Thrombosis

Experience with the management of valve thrombosis in pregnant women is limited to mostly case series. Heparin may be considered for small nonobstructive thrombi. However, for obstructive valve thrombosis, the treatment options are surgical thrombectomy and thrombolysis, both of which carry substantial fetal and maternal risks.

- In a series of 10 women treated for 12 episodes of valve thrombosis with surgery (n = 4), thrombolysis (n = 7), and heparin (n = 1),[87] one maternal death and one additional fetal death occurred in the surgical group, and two maternal deaths and one bleeding event requiring surgical drainage, but no fetal mortality in the surviving women, occurred in the thrombolysis group.
- In a review of thrombolysis during pregnancy included 172 patients[88] over 34 years, rates of maternal mortality, hemorrhagic complications, and fetal mortality were 1.2%, 8%, and 5.8%, respectively. These data should be interpreted with caution, because they included patients treated with thrombolysis for a variety of conditions, including prosthetic valve thrombosis at several centers over an extended period.

REFERENCES

1. Mackenzie J. Heart disease and pregnancy. London: (Oxford Medical Publications) Henry Frowde and Hodder and Stoughton; 1921.
2. Burwell CS, Metcalfe J. Heart disease and pregnancy: physiology and management. Boston: Little Brown & Co; 1958.
3. Bastos Barbosa PJ, Lopes AA, Feitosa GS, et al. Prognostic factors of rheumatic mitral stenosis during pregnancy and puerperium. Arq Bras Cardiol 2000;75:220–4.
4. Diao M, Kane A, Bamba Ndiaye M, et al. Pregnancy in women with heart disease in sub-Saharan Africa. Arch Cardiovasc Dis 2011;104:370–4.
5. Lesniak-Sobelga A, Tracz W, Kostkiewicz M, et al. Clinical and echocardiographic assessment of pregnant women with valvular heart diseases— maternal and fetal outcome. Int J Cardiol 2004;94: 15–23.
6. Sawhney H, Aggarwal N, Suri V, et al. Maternal and perinatal outcome in rheumatic heart disease. Int J Gynaecol Obstet 2003;80:9–14.
7. Bhatla N, Lal S, Behera G, et al. Cardiac disease in pregnancy. Int J Gynec Obst 2003;82:153–9.
8. Hameed A, Karaalp IS, Tummala PP, et al. The effect of valvular heart disease on maternal and fetal outcome of pregnancy. J Am Coll Cardiol 2001;37: 893–9.
9. Elkayam U, Bitar F. Valvular heart disease and pregnancy, part 1: native valves. J Am Coll Cardiol 2005; 46:223–30.
10. Silversides CK, Colman JM, Sermer M, et al. Cardiac risk in pregnant women with rheumatic mitral stenosis. Am J Cardiol 2003;91:1382–5.
11. Bonow RO, Carabello BA, Chatterjee K, et al. 2008 Focused update incorporated into the ACC/AHA 2006 guidelines for the management of patients with valvular heart disease: a report of the American College of Cardiology/American Heart Association Task Force on Practice Guidelines (Writing Committee to Revise the 1998 Guidelines for the Management of Patients With Valvular Heart Disease): endorsed by the Society of Cardiovascular Anesthesiologists, Society for Cardiovascular Angiography and Interventions, and Society of Thoracic Surgeons. Circulation 2008;118(15):e523.
12. Morley CA, Lim BA. The risks of delay in diagnosis of breathlessness in pregnancy. BMJ 1995;311: 1083–4.
13. Al Kasab SM, Sabag T, Al Zaibag M, et al. β-adrenergic receptor blockade in the management of pregnant women with mitral stenosis. Am J Obstet Gynecol 1990;163:37–40.
14. Wisenbaugh T, Essop R, Middlemost S, et al. Pulmonary hypertension is a contraindication to β-blockade in patients with severe mitral stenosis. Am Heart J 1993;125:786–90.
15. Hameed A, Akhter MW, Bitar F, et al. Left atrial thrombosis in pregnant women with mitral stenosis and sinus rhythm. Am J Obstet Gynecol 2005;193: 501–4.
16. Logan A, Turner R. Mitral valvotomy in pregnancy. Lancet 1952;1:1286.
17. Brock RC. Valvotomy in pregnancy. Proc R Soc Med 1952;45:538–40.
18. Cooley DA, Chapman DW. Mitral commissurotomy during pregnancy. JAMA 1952;150:1113–4.
19. Ueland K. Cardiac surgery and pregnancy. Am J Obstet Gynecol 1965;92:148–62.
20. Bernal JM, Miralles PJ. Cardiac surgery with cardiopulmonary bypass during pregnancy. Obstet Gynecol Surv 1986;41:1–6.
21. Vosloo S, Reichart B. The feasibility of closed mitral valvotomy in pregnancy. J Thorac Cardiovasc Surg 1987;93:675–9.
22. Leyse R, Ofstun M, Dillard DH, et al. Congenital aortic stenosis in pregnancy, corrected by extracorporeal circulation. JAMA 1961;176:1009–12.
23. Mannix EP, Mahajan DR. Open-heart surgery during pregnancy: a report of three cases. J Thorac Cardiovasc Surg 1967;53:592–601.

24. Weiss BM, von Segesser LK, Alon E, et al. Outcome of cardiovascular surgery and pregnancy: a systematic review of the period 1984-1996. Am J Obstet Gynecol 1998;179:1643–53.

25. Jafferani A, Malik A, Khawaja RD, et al. Surgical management of valvular heart diseases in pregnancy. Eur J Obstet Gynecol Reprod Biol 2011; 159:91–4.

26. Safian RD, Berman AD, Sachs B, et al. Percutaneous balloon mitral valvuloplasty in a pregnant woman with mitral stenosis. Cathet Cardiovasc Diagn 1988;15:103–8.

27. Palacios IF, Block PC, Wilkins GT, et al. Percutaneous mitral balloon valvuloplasty during pregnancy in a patient with severe mitral stenosis. Cathet Cardiovasc Diagn 1988;15:109–11.

28. Smith R, Brender D, McRedie M. Percutaneous transluminal balloon dilatation of the mitral valve in pregnancy. Br Heart J 1989;61:551–3.

29. Hameed AB, Mehra A, Rahimtoola SH. The role of catheter balloon commissurotomy for severe mitral stenosis in pregnancy. Obstet Gynecol 2009;114: 1136–40.

30. Carabello BA. Modern management of mitral stenosis. Circulation 2005;112(3):432.

31. Clark SL, Phelan JP, Greenspoon J, et al. Labor and delivery in the presence of mitral stenosis: central hemodynamic observations. Am J Obstet Gynecol 1985;152:984–8.

32. Biswas RG, Bandyopadhyay BK, Sarkar M, et al. Perioperative management of pregnant patients with heart disease for caesarian section under anaesthesia. J Indian Med Assoc 2003;101:632–4.

33. Arias F, Pineda J. Aortic stenosis and pregnancy. J Reprod Med 1978;20:229–32.

34. Jewett JF. Committee on maternal welfare: aortic stenosis with sudden death. N Engl J Med 1972; 286:45–6.

35. Avila WS, Hajjar LA, da Rocha e Souza T, et al. Aortic valvuloplasty with balloon catheter in maternal-fetal emergency in adolescence. Arq Bras Cardiol 2009; 93:e76–9.

36. Lao TT, Sermer M, MaGee L, et al. Congenital aortic stenosis and pregnancy - a reappraisal. Am J Obstet Gynecol 1993;169:540–5.

37. Yap SC, Drenthen W, Pieper PG, et al. Risks of complications during pregnancy in women with congenital aortic stenosis. Int J Cardiol 2008;126: 240–6.

38. Seeliger T, Schild RL, Koch A, et al. Kongenitale aortenklappenstenose mit sehr hohem druckgradienten bei einer schwangeren patientin. [congenital aortic valve stenosis with very high pressure gradient in a pregnant patient]. Dtsch Med Wochenschr 2008; 133:2272–4 [in German].

39. Silversides CK, Colman JM, Sermer M, et al. Early and intermediate-term outcomes of pregnancy with congenital aortic stenosis. Am J Cardiol 2003;91: 1386–9.

40. McIvor RA. Percutaneous balloon aortic valvuloplasty during pregnancy. Int J Cardiol 1991;32:1–4.

41. Angel JL, Chapman C, Knuppel RA, et al. Percutaneous balloon valvuloplasty in pregnancy. Obstet Gynecol 1988;72:438–40.

42. Tzemos N, Silversides CK, Colman JM, et al. Late cardiac outcomes after pregnancy in women with congenital aortic stenosis. Am Heart J 2009;157: 474–80.

43. Huntington K, Hunter AG, Chan KL. A prospective study to assess the frequency of familial clustering of congenital bicuspid aortic valve. J Am Coll Cardiol 1997;30(7):1809.

44. Cripe L, Andelfinger G, Martin LJ, et al. Bicuspid aortic valve is heritable. J Am Coll Cardiol 2004; 44(1):138.

45. Drenthen W, Pieper PG, Roos-Hesselink JW, et al. ZAHARA Investigators Outcome of pregnancy in women with congenital heart disease: a literature review. J Am Coll Cardiol 2007; 49(24):2303.

46. Anderson RA, Fineron PW. Aortic dissection in pregnancy: importance of pregnancy-associated changes in the vessel wall and bicuspid aortic valve in pathogenesis. Br J Obstet Gynaecol 1994;101: 1085–8.

47. Hume M, Krosnick G. Dissecting aneurysm in pregnancy associated with aortic insufficiency: report of a case with successful surgical repair. N Engl J Med 1963;268:174–8.

48. Aziz F, Penupolu S, Alok A, et al. Peripartum aortic dissection: a case report and review of literature. J Thorac Dis 2011;3:65–7.

49. Warnes CA, Williams RG, Bashore TM, et al. ACC/AHA 2008 Guidelines for the Management of Adults with Congenital Heart Disease: a report of the American College of Cardiology/American Heart Association Task Force on Practice Guidelines (writing committee to develop guidelines on the management of adults with congenital heart disease). Circulation 2008;118(23):e714.

50. Hiratzka LF, Bakris GL, Beckman JA, et al. 2010 ACCF/AHA/AATS/ACR/ASA/SCA/SCAI/SIR/STS/SVM guidelines for the diagnosis and management of patients with Thoracic Aortic Disease: a report of the American College of Cardiology Foundation/American Heart Association Task Force on Practice Guidelines, American Association for Thoracic Surgery, American College of Radiology, American Stroke Association, Society of Cardiovascular Anesthesiologists, Society for Cardiovascular Angiography and Interventions, Society of Interventional Radiology, Society of Thoracic Surgeons, and Society for Vascular Medicine. Circulation 2010; 121(13):e266.

51. Fedak PW, Verma S, David TE, et al. Clinical and pathophysiological implications of a bicuspid aortic valve. Circulation 2002;106(8):900.

52. McKellar SH, MacDonald RJ, Michelena HI, et al. Frequency of cardiovascular events in women with a congenitally bicuspid aortic valve in a single community and effect of pregnancy on events. Am J Cardiol 2011;107:96–9.

53. Dore A, Somerville J. Pregnancy in patients with pulmonary autograft valve replacement. Eur Heart J 1997;18(10):1659.

54. Tilak M, Smith J, Rogers D, et al. Successful near-term pregnancy outcome after repair of a dissecting thoracic aortic aneurysm at 14 weeks gestation. Canad J Anesth 2005;52:1071–5.

55. Sakaguchi M, Kitahara H, Watanabe T, et al. Successful surgical treatment for acute aortic dissection in pregnancy with Marfan's syndrome. Jpn J Thorac Cardiovasc Surg 2005;53:220–2.

56. Williams A, Child A, Rowntree J, et al. Marfan's syndrome: successful pregnancy after aortic root and arch replacement. BJOG 2002;109:1187–8.

57. Lunel A, Audra P, Plauchu H, et al. Syndrome de Marfan et grossesse. [Marfan's syndrome and pregnancy]. J Gynecol Obstet Biol Reprod 2006;35:607–13 [in French].

58. Rossiter JP, Repke JT, Morales AJ, et al. A prospective longitudinal evaluation of pregnancy in the Marfan syndrome. Am J Obstet Gynecol 1995;173:1599–606.

59. Lipscomb KJ, Clayton Smith J, Clarke B, et al. Outcome of pregnancy in women with Marfan's syndrome. Br J Obstet Gynaecol 1997;104:201–6.

60. Lind J, Wallenburg HC. The Marfan syndrome and pregnancy: a retrospective study in a Dutch population. Eur J Obstet Gynecol Reprod Biol 2001;98:28–35.

61. Pacini L, Digne F, Boumendil A, et al. Maternal complication of pregnancy in Marfan syndrome. Int J Cardiol 2009;136:156–61.

62. Meijboom LJ, Vos FE, Timmermans J, et al. Pregnancy and aortic root growth in the Marfan syndrome: a prospective study. Eur Heart J 2005;26:914–20.

63. Blaszczyk A, Tang YX, Dietz HC, et al. Preimplantation genetic diagnosis of human embryos for Marfan's syndrome. J Assist Reprod Genet 1998;15:281–4.

64. Lacassie HJ, Millar S, Leithe LG, et al. Dural ectasia: a likely cause of inadequate spinal anaesthesia in two parturients with Marfan's syndrome. Br J Anaesth 2005;94(4):500.

65. Hameed AB, Goodwin TM, Elkayam U. Effect of pulmonary stenosis on pregnancy outcomes - a case-control study. Am Heart J 2007;154:852–4.

66. Drenthen W, Pieper PG, Roos Hesselink JW, et al. Non-cardiac complications during pregnancy in women with isolated congenital pulmonary valve stenosis. Heart 2006;92:1838–43.

67. Turner GM, Oakley CM, Dixon HG. Management of pregnancy complicated by hypertrophic cardiomyopathy. BMJ 1968;4:281.

68. Oakley CD, McGarry K, Limb DG, et al. Management of pregnancy in patients with hypertrophic cardiomyopathy. BMJ 1979;1:1749–50.

69. Thaman R, Varnava A, Hamid MS, et al. Pregnancy related complications in women with hypertrophic cardiomyopathy. Heart 2003;89:752–6.

70. Autore C, Conte MR, Piccininno M, et al. Risk associated with pregnancy in hypertrophic cardiomyopathy. J Am Coll Cardiol 2002;40:1864–9.

71. Kolibash AJ, Ruiz DE, Lewis RP. Idiopathic hypertrophic subaortic stenosis in pregnancy. Ann Intern Med 1975;82:791–4.

72. Shah DM, Sunderji SG. Hypertrophic cardiomyopathy and pregnancy: report of a maternal mortality and review of literature. Obstet Gynecol Surv 1985;40:444–8.

73. Pelliccia F, Cianfrocca C, Gaudio C, et al. Sudden death during pregnancy in hypertrophic cardiomyopathy. Eur Heart J 1992;13:421–3.

74. Tessler MJ, Hudson R, Naugler-Colville M, et al. Pulmonary oedema in two parturients with hypertrophic obstructive cardiomyopathy (HOCM). Can J Anaesth 1990;37:469–73.

75. Avila WS, Amaral FM, Ramires JAF, et al. Influence of pregnancy on clinical course and fetal outcome of women with hypertrophic cardiomyopathy. Arq Bras Cardiol 2007;88:423–8.

76. Joslar JA, Page RL. Antiarrhythmic drugs in pregnancy. Curr Opin Cardiol 2001;16:40–5.

77. Piacenza JM, Kirkorian G, Audra PH, et al. Hypertrophic cardiomyopathy and pregnancy. Eur J Obstet Gynecol Reprod Biol 1998;80:17–23.

78. Paula LJ, Ribeiro HB, Oliveira Júnior RM, et al. Implantable cardioverter-defibrillator in pregnant women with hypertrophic cardiomyopathy. Rev Bras Cir Cardiovasc 2010;25:406–9.

79. Minnich ME, Quirk JG, Clark RB. Epidural anesthesia for vaginal delivery in a patient with idiopathic hypertrophic subaortic stenosis. Anesthesiology 1987;67:590–2.

80. Autore C, Brauneis S, Apponi F, et al. Epidural anesthesia for cesarean section in patients with hypertrophic cardiomyopathy: a report of three cases. Anesthesiology 1999;90:1205–7.

81. Sbarouni E, Oakley CM. Outcome of pregnancy in women with valve prostheses. Br Heart J 1994;71:196–201.

82. Pieper PG, Balci A, Van Dijk AP. Pregnancy in women with prosthetic heart valves. Neth Heart J 2008;16:406–11.

83. Elkayam U, Bitar F. Valvular heart disease and pregnancy. Part II: prosthetic valves. J Am Coll Cardiol 2005;46:403–10.

84. Avila WS, Rossi FG, Grinberg M, et al. Influence of pregnancy after bioprosthetic valve replacement in young women: a prospective five-year study. J Heart Valve Dis 2002;11: 864–9.

85. Cleuziou J, Hörer J, Kaemmerer H, et al. Pregnancy does not accelerate biological valve degeneration. Int J Cardiol 2010;145:418–21.

86. Salazar E, Espinola N, Roman L, et al. Effect of pregnancy on the duration of bovine pericardial prostheses. Am Heart J 1999;137:714–20.

87. Sahnoun-Trabelsi I, Jimenez M, Choussat A, et al. Prosthetic valve thrombosis in pregnancy. A single-center study of 12 cases. Arch Mal Coeur Vaiss 2004;97:305 [in French].

88. Turrentine MA, Braems G, Ramirez MM. Use of thrombolytics for the treatment of thromboembolic disease during pregnancy. Obstet Gynecol Surv 1995;50:534.

Congenital Heart Disease in Pregnancy

Wayne J. Franklin, MD[a],*, Manisha Gandhi, MD[b]

KEYWORDS

- Pregnancy • Congenital heart disease • CARPREG score • Contraindications
- Infective endocarditis • Eisenmenger syndrome • Pulmonary hypertension • Tetralogy of Fallot

KEY POINTS

- For cardiac patients, prepregnancy counseling before conception is strongly recommended.
- It is important for the clinician to understand the normal hemodynamic changes during pregnancy.
- Pregnant patients can be risk-stratified into low, medium, and high cardiac risk based on the CARPREG Risk Score.
- Cardiac absolute contraindications against pregnancy include: pulmonary hypertension, Marfan syndrome with dilated aortic root (4 cm), severe left heart obstruction, and systemic ventricular function less than 30%.
- Medications to avoid or use with caution in pregnancy include: angiotensin converting enzyme inhibitors, angiotension-II receptor blockers, amiodarone, warfarin, spironolactone.
- Pregnant patients with congenital heart disease can be managed successfully with collaboration between the maternal–fetal medicine specialist and an adult congenital heart disease cardiologist.

INTRODUCTION

Each patient with known congenital heart disease (CHD) should ideally be seen before pregnancy by a cardiologist who is experienced in adult CHD and a maternal–fetal medicine specialist for a preconception consult.[1,2] The discussion should include the effect of pregnancy on the mother and the impact of the mother's heart disease on the fetus. However, in many circumstances, this discussion does not occur. Drenthen showed that while 69% of Fontan patients discussed pregnancy with their cardiologist, and 49% had pregnancy discouraged, 77% were still considering pregnancy.[3]

MATERNAL RISK

Risk stratification of the mother based upon her cardiac diagnosis can be helpful in the preconception evaluation. In general, regurgitant lesions are well-tolerated, while stenotic lesions convey higher risk. The risk varies from very low (eg, similar to the general population), as in mild mitral regurgitation, to very high, as in severe coarctation. Siu and colleagues,[4] as part of the Cardiac disease in Pregnancy (CARPREG) investigators found that, in their cohort of 599 women with heart disease, there was a 13% incidence of a cardiac event, notably pulmonary edema, arrhythmia, stroke, or cardiac death. The authors developed a score to predict adverse maternal outcomes (Box 1).

Functional capacity assessment by history and physical examination, and hemodynamic status with an echocardiogram and electrocardiogram are recommended as part of the prepregnancy clinic visit. Recent data also suggest that cardiopulmonary exercise testing should be performed,

[a] Texas Adult Congenital Heart Disease Program, Texas Children's Hospital, Departments of Pediatrics and Medicine, Baylor College of Medicine, 6621 Fannin Street, 20th Floor West Tower, MC 19-345C, Houston, TX 77030, USA; [b] Departments of Obstetrics and Gynecology, Baylor College of Medicine, Houston, TX 77030, USA
* Corresponding author.
E-mail address: wjfranklinmd@gmail.com

Cardiol Clin 30 (2012) 383–394
doi:10.1016/j.ccl.2012.04.003

Box 1
CARPREG Risk Score: Predictors of maternal cardiovascular events

New York Heart Association (NYHA) functional class >II

Cyanosis (room air saturation <90%)

Prior cardiovascular event

Systemic ventricular ejection fraction <40%

Left heart obstruction (eg, mitral valve area <2 cm^2 or aortic valve area <1.5 cm^2, or left ventricular [LV] outflow gradient of >30 mm Hg)

CARPREG risk score: for each CARPREG predictor that is present, a point is assigned. Risk estimation of cardiovascular maternal complications.

0 points-5%

1 point-27%

>2 points-75%

Data from Siu SC, Sermer M, Colman JM, et al, Cardiac Disease in Pregnancy (CARPREG) Investigators. Prospective multicenter study of pregnancy outcomes in women with heart disease. Circulation 2001;104(5): 515–21.

Box 2
Contraindications to pregnancy

- Pulmonary arterial hypertension of any cause
- Marfan syndrome with dilated aortic root >40 mm
- Aortic dilatation >50 mm in aortic disease associated with bicuspid aortic valve
- Severe left heart obstructive lesions (severe mitral stenosis, severe symptomatic aortic stenosis (AS), or native severe coarctation)
- Severe systemic ventricular dysfunction (LV ejection fraction [LVEF] <30%, NYHA III-IV)
- Previous peripartum cardiomyopathy with any residual impairment of LV function

Data from Refs.[4,6,7]

since an abnormal chronotropic response is predictive of maternal and neonatal events.[5] If indicated, cardiac catheterization or cardiac magnetic resonance imaging should be performed in moderate to high-risk pregnancy patients. In patients who are found to be very high risk, other options should be recommended, such as adoption, surrogacy, and appropriate contraception or sterilization.

Contraindications to Pregnancy

In conditions where the maternal risk of death exceeds 10%, pregnancy should be routinely avoided. Due to the prohibitively high risk to the mother and/or fetus, pregnancy should be avoided in the conditions listed in **Box 2**.

FETAL RISK

Maternal heart disease is associated with fetal and neonatal complications, such as intrauterine growth restriction, fetal loss, and prematurity. These complications are more common in cases of maternal cyanosis, anticoagulation, poor NYHA functional class, left heart obstructive lesions, maternal smoking, or multifetal gestation.[8] In women who have CHD, the risk of CHD in the offspring is 7% to 8%, for conditions with no chromosomal abnormality or family history.[3] When the father

has CHD, the risk of CHD in the fetus is roughly 3% to 4%.[6] Nonetheless, CHD in the fetus approaches 50% in single gene disorders such as Marfan syndrome. Genetic counseling is recommended if there is a dysmorphism or a chromosomal abnormality suggested.[9]

PRECONCEPTION MEDICAL MANAGEMENT

Medical or surgical intervention may be necessary before conception in order to optimize cardiac function and to minimize the risks of pregnancy. This should include a review of all cardiac medications, with cessation of any contraindicated drugs and substitution of suitable alternatives (**Box 3**). Comorbidities should also be well-controlled, including hypertension, diabetes, and obesity. Surgery or percutaneous intervention (eg, balloon dilation or transcatheter septal defect closure) should be strongly considered for significant valve disease, and any arrhythmias should be well-controlled.

Box 3
Cardiac drugs to avoid/use with caution

Angiotensin converting enzyme (ACE) inhibitors

Angiotension-II receptor blockers (ARBs)

Amiodarone

Warfarin[a]

Spironolactone

[a] Use during first trimester is contraindicated. Warfarin may be used from weeks 13–35, and then heparin may be used until delivery.[10]

GENERAL APPROACH TO PATIENTS WITH CHD

All women with CHD who are pregnant should be referred to a cardiologist as early as possible to risk stratify and to develop a management strategy with the obstetrician and/or maternal–fetal medicine specialist. Ideally, a multidisciplinary team should participate, including a maternal-fetal medicine specialist, adult CHD (ACHD) cardiologist, and obstetric anesthesiologist. In some cases, an adult intensivist should be consulted if the mother is very high risk, and a neonatologist should be consulted if the baby is considered at risk. Cardiology office visits are recommended during the first trimester to establish the pregnancy plan, at weeks 18 to 22 with a fetal echocardiogram due to increased risk of fetal CHD, and at weeks 28 to 30 (when maternal plasma volume is highest) to confirm the delivery plan (eg, hospital location, mode of delivery, anesthesia type, bacterial endocarditis prophylaxis plan, and other parts of the plan). Close communication between the cardiologist and maternal–fetal medicine physician is important after every clinic visit, but specifically after the third trimester visit so the plan for delivery is well-outlined. In some cases, the woman may be asked to temporarily relocate closer to the tertiary hospital at 35 weeks gestation in order to be nearby when labor begins. Oxytocin administration and artificial rupture of membranes should follow routine obstetric guidelines. While there is no absolute contraindication to misoprostol or dinoprostone, there is a theoretical risk of coronary vasospasm and a low risk of arrhythmias.[11]

Percutaneous Cardiovascular Intervention

If percutaneous cardiac catheterization and intervention are necessary, the preferred time is after the fourth month in the second trimester. By this gestational age, organogenesis is complete; the fetal thyroid is still inactive, and the volume of the uterus is small, so there is greater distance between the fetus and mother's chest than in later weeks. The gravid uterus should be double-shielded from direct radiation, and unfractionated heparin should be used (generally 40–70 U/kg), with an activated clotting time of at least 200 seconds, but not exceeding 300 seconds.

Cardiac Surgery and Cardiopulmonary Bypass

For cardiac surgery and cardiopulmonary bypass, maternal mortality is now similar to that of nonpregnant women. However, there is significant morbidity including late neurologic impairment in 3% to 6% of children, and fetal mortality remains high.[12] Thus, cardiac surgery is recommended only when medical or interventional procedures fail, and the mother's life is threatened. The recommended time for surgery is between the 13th and 28th week.[13,14] During cardiopulmonary bypass, fetal heart rate and uterine tone should be followed closely in addition to standard monitoring. Pump flow greater than 2.5 L/min/m^2 and perfusion pressure greater than 70 mm Hg are necessary to attain adequate uteroplacental perfusion. Cardiopulmonary bypass time should be minimized.[15] Maintenance of the maternal hematocrit greater than 28% is recommended to optimize oxygen delivery. If possible, normothermic perfusion is best, and careful management of pH is recommended to avoid hypocapnia, which can lead to uteroplacental vasoconstriction and fetal hypoxia. In general, neonatal survival at 26 weeks is approximately 80%, with 20% of newborns having a significant neurologic abnormality. Thus, cesarean section may be considered before cardiopulmonary bypass if gestational age is beyond 26 weeks.[9,16]

Delivery and Postpartum Care

The mode of delivery is usually determined by obstetric instead of cardiac conditions. Spontaneous vaginal delivery is preferred in most cases. Assistance in the second stage via forceps or vacuum should be considered in cases where the effects of Valsalva need to be minimized, such as in maternal AS. Exceptions to vaginal delivery include warfarin treatment, Marfan syndrome, aortic aneurysm, and a critically ill mother. In these cases, labor should generally be avoided and cesarean section is recommended. However, vaginal delivery is associated with lower risk of maternal and neonatal complications, less blood loss, fewer acute hemodynamic changes, and lower peripartum infection risk compared with cesarean section. Recommendations for vaginal delivery may be more difficult to follow since the rates of first-time cesarean section in the United States have increased from 27% in 2003 to 32% in 2007.[17,18]

Infective Endocarditis

There are few prospective data on bacterial infective endocarditis (IE) prophylaxis during delivery. Retrospective studies have shown that the estimated overall incidence of IE is 0.006% (approximately 1 case per 100,000 pregnancies) and an incidence of 0.5% in patients with known valvular or CHD. In general, the rate of bacteremia with uncomplicated vaginal or cesarean delivery is low, and routine subacute bacterial endocarditis (SBE) prophylaxis is not recommended by the

American Heart Association or American Dental Association except in cases with prior history of IE. However, many maternal-fetal medicine practitioners still administer peripartum SBE prophylaxis for most cardiac patients.[7,19]

Anesthetic Considerations

Effective anesthesia to limit the cardiac stress and workload from contractions is important. Regional anesthesia techniques such as spinal or epidural administration are commonly used, but these have a risk of vasodilation and hypotension due to autonomic paralysis. For regional anesthesia in high-risk cardiac patients, slow and incremental dose epidurals with invasive monitoring are recommended, since these have a lower risk of cardiovascular collapse than spinal anesthesia, due to the lower doses of analgesics used.

Continuous electrocardiographic and intermittent blood pressure monitoring during labor and delivery should be routinely performed for all CHD patients. Invasive blood pressure and central venous pressure should be implemented in lesions where large or acute fluid changes are poorly tolerated, such as left-sided obstructive lesion or severely depressed ventricular function. Pulmonary artery catheters are rarely indicated and have not been proven to be helpful.

The risk of cardiopulmonary decompensation exists after delivery (and up until 6 weeks after delivery) due to changes in circulating plasma volume, elevated cardiac output, stroke volume, and heart rate. LV dimensions also return gradually to their prepregnancy state. Thus, it is recommended to monitor the patient closely after delivery and not immediately discharge her to the general postpartum ward where telemetry and acute nursing care may not be available.[9]

Methods of Termination of Pregnancy in the ACHD Patient

Pregnancy termination should be considered in women whose gestation represents a major risk to the mother or fetus. The first trimester is the safest time for elective termination, which should be performed at a hospital instead of an outpatient facility, in order for emergency medical support to be readily available. Anesthesia and method of termination should be individualized. High-risk cardiac conditions should be treated at an experienced center with on-site intensivists and cardiac surgery. Endocarditis prophylaxis is generally not recommended, but gynecologists often give antibiotic prophylaxis to prevent postabortal endometritis, which can occur in 5% to 20% of women who do not receive antibiotics.[20]

Dilatation with evacuation is the safest termination procedure within the first and second trimesters. If surgical evacuation is not possible, prostaglandin E1 or E2 or misoprostol can be given to evacuate the uterus. Caution is advised, since these medications are absorbed into the systemic circulation and can decrease systemic vascular resistance and blood pressure, and can increase heart rate. Prostaglandin F should be avoided, because it can increase the maternal pulmonary vascular resistance and decrease coronary perfusion.[21] Within the first 7 weeks gestation, mifepristone may also be used as an alternative to surgery. Saline abortion should not be performed, because saline absorption can cause rapid expansion of intravascular volume, and can lead to maternal heart failure and clotting disorders.

PREGNANCY IN SPECIFIC CHD CONDITIONS
Pulmonary Hypertension

Maternal risk
Pulmonary arterial hypertension (PAH) is the result of progressive pulmonary vascular changes that arise from a variety of causes. Patients with CHD are particularly predisposed to its development, with an incidence of 4% in all patients with CHD.[22] PAH is defined as a mean pulmonary artery pressure greater than 25 mm Hg with a normal left atrial or pulmonary capillary wedge pressure (<15 mm Hg). Some definitions also include a pulmonary vascular resistance of >2 to 3 Wood units.[23] A high maternal mortality risk (ranging from 17% to 50%) exists in patients with PAH and Eisenmenger syndrome. Maternal death occurs in the third trimester and the first few post-natal months due to pulmonary hypertensive crises, pulmonary vascular thrombosis, and/or advanced right heart failure.[24] This can develop even in patients who are highly functional with few symptoms before pregnancy. However, even moderate forms of PAH can progress during pregnancy due to the result of the decrease in systemic vascular resistance and volume overload of the right ventricle. For PAH in pregnancy, no safe pulmonary artery pressure is known.

Obstetric and offspring risk
In successful deliveries, neonatal survival rates are reported to be as high as 89%.[24]

Clinical management
In advanced PAH cases (eg, World Health Organization [WHO] class 3 or 4), if pregnancy occurs, termination should be strongly considered. Due to the risks of anesthesia, this should be done at a tertiary care center with experienced anesthesiologists and gynecologists. If patients are taking endothelin receptor antagonists prior to pregnancy,

they should stop immediately after conception, since these are teratogenic. Peripartum management includes maintenance of plasma volume and avoidance if systemic hypotension, hypoxemia, and acidemia that may lead to refractory heart failure. Supplemental oxygen should be used with maternal oxygen desaturation less than 92%. Prostacyclin analogs (such as intravenous prostacyclin or inhaled iloprost) have been used to improve intrapartum hemodynamics.

Medical therapy In patients who are on warfarin for anticoagulation, this should be stopped at least during the first trimester due to embryopathy risks. Warfarin may be continued until week 35, at which time the patient should changed to unfractionated or low molecular weight heparin. In patients with connective tissue associated PAH, anticoagulation should be considered. In PAH with subsequent portal hypertension, anticoagulation should not be used due to increased risk of bleeding. Oxygen may be used for desaturated patients with PAH throughout pregnancy for severe cyanosis or symptomatic relief.

Delivery The mode of delivery should be individualized. Planned cesarean section or vaginal delivery are recommended over emergency cesarean section; thus close intrapartum monitoring is paramount.

Eisenmenger Syndrome

Eisenmenger patients are some of the highest-risk pregnant patients with heart disease. Maternal–fetal mortality is nearly 50%, most often in the peripartum or postpartum period.[25] Systemic vasodilation increases the right-to-left shunt, leading to worsening cyanosis and an eventual low cardiac output state.

Obstetric and offspring risk
Cyanosis poses a notable risk to the fetus, with a live birth unlikely (<12%) if oxygen saturation is below 85%.

Management
Follow-up When pregnancy occurs, the elevated maternal and fetal risks should be communicated and the termination of pregnancy offered. However, termination also carries its own risks.[7] If the patient elects to continue, care should be based with a specialized high-risk obstetric and cardiac team. Bed rest may be helpful. Thromboembolism is a significant risk for cyanotic patients, thus, these patients should be considered for thrombo-embolic prophylaxis. However, anticoagulation should be used with caution, since these patients are at high risk for hemoptysis and

thrombocytopenia. The risks and benefits of anticoagulation should be discussed and considered on an individual basis. Microcytosis and iron deficiency anemia are frequent and should be treated with supplemental oral or intravenous iron. At least monthly cardiology clinic visits with oxygen saturation measurement and complete blood count are recommended.

Delivery If the maternal or fetal conditions worsen, an early cesarean section should be undertaken. Due to high anesthetic risks, delivery should be performed at an experienced tertiary care center.[7]

Cyanotic Heart Disease Without Pulmonary Arterial Hypertension

Maternal risk
Cyanotic CHD is usually addressed before pregnancy, but many unrepaired or palliated patients survive into adulthood. Medical complications (eg, heart failure, pulmonary or systemic thrombosis, arrhythmias, or endocarditis) occur in 30% of pregnant patients with cyanosis. If resting room air oxygen saturation is less than 85%, a significant maternal and fetal mortality exists, and pregnancy should be avoided. If maternal resting oxygen saturation is 85% to 90%, measurement during exercise (eg, treadmill test or 6-minute walk) is recommended. If the patient desaturates substantially and early, this portends a poor prognosis, and the patient should be counseled against pregnancy.

Obstetric and offspring risk
The amount of maternal hypoxia is the most important predictor of fetal outcome. When resting room air oxygen saturation is greater than 90%, the fetal outcome is very good (<10% fetal loss). If maternal saturation is less than 85%, the chance of a live birth is approximately 12%, and pregnancy should thus be avoided.[25]

Clinical management
Follow-up During pregnancy, restriction of physical activity and supplemental oxygen are recommended. Due to the increased risk of paradoxic embolism, the avoidance of venous stasis is important. This can be done through the use of compression stockings and the avoidance of the supine position for prolonged periods. In cases of prolonged bed rest, prophylactic subcutaneous heparin should be considered. Thromboembolic disease remains a major concern, and so these patients should be considered for prophylaxis after hematology consultation.

Medical therapy Low molecular weight heparin for thromboprophylaxis should considered if hemostasis and coagulation are normal. Diuretics and iron therapy may also be used in the same manner as polycythemia associated with Eisenmenger syndrome.

Delivery Vaginal delivery is recommended in most cases. If the condition of the mother or the fetus worsens, early cesarean section should be undertaken. Due to the risk of anesthesia and cardiopulmonary disease, this should be performed in a tertiary care center experienced in the management of these complex cyanotic patients.[7]

LV Outflow Tract Obstruction and AS

Patients with symptoms from known severe LV outflow tract obstruction (LVOTO) should be advised against pregnancy, and this condition should be addressed before conception. Management of supravalvular and subvalvular stenosis is only described in case reports during pregnancy, but the management is most likely similar to valvular aortic stenosis, even though balloon valvuloplasty is generally not an effective option.[26] In women of childbearing age, the main cause of AS is congenital bicuspid aortic valve. Many patients can be asymptomatic and have very few symptoms, even when the AS is severe. The patient's first symptoms may occur during pregnancy. Echocardiography is the mainstay for diagnosis, and exercise testing is recommended in asymptomatic patients prior to conception to evaluate the valve morphology, measure the gradient severity, assess the exercise tolerance, and determine the amount of aortic insufficiency (AI). The thoracic aorta should also be evaluated prior to conception to assess for aneurysm and coarctation.

Maternal risk

Cardiac complications during pregnancy are related to the severity of the left heart obstruction and symptoms. Pregnancy is usually well-tolerated each trimester with asymptomatic mild or moderate AS. Some patients with severe AS may also tolerate pregnancy well, and these can generally be risk stratified with exercise testing prior to conception. Some patients with AS can have no symptoms with exercise and can display a normal blood pressure response during exercise. With pregnancy, the increase in cardiac output can lead to a significant increase in valve gradient. In severe AS, heart failure and pulmonary edema occur in 10% of patients, and arrhythmias (predominantly supraventricular tachycardia) occur in 3% to 25% of patients. Mortality is now uncommon with close monitoring. Patients with bicuspid aortic valve continue to have a risk of aortic root dilation and dissection.[27,28]

Obstetric and neonatal risk

Obstetric complications (such as hypertension and preterm labor) can be increased in patients with severe AS. Preterm birth, intrauterine growth restriction, and low birth weight are noted in up to 25% of neonates born to mothers with moderate and severe AS.

Clinical management

All symptomatic patients with severe AS or asymptomatic AS patients with impaired LV systolic function or an abnormal exercise test should be advised against pregnancy. In these cases, valvuloplasty or surgery should done before conception. Pregnancy is permissible in asymptomatic patients, even with severe cases, when LV dimension, function, and the prepregnancy exercise test are normal and severe LV hypertrophy has been excluded. Irrespective of symptoms, prepregnancy surgery should be strongly considered in women with at least moderate AS and who have an ascending aorta greater than 5.0 cm.[7]

Follow-up Regular follow-up is required by an experience team of cardiologists and obstetricians. In severe AS, monthly or bimonthly cardiology evaluations with echocardiography are recommended to assess symptom status and degree of progression of AS.

Medical therapy Medical treatment and exercise restriction are indicated for patients with advancing signs or symptoms of heart failure. Thiazide or loop diuretics can be given for pulmonary congestion.

Interventions during pregnancy During pregnancy in patients with severe symptoms who are not responding to medical therapy, percutaneous valvuloplasty can performed in noncalcified valves with mild insufficiency. If this is not possible and patients have life-threatening symptoms, surgical aortic valve replacement should be considered after early delivery (ideally at 28 weeks or after) by cesarean section.

Delivery In severe AS, especially in severely symptomatic patients beyond 28 weeks, cesarean section should be considered with general anesthesia. In mild or moderate AS, vaginal delivery is recommended, thus avoiding a decrease in systemic vascular resistance by employing regional anesthesia.

Atrial Septal Defect

Maternal risk

Women with atrial septal defects (ASDs) usually tolerate pregnancy very well. The only contraindication to conception is PAH or Eisenmenger Syndrome (discussed earlier). Patients with symptomatic or hemodynamically significant lesions with left-to-right shunt should have this closed percutaneously, if possible, or surgically. Arrhythmias (usually supraventricular tachycardia) occur more frequently in unrepaired ASDs or when closed at an older age, or when the woman is older than 30 years of age. Unrepaired patients have a 5% risk of thromboembolism.[29]

Obstetric and offspring risk
In patients with unrepaired ASD, preeclampsia and small for gestational age newborns are more common. In repaired defects, no increased maternal risk has been noted.

Clinical management
Cardiology evaluation in the first and third trimesters is usually adequate. For secundum ASDs, percutaneous device closure may be performed in pregnancy, but this is usually reserved for when the mother shows clinical decompensation. Closure of a small ASD or patent foramen ovale in an otherwise well woman is not indicated. Due to the increased risk of paradoxic embolism in women with atrial level shunts, air filters to all intravenous lines, prevention of venous stasis with compression stockings, and early ambulation after delivery should be undertaken. Vaginal delivery is recommended in most cases.

Ventricular Septal Defect

Maternal risk
For large ventricular septal defects (VSDs) with pulmonary hypertension, the guidelines for pulmonary hypertension should be followed. Small VSDs without evidence of left heart enlargement have a low risk of cardiovascular complications during pregnancy. Repaired VSDs have an excellent prognosis, especially when LV function is normal. When a VSD is present, a preconception echocardiogram to characterize the defect and estimate pulmonary pressures is necessary.

Obstetric and offspring risk
Preeclampsia may occur more frequently than in women with normal hearts.[30]

Clinical management
Cardiology evaluation in the first and third trimesters is usually adequate. Vaginal delivery is recommended in most cases, unless pulmonary hypertension is present. Air filters to all intravenous lines should be used to minimize the risk of paradoxic embolism.

Atrioventricular Canal or Atrioventricular Septal Defect

Maternal risk
In any hemodynamically significant unrepaired atrioventricular canal (AVC) defect, surgical correction should be considered prior to pregnancy. If there is no significant pulmonary hypertension, patients with AVC defects usually do well after surgical repair. The maternal risk during pregnancy is related to the degree of right and left atrioventricular (AV) valve regurgitation and the presence of any intracardiac shunting from residual septal defects. Women with symptoms from severe residual left AV valve regurgitation should have their defect surgically repaired before conception. Patients are at risk of rhythm disturbances, advancement of NYHA class, and exacerbation of AV valve regurgitation throughout pregnancy. The risk of pulmonary edema is low and is related to degree of AV valve regurgitation and ventricular dysfunction. As with other mitral valve operations, AV valve repair is preferred over valve replacement.[31,32] If pulmonary hypertension is present with an AVC defect, the general pulmonary hypertension management guidelines should be followed.

Obstetric and offspring risk
Obstetric complications are generally dependent on the risk of acute heart failure in the peripartum period, and they relate to symptoms and pulmonary artery pressure during pregnancy. Offspring mortality as high as 6% has been reported, related to the incidence of a complex congenital cardiac defect.[31]

Management
Follow-up A clinic visit once per trimester is generally recommended. In cases of moderate or severe AV valve regurgitation or depressed ventricular function, an echocardiogram should be performed at each visit. In the presence of an intracardiac shunt from a residual septal defect, the risk of paradoxic embolism exists, and thus air filters to intravenous lines and thromboembolism prophylaxis should be undertaken.

Delivery Vaginal delivery is advisable in most uncomplicated cases.

Coarctation of the Aorta

Maternal risk
Pregnancy is usually well tolerated in patients after prior repair of coarctation of the aorta (CoA). Significant native or re-coarctation should be repaired prior to conception. Women with unrepaired native CoA and those patients with repaired

CoA who have residual hypertension, residual CoA, or aortic aneurysm have an elevated risk of aortic or cerebral aneurysm rupture during pregnancy and delivery. Additional risk factors for rupture include aortic dilation and bicuspid aortic valve; thus assessment for these defects in the prepregnancy evaluation is important.

Obstetric and offspring risk

An increased risk of hypertension and spontaneous abortion has been noted.[33]

Clinical management

Frequent assessment of blood pressure is indicated with clinical evaluation at least once per trimester. Hypertension should be treated with standard therapies in pregnancy, although very aggressive treatment in women with residual significant CoA (ie, gradient of >20 mm Hg) should be avoided to prevent placental hypoperfusion. Transcathether dilation for recurrent CoA during pregnancy is associated with a higher risk of dissection than in the nonpregnant patient, and intervention thus should be reserved for cases of severe hypertension or maternal or fetal compromise. Covered stents may decrease the risk of dissection.

Delivery Close peripartum blood pressure monitoring is mandatory. Vaginal delivery is preferred with epidural anesthesia, especially in hypertensive patients.

Pulmonary Valve Stenosis and Pulmonary Insufficiency

Maternal risk

Pulmonary valve stenosis (PS) is usually well tolerated during pregnancy. Nonetheless, severe PS (peak Doppler gradient >64 mm Hg) may lead to right ventricular (RV) dysfunction and arrhythmias. Intervention, most frequently via balloon valvuloplasty, to relieve the severe PS should be done before conception.

Severe pulmonary insufficiency (PI) has been listed as an independent risk factor for maternal complications, especially in cases of RV dysfunction.[7] In symptomatic women or in abnormal RV function due to PI, prepregnancy pulmonary valve replacement should be offered. Surgical pulmonary valve replacement has been the traditional option, but now percutaneous pulmonary valve implantation should be considered in favorable cases, notably in RV-to-pulmonary artery conduit failure or when the native pulmonary annulus was spared during a prior operation.[33]

Obstetric and offspring risk

Women with PS may have increased risk of hypertension-related disorders. The incidence of

complications in the newborns appears to be increased, even if the mothers are fully saturated with normal ventricular function. Isolated PI (ie, without prior PS or repaired tetralogy of Fallot) generally adds no additional risk to the offspring.[34]

Management

Follow-up Mild PS and moderate PS are considered to be low-risk defects, and follow-up once per trimester is reasonable. For severe PS, these patients should be seen monthly or bimonthly, with an echocardiogram, evaluation of clinical status, and assessment of RV function. In women with symptomatic severe PS who are refractory to medical therapy and bed rest, transcatheter valvuloplasty may be performed with concerted efforts to minimize fetal radiation exposure.

Delivery Vaginal delivery is recommended in patients with mild or moderate PS and in severe PS in NYHA Class 1/2 symptoms. Cesarean section should be considered in women with severe PS in NYHA Class 3/4 despite medical therapy and bed rest, or where transcatheter valvuloplasty cannot be performed or has failed.

Tetralogy of Fallot

Maternal risk

In unrepaired tetralogy of Fallot (ToF) patients, surgical repair is recommended before conception. Women with repaired ToF and PI usually tolerate pregnancy well. Arrhythmias and heart failure have been shown to occur in up to 12% of patients. Other complications include thromboembolism, progressive aortic root dilation, and endocarditis. Dysfunction of the RV and moderate to severe PI are risk factors for cardiac complications, and pregnancy may be associated with an increase in RV size. In symptomatic patients with a marked dilation of the RV from PI, preconception pulmonary valve replacement with a bioprosthesis should be considered.

Offspring risk

The risk of CHD in offspring is increased. In a recent study at the authors' institution of 126 pregnancies in 95 women with congenital heart defects, the incidence of ToF or its variants was 18%.[35] This is similar to other large retrospective studies.[36,37]

Clinical management

Follow-up Cardiology assessment every trimester is indicated for the majority of patients. Echocardiography at each visit is recommended with special attention to RV size and assessment of the RV outflow tract. In cases with severe PI, monthly or bimonthly cardiac is recommended. If signs or symptoms of RV dysfunction occur during pregnancy, treatment with diuretics should ensue, and bed rest is advised. In those who do not respond to therapy, transcatheter pulmonary valve implantation or early delivery should be strongly considered.

Delivery The recommended mode of delivery is vaginal in most cases.

Ebstein Anomaly

Maternal risk

In patients with Ebstein anomaly without cyanosis and heart failure, pregnancy is well-tolerated. Symptomatic women with cyanosis and/or heart failure should be treated prior to conception, or they should be warned against pregnancy. In severe symptomatic triscuspid regurgitation (TR), repair should is recommended before pregnancy, especially since the clinical problems encountered depend on the severity of TR, the amount of right-to-left atrial shunting, and the status of the RV. Pre-excitation is a common association, and supraventricular tachycardia during pregnancy is associated with a worse prognosis.

Obstetric and offspring risk

The risk of preterm delivery and fetal mortality is increased.[38]

Clinical management

Follow-up Even with severe TR with clinical heart failure during pregnancy, these cases can generally be treated medically. Women with Ebstein anomaly and left-to-right interatrial shunting at baseline can develop right-to-left shunting and cyanosis during pregnancy. Paradoxic emboli risk is also increased.

Delivery The recommended mode of delivery is vaginal in the majority of patients.

Dextro-Transposition of the Great Arteries

Maternal risk

Although many patients tolerate pregnancy well many years after an atrial switch operation (Senning or Mustard repair), they have increased risk of arrhythmias, which can be life-threatening, and heart failure (WHO class 3). Some patients will have bradycardia or junctional rhythm, which can impact the use of certain medications, such as beta-blockers, that may be beneficial in cardiomyopathy. A decline in systemic RV function is expected, as early as the third decade, and generally occurs by the fourth decade of life. Women with severe impairment of the systemic RV function or severe systemic TR should be counseled against pregnancy.

Obstetric and offspring risk

Pregnancy-induced hypertension and preeclampsia and offspring complications occur more often than in normal pregnancy.[39]

Clinical management

Follow-up Patients who have undergone the atrial switch operation should have cardiology visits and echocardiographic evaluation at least every trimester. Symptoms, systemic RV function, and cardiac rhythm should be assessed.

Delivery In asymptomatic patients with low–normal to moderate RV function, vaginal delivery is recommended. If RV function worsens or advanced symptoms arise, an early cesarean section should be considered to avoid pulmonary edema or progressive heart failure.

Arterial switch (of Jatene) operation

Worldwide, a few dextro-transposition of the great arteries (D-TGA) patients who have undergone the arterial switch operation are now of childbearing age. However, this population will certainly increase, since this operation (and no longer the atrial switch operation) is now the preferred operation for D-TGA newborns. Currently, many of these patients have reached their childbearing years, and many will choose to conceive. If the patients are in good clinical condition before pregnancy, the cardiac risk of pregnancy appears low. Vaginal delivery is advised. More studies are needed in this population.

Levo-Transposition of the Great Arteries, Also Known as Congenitally Corrected TGA

Maternal risk

In women with congenitally corrected TGA (cc-TGA) (also called atrioventricular and ventriculoarterial discordance or ventricular inversion), risk depends on functional class, systemic RV function, presence of arrhythmias, and associated lesions. An irreversible cardiomyopathy develops in 40% of these patients by age 30; thus patients are at increased risk of arrhythmias (some life-threatening) and heart failure. Since complete AV block can develop in these patients, beta-blockers should be used with extreme caution. Women with NHYA functional class 3 or 4, moderate-to-severe or severe systemic RV dysfunction, or severe TR should be advised against conception.

Obstetric and offspring risk

The rate of fetal loss is increased.

Management

Follow-up Patients should have a full clinical evaluation at least every trimester, including echo measurement of systemic RV function and TR, electrocardiogram, and symptom assessment.[7,40]

Delivery In asymptomatic patients with normal or mild depressed systemic RV function, vaginal delivery is advised. If RV function deteriorates, an early cesarean section should be scheduled in an attempt to avoid the development or exacerbation of heart failure.

Fontan Physiology

Maternal risk

Although successful pregnancies have been reported in Fontan patients, these are all high-risk pregnancies. Thus, preconception counseling should be explicit, and women should be counseled accordingly, preferably with a maternal–fetal medicine specialist. Maternal risk is likely even higher if the Fontan circulation is suboptimal, such as with signs of decreased cardiac output, recurrent tachycardia, or hepatic disease. Patients with a resting oxygen saturation of less than 85%, moderate-to-severe AV regurgitation, depressed ventricular function, or with protein-losing enteropathy should be counseled against pregnancy.

Obstetric and offspring risk

The offspring risk includes premature birth, low birthweight infants, and intrauterine fetal demise in up to 50% of cases.[3,8]

Management

Follow-up These patients require frequent surveillance during pregnancy and the first 4 postpartum weeks. Angiotensin-converting enzyme inhibitors must be discontinued, and anticoagulation must be adjusted. Even though anticoagulants have been discussed intermittently in pregnancy reviews, the risk for thromboembolism in pregnant Fontan patients remains elevated.

Delivery In general, vaginal delivery is preferred. If ventricular systolic function deteriorates, an early cesarean section should be scheduled in an experienced center to minimize complications and further progression of heart failure.

SUMMARY

In most cases, pregnancy can be successfully managed in the mother with congenital heart disease. However, there are a several cardiac contraindications to pregnancy. In order to optimize maternal and neonatal outcomes, close colloboration between the maternal-fetal medicine specialist and the cardiologist with expertise in ACHD is important.

REFERENCES

1. Royal College of Obstetrics and Gynecology. Saving mothers' lives: reviewing maternal deaths to make motherhood safer. 7th report of the Confidential Inquiries into Maternal Deaths in the UK. London: CEMACH; 2007.
2. Warnes CA, Liberthson R, Danielson GK, et al. Task force 1: the changing profile of congenital heart disease in adult life. J Am Coll Cardiol 2001;37(5):1170–5.
3. Drenthen W, Pieper PG, Roos-Hesselink JW, et al. Outcome of pregnancy in women with congenital heart disease: a literature review. J Am Coll Cardiol 2007;49:2303–11.
4. Siu SC, Sermer M, Colman JM, et al, Cardiac Disease in Pregnancy (CARPREG) Investigators. Prospective multicenter study of pregnancy outcomes in women with heart disease. Circulation 2001;104(5):515–21.
5. Lui GK, Silversides CK, Khairy P, et al, Alliance for Adult Research in Congenital Cardiology (AARCC). Heart rate response during exercise and pregnancy outcome in women with congenital heart disease. Circulation 2011;123(3):242–8.
6. Thorrne SA. Pregnancy in heart disease. Heart 2004;90(4):450–6.
7. Warnes CA, Williams RG, Bashore TM, et al, American College of Cardiology, American Heart Association Task Force on Practice Guidelines (Writing Committee to Develop Guidelines on the Management of Adults With Congenital Heart Disease), American Society of Echocardiography; Heart Rhythm Society, International Society for Adult Congenital Heart Disease, Society for Cardiovascular Angiography and Interventions, Society of Thoracic Surgeons. ACC/AHA 2008 guidelines for the management of adults with congenital heart disease: a report of the American College of Cardiology/American Heart Association Task Force on Practice Guidelines (Writing Committee to Develop Guidelines on the Management of Adults With Congenital Heart Disease). Developed in collaboration with the American Society of Echocardiography, Heart Rhythm Society, International Society for Adult Congenital Heart Disease, Society for Cardiovascular Angiography and Interventions, and Society of Thoracic Surgeons. J Am Coll Cardiol 2008;52(23):e143–263.
8. Khairy P, Ouyang DW, Fernandes SM, et al. Pregnancy outcomes in women with congenital heart disease. Circulation 2006;113(4):517–24.
9. European Society of Gynecology, Association for European Paediatric Cardiology, German Society for Gender Medicine, Authors/Task Force Members, Regitz-Zagrosek V, Blomstrom Lundqvist C, Borghi C, et al. ESC guidelines on the management of

cardiovascular diseases during pregnancy: the Task Force on the Management of Cardiovascular Diseases during Pregnancy of the European Society of Cardiology (ESC). Eur Heart J 2011;32(24):3147–97.

10. Bates SM, Greer IA, Pabinger I, et al, American College of Chest Physicians. Venous thromboembolism, thrombophilia, antithrombotic therapy, and pregnancy: American College of Chest Physicians evidence-based clinical practice guidelines (8th edition). Chest 2008;133(Suppl 6):844S–86S.

11. Perloff JK. Congenital heart disease in adults. 2nd edition. Philadelphia: WB Saunders; 1998. p. 93–7.

12. Chambers CE, Clark SL. Cardiac surgery during pregnancy. Clin Obstet Gynecol 1994;37(2):316–23.

13. Salazar E, Zajarias A, Gutierrez N, et al. The problem of cardiac valve prostheses, anticoagulants, and pregnancy. Circulation 1984;70(3 Pt 2): I169–77.

14. Becker RM. Intracardiac surgery in pregnant women. Ann Thorac Surg 1983;36(4):453–8.

15. Chandrasekhar S, Cook CR, Collard CD. Cardiac surgery in the parturient. Anesth Analg 2009; 108(3):777–85.

16. Parry AJ, Westaby S. Cardiopulmonary bypass during pregnancy. Ann Thorac Surg 1996;61(6): 1865–9 Review.

17. United States ceserean section rate. 2003. Available at: http://www.cdc.gov/nchs/data/nvsr/nvsr54/nvsr54_04.pdf. Accessed March 2012.

18. United States ceserean section rate. 2005. Available at: http://www.nytimes.com/2010/03/24/health/24birth.html. Accessed March 2012.

19. Habib G, Hoen B, Tornos P, et al, ESC Committee for Practice Guidelines. Guidelines on the prevention, diagnosis, and treatment of infective endocarditis (new version 2009): the Task Force on the Prevention, Diagnosis, and Treatment of Infective Endocarditis of the European Society of Cardiology (ESC). Endorsed by the European Society of Clinical Microbiology and Infectious Diseases (ESCMID) and the International Society of Chemotherapy (ISC) for Infection and Cancer. Eur Heart J 2009;30(19): 2369–413.

20. ACOG Committee on Practice Bulletins. ACOG Practice Bulletin No. 74. Antibiotic prophylaxis for gynecologic procedures. Obstet Gynecol 2006;108:225–34.

21. Secher NJ, Thayssen P, Arnsbo P, et al. Effect of prostaglandin E2 and F2alpha on the systemic and pulmonary circulation in pregnant anesthetized women. Acta Obstet Gynecol Scand 1982;61(3):213–8.

22. Duffels MG, Engelfriet PM, Berger RM, et al. Pulmonary arterial hypertension in congenital heart disease: an epidemiologic perspective from a Dutch registry. Int J Cardiol 2007;120(2):198–204.

23. Humbert M, McLaughlin VV. The 4th World Symposium on Pulmonary Hypertension. Dana Point, California; 2008.

24. Bédard E, Dimopoulos K, Gatzoulis MA. Has there been any progress made on pregnancy outcomes among women with pulmonary arterial hypertension? Eur Heart J 2009;30(3):256–65.

25. Presbitero P, Somerville J, Stone S, et al. Pregnancy in cyanotic congenital heart disease. Outcome of mother and fetus. Circulation 1994;89(6): 2673–6.

26. van der Tuuk K, Drenthen W, Moons P, et al. Three live-birth pregnancies in a woman with Williams syndrome. Congenit Heart Dis 2007;2(2):139–42.

27. Yap SC, Drenthen W, Pieper PG, et al, ZAHARA investigators. Risk of complications during pregnancy in women with congenital aortic stenosis. Int J Cardiol 2008;126(2):240–6.

28. Bhargava B, Agarwal R, Yadav R, et al. Percutaneous balloon aortic valvuloplasty during pregnancy: use of the Inoue balloon and the physiologic antegrade approach. Cathet Cardiovasc Diagn 1998;45(4):422–5.

29. Webb G, Gatzoulis MA. Atrial septal defects in the adult: recent progress and overview. Circulation 2006;114(15):1645–53.

30. Yap SC, Drenthen W, Pieper PG, et al, ZAHARA investigators. Pregnancy outcome in women with repaired versus unrepaired isolated ventricular septal defect. BJOG 2010;117(6):683–9.

31. Drenthen W, Pieper PG, van der Tuuk K, et al, Zahara Investigators. Cardiac complications relating to pregnancy and recurrence of disease in the offspring of women with atrioventricular septal defects. Eur Heart J 2005;26(23):2581–7.

32. Vriend JW, Drenthen W, Pieper PG, et al. Outcome of pregnancy in patients after repair of aortic coarctation. Eur Heart J 2005;26(20):2173–8.

33. Feltes TF, Bacha E, Beekman RH 3rd, et al, American Heart Association Congenital Cardiac Defects Committee of the Council on Cardiovascular Disease in the Young, Council on Clinical Cardiology, Council on Cardiovascular Radiology and Intervention. Indications for cardiac catheterization and intervention in pediatric cardiac disease: a scientific statement from the American Heart Association. Circulation 2011;123(22):2607–52.

34. Drenthen W, Pieper PG, Roos-Hesselink JW, et al, ZAHARA investigators. Non-cardiac complications during pregnancy in women with isolated congenital pulmonary valvar stenosis. Heart 2006;92(12): 1838–43.

35. Saraf AP, Franklin WJ, Ananaba I, et al. Pregnancy outpatient study: a review of pregnant patients at Texas Children's Hospital [oral abstract]. Orlando (FL): Presented at American Heart Association Scientific Sessions; 2011.

36. Veldtman GR, Connolly HM, Grogan M, et al. Outcomes of pregnancy in women with tetralogy of Fallot. J Am Coll Cardiol 2004;44(1):174–80.

37. Balci A, Drenthen W, Mulder BJ, et al. Pregnancy in women with corrected tetralogy of Fallot: occurrence and predictors of adverse events. Am Heart J 2011; 161(2):307–13.

38. Connolly HM, Warnes CA. Ebstein's anomaly: outcome of pregnancy. J Am Coll Cardiol 1994; 23(5):1194–8.

39. Canobbio MM, Morris CD, Graham TP, et al. Pregnancy outcomes after atrial repair for transposition of the great arteries. Am J Cardiol 2006;98(5):668–72.

40. Therrien J, Barnes I, Somerville J. Outcome of pregnancy in patients with congenitally corrected transposition of the great arteries. Am J Cardiol 1999; 84(7):820–4.

Anticoagulation in Pregnancy

Sorel Goland, MD[a],[*], Uri Elkayam, MD[b]

KEYWORDS

- Pregnancy • Anticoagulation • Mechanical prosthetic valves • Thromboembolism
- Antithrombotic therapy

KEY POINTS

- Normal pregnancy is accompanied by changes in hemostasis that produce a hypercoagulable state that helps to prevent possible hemorrhage during delivery or miscarriage. Most clotting factors usually increase in pregnancy, whereas several anticoagulants and fibrinolytic activity decrease.
- In pregnant patients with prosthetic valves, therapy with low-molecular-weight heparin is an attractive alternative to vitamin K antagonists (which can have harmful fetal effects) and unfractionated heparin, which has several disadvantages, including heparin-induced thrombocytopenia and osteopenia.
- Mitral stenosis (MS), the most common valvular heart disease in pregnancy with a significant impact on both maternal and fetal outcome, carries a significant risk of thromboembolism. Prophylactic anticoagulation is indicated in patients with MS with atrial fibrillation or a previous history of an embolic event because these patients have the highest risk for thromboembolic events.
- Anticoagulation therapy is not required in pregnant women with a short episode of lone atrial fibrillation.

THE HYPERCOAGULABLE STATE OF PREGNANCY

Normal pregnancy is accompanied by changes in hemostasis that produce a hypercoagulable state that helps to prevent possible hemorrhage at the time of delivery or miscarriage. Most clotting factors usually increase in pregnancy, together with a decrease in several anticoagulants and fibrinolytic activity. Specifically, there is an increased concentration of factors VII, VIII, X, and von Willebrand factor.[1] Concomitantly, there is a decrease in anticoagulant factors, including free and total protein S, as well as decreased activity during early pregnancy. Although protein C levels remain unchanged,[2,3] there is an increase in activated protein C resistance, partly because of several modifiers such as the presence of factor V Leiden mutation, thrombin generation, and the presence

of antiphospholipid antibodies.[4] Fibrinolysis is decreased, predominantly because of diminished tissue plasminogen activator activity. Plasminogen activator inhibitor type 1 (PAI-1) levels are increased as well as levels of PAI-2, produced by the placenta. Other markers of thrombin generation include increased thrombin-antithrombin complexes, prothrombin fragments 1 and 2, peak thrombin generation, and increased D-dimer levels.[2,3,5] All these changes result in a hypercoagulable state of pregnancy and may not return to normal ranges for at least 8 weeks after delivery,[6] and result in a 3-fold to 4-fold and 4-fold to 5-fold increase in arterial thromboembolism (strokes and myocardial infarction) and venous thromboembolism, respectively, during gestation, and a further increased risk (20-fold) post partum[7] compared with that of nonpregnant women.[7–9] The overall prevalence of thromboembolic events during

Disclosures.

[a] Department of Cardiology, Kaplan Medical Center, PO Box 1, Rehovot, Israel 76100; [b] Division of Cardiovascular Disease, Department of Medicine, University of Southern California, 1200 North State Street, Los Angeles, CA 90033, USA

* Corresponding author. Kaplan Medical Center, PO Box 1, Rehovot, Israel 76100.

E-mail address: sorelgoland@yahoo.com

doi:10.1016/j.ccl.2012.05.003
0733-8651/12/$ – see front matter © 2012 Elsevier Inc. All rights reserved.

pregnancy is approximately 2 per 1000 deliveries[8-10]; most (up to 80%) are venous and the rest of these events are arterial.[9]

Because of alterations in hemostasis and coagulability[11,12] pregnancy in women with mechanical heart valves (MHVs) carries a high rate of thromboembolic complications. Earlier published studies reported thromboembolic events in 7% to 23% of such cases[12-14]; half of them had valve thrombosis, leading to a high mortality of up to 40%. More recent reports, including mostly women with new-generation, less thrombogenic MHVs, have described maternal mortality between 1% and 4%, with most deaths attributable to thrombotic complications.[15,16] Prepregnancy counseling and education of the patient and her family regarding appropriate anticoagulation strategy planning are of paramount importance. However, women receiving suboptimal therapy often come to medical attention already pregnant. Because of the increased risk of severe thromboembolic complications in pregnancy, effective anticoagulation is critical in such patients, but remains problematic because both vitamin K antagonists (VKAs) and unfractionated heparin (UFH) can be associated with important fetal and maternal complications.

ANTICOAGULATION IN PATIENTS WITH PROSTHETIC VALVES
VKAs

VKAs are the preferred agents for long-term anticoagulation in nonpregnant women with MHV, but can have harmful fetal effects. When used during the critical period for organogenesis, the fourth to the eighth week after conception, there is a 15% to 56% reported risk of miscarriage[17-23] and, depending on the case series, a 5% to 30% risk of congenital anomalies.[17-19] Placental transfer of warfarin later in pregnancy can result in fetal bleeding or stillbirth[20-22] and long-term sequelae include an increased risk of adverse neurologic outcome.[15] Vitale and colleagues[24] reported a high frequency of fetal complications (88%), including spontaneous abortions, congenital heart disease, growth retardation, and warfarin embryopathy in women with MHV when treated with warfarin at a dose exceeding 5 mg/d throughout the pregnancy. Sadler and colleagues[25] described similar results, regardless of the warfarin dose. Long-term effects included an adverse neurologic outcome in 14% of cases and low IQ in 4%.[22]

UFH

UFH has traditionally been considered the drug of choice for the prevention and treatment of thrombotic disorders during pregnancy.[23] This drug does not cross the placenta and therefore offers little direct risk to the fetus.[26,27] However, UFH has several disadvantages including heparin-induced thrombocytopenia (HIT) and osteopenia,[26] and the latter may lead to symptomatic vertebral fracture in approximately 2% of women.[28,29] In addition, an increase in the volume of distribution caused by a 40% to 50% increase in maternal blood volume, as well as an increase in glomerular filtration,[12,30] which lead to an increase in renal excretion of heparin compounds, results in a shorter half-life and lower peak plasma concentration of heparin compounds, and the need to use higher doses and more frequent administration.[31] The incidence of HIT is low in pregnancy, but the risk is unknown.[23] In HIT, fondaparinux, a new selective factor Xa inhibitor, is the anticoagulant of choice, although data on its use in pregnancy are limited.[32]

Low-Molecular-Weight Heparin

Therapy with low-molecular-weight heparin (LMWH) in pregnancy is an attractive alternative to VKAs and UFH. LMWH has superior subcutaneous absorption and bioavailability[28] (90% vs 10%), and a 2-fold to 4-fold longer half-life. Because LMWH does not bind to plasma proteins, it may be associated with a more predictable dose response compared with UFH.[33] Similar to UFH and because of accelerated clearance, LMWH has a shorter half-life and lower peak plasma concentration during pregnancy than in nonpregnant women, and therefore requires higher doses and sometimes more frequent administration.[34] In nonpregnant patients, LMWH has been associated with fewer side effects than UFH.[23] Potential advantages of LMWH include less bleeding, a more predictable and stable response, and a lower risk of HIT.[35,36] However, in a randomized trial of low-dose UFH versus LMWH for thromboprophylaxis in pregnancy, there was no difference in the incidence of clinically significant bone loss (2%–2.5%) between women on UFH compared with those on enoxaparin.[37] Disadvantages of LMWH are its longer half-life and the inability to fully reverse its effect, issues that may increase the risk of bleeding at the time of delivery.[38]

GUIDELINES FOR ANTICOAGULATION REGIMENS IN PREGNANT PATIENTS WITH PROSTHETIC HEART VALVES

The 2008 American College of Cardiology (ACC)/ American Heart Association (AHA) guidelines (**Box 1**) state that there are insufficient grounds to make definitive recommendations about optimal

Box 1
ACC/AHA 2006 recommendation for anticoagulation during pregnancy in patients with mechanical prosthetic valves

Class I

1. All pregnant patients with mechanical prosthetic valves must receive continuous therapeutic anticoagulation with frequent monitoring (level of evidence: B).

2. For women requiring long-term warfarin therapy who are attempting pregnancy, pregnancy tests should be monitored, with discussions about subsequent anticoagulation therapy, so that anticoagulation can be continued uninterrupted when pregnancy is achieved (level of evidence: C).

3. Pregnant patients with mechanical prosthetic valves who elect to stop warfarin between weeks 6 and 12 of gestation should receive continuous intravenous UFH, dose-adjusted UFH, or dose-adjusted subcutaneous LMWH (level of evidence: C).

4. For pregnant patients with mechanical prosthetic valves, up to 36 weeks of gestation, the therapeutic choice of continuous intravenous or dose-adjusted subcutaneous UFH, dose-adjusted LMWH, or warfarin should be discussed fully. If continuous intravenous UFH is used, the fetal risk is lower, but the maternal risks of prosthetic valve thrombosis, systemic embolization, infection, osteoporosis, and HIT are higher (level of evidence: C).

5. In pregnant patients with mechanical prosthetic valves who receive dose-adjusted LMWH, the LMWH should be administered twice daily subcutaneously to maintain the anti-Xa level between 0.7 and 1.2 U per mL 4 hours after administration (level of evidence: C).

6. In pregnant patients with mechanical prosthetic valves who receive dose-adjusted UFH, the aPTT should be at least twice control (level of evidence: C).

7. In pregnant patients with mechanical prosthetic valves who receive warfarin, the international normalized ratio (INR) goal should be 3.0 (range 2.5–3.5) (level of evidence: C).

8. In pregnant patients with mechanical prosthetic valves, warfarin should be discontinued and continuous intravenous UFH given starting 2 to 3 weeks before planned delivery (level of evidence: C).

Class IIa

1. In patients with mechanical prosthetic valves, it is reasonable to avoid warfarin between weeks 6 and 12 of gestation because of the high risk of fetal defects (level of evidence: C).

2. In patients with mechanical prosthetic valves, it is reasonable to resume UFH 4 to 6 hours after delivery and begin oral warfarin in the absence of significant bleeding (level of evidence: C).

3. In patients with mechanical prosthetic valves, it is reasonable to give low-dose aspirin (75–100 mg per day) in the second and third trimesters of pregnancy in addition to anticoagulation with warfarin or heparin (level of evidence: C).

Adapted from Bonow RO, Carabello BA, Chatterjee K, et al. American College of Cardiology/American Heart Association Task Force on Practice Guidelines. 2008 focused update incorporated into the ACC/AHA 2006 guidelines for the management of patients with valvular heart disease: a report of the American College of Cardiology/American Heart Association Task Force on Practice Guidelines (Writing Committee to revise the 1998 guidelines for the management of patients with valvular heart disease). Endorsed by the Society of Cardiovascular Anesthesiologists, Society for Cardiovascular Angiography and Interventions, and Society of Thoracic Surgeons. J Am Coll Cardiol 2008;52(13): e1–142.

antithrombotic therapy in pregnant patients with MHVs, because properly designed studies have not been performed.[39] Generally, both the ACC/AHA and the European Society of Cardiology (ESC)[39–40] guidelines recommend discussing the risks of available anticoagulation regimens with the pregnant patient. Antithrombotic preventive therapy options during pregnancy include continuation of VKAs throughout the second trimester of pregnancy as well as dose-adjusted subcutaneous or intravenous UFH between the sixth and the twelfth week or throughout pregnancy with an activated partial thromboplastin time (aPTT) at least twice the control level. The ACC/AHA guidelines include the option of LMWH instead of UFH with peak anti-Xa factor levels between 0.7 and 1.2 U/mL 4 hours after administration.

The American College of Chest Physicians (ACCP) Conference on Antithrombotic and Thrombolytic Therapy (**Box 2**) concluded that it is reasonable to use one of the following 3 regimens: (1) either LMWH or UFH between 6 and 12 weeks

Box 2
Recommendations of the 2008 ACCP Consensus Conference on antithrombotic therapy in patients with MHVs

Adjusted-dose twice a day LMWH throughout pregnancy (grade 1C). We suggest that doses be adjusted to achieve the manufacturer's peak anti-Xa LMWH 4 hours after subcutaneous injection (grade 2C)

or

Adjusted-dose UFH throughout pregnancy administered subcutaneously every 12 hours in doses adjusted to keep the midinterval aPTT at least twice control or attain an anti-Xa heparin level of 0.35 to 0.70 U/mL (grade 1C)

or

UFH or LMWH (as above) until the thirteenth week with warfarin substitution until close to delivery when UFH or LMWH is resumed (grade 1C).

Data from Bates SM, Greer IA, Pabinger I, et al. Venous thromboembolism, thrombophilia, antithrombotic therapy and pregnancy: American College of Chest Physicians Evidence-Based Clinical Practice Guidelines (8th edition). Chest 2008;133(Suppl 6):844S–86S.

and close to term only, with warfarin used at other times; (2) aggressive dose-adjusted UFH throughout pregnancy; or (3) aggressive adjusted-dose LMWH throughout pregnancy aiming to attain a peak anti-Xa level of 0.7 to 1.2 U/mL at 4 to 6 hours after injection.[23] UFH or LMWH throughout pregnancy is not recommended by the recent ESC guidelines, considering continuation of VKAs throughout pregnancy when the warfarin dose is less than 5 mg daily (**Table 1**).[40] Discontinuation of VKAs and a switch to UFH or LMWH is recommended between weeks 6 and 12 under strict dose control and supervision. When a higher dose of VKAs is required, discontinuation of VKAs between weeks 6 and 12 and replacement by adjusted-dose UFH (aPTT $\geq$2 times the control, in high-risk patients applied as an intravenous fusion) or LMWH twice daily (dose adjusted according to weight) is recommended (the anti-Xa level should be maintained between 0.8 and 1.2 U/mL [4–6 hours after application]) (**Table 2**).

REVIEW OF DATA AND RECOMMENDATIONS ON ANTICOAGULATION REGIMENS IN PREGNANT PATIENTS WITH PROSTHETIC HEART VALVES

In the absence of controlled clinical trials, current recommendations are based on limited, observational data. Only a few and mostly small

series[14,24,41–43] comprise the basis from which current guidelines and recommendations are derived.[39,40] Maternal mortality in patients with MHV remains the most devastating complication, and even contemporary series confirm that mortality and complications may not necessarily be avoided.[12–16]

In the largest literature review before 1998, which included more than 900 pregnant women with MHV, Chan and colleagues[15] evaluated maternal and fetal outcomes according to the type of anticoagulation used during pregnancy: VKAs alone, VKAs with UFH during the first trimester, UFH throughout pregnancy, and antiplatelet agents alone. Rates of maternal thromboembolic complications in women who received UFH alone, VKAs with heparin substitution during the first trimester, and warfarin alone were 33.3%, 9.2%, and 3.9%, respectively. However, the rates of congenital fetal anomalies were 0%, 3.4%, and 6.4%, respectively. These results suggest that heparin alone is insufficient to prevent thromboembolism among pregnant women with MHV compared with VKA regimens. Compared with regimens using warfarin alone, substitution with UFH during the first trimester was associated with a reduction in embryopathy from 6.4% to 3.4%, but also with an increase in maternal thromboembolic risk from 3.9% to 9.2%.

Reports by one group suggested that the risk of fetal damage was reduced although not eliminated if the daily warfarin dose was less than 5 mg.[24] However, several reports described the development of warfarin embryopathy and fetal loss with low-dose warfarin.[19,25,44,45] For this reason, pregnancy without fetal complications cannot be guaranteed even to women who are well anticoagulated on less than 5 mg/d of warfarin during pregnancy. The risk of fetal malformation and other effects associated with use of VKAs throughout pregnancy suggests that these drugs should be considered only in women with a high risk of thrombosis, such as highly thrombogenic MHVs or a history of thromboembolic complications on a therapeutic dose of heparin.[16,23]

Supporting the published review by Chan and colleagues,[15] Silissen and colleagues[46] recently described 79 women who had 155 pregnancies after valve replacement. Two women died during pregnancy: one from heart failure and one from postpartum bleeding. There were 4 thromboembolic episodes in the early study period in women with a mitral prosthesis on UFH. Detailed information on the UFH regimen and monitoring results at the time of the episodes were not available. Because of a lack of information related to the level of anticoagulation and its monitoring, these reports

Table 1
ESC 2011 recommendation for anticoagulation during pregnancy in patients with mechanical prosthetic valves

Recommendations	Class[a]	Level[b]
OACs are recommended during the second and third trimesters until the 36th week	I	C
Change of anticoagulation regimen during pregnancy should be implemented in hospital	I	C
If delivery starts while on OACs, cesarean delivery is indicated	I	C
OAC should be discontinued and dose-adjusted UFH (a PTT ≥2× control) or adjusted-dose LMWH (target anti-Xa level 4–6 h after dose 0.8–1.2 U/mL) started at the 36th wk of gestation	I	C
In pregnant women managed with LMWH, the post-dose anti-Xa level should be assessed weekly	I	C
LMWH should be replaced by intravenous UFH at least 36 h before planned delivery. UFH should be continued until 4–6 h before planned delivery and restarted 4–6 h after delivery if there are no bleeding complications	I	C
Immediate echocardiography is indicated in women with mechanical valves presenting with dyspnea or an embolic event	I	C
Continuation of OACs should be considered during the first trimester if the warfarin dose required for therapeutic anticoagulation is <5 mg/d (or phenprocoumon <3 mg/d or acenocoumarol <2 mg/d), after patient information and consent	IIa	C
Discontinuation of OAC between weeks 6 and 12 and replacement by adjusted-dose UFH (aPTT ≥2× control; in high-risk patients applied as intravenous infusion) or LMWH twice daily (with dose adjustment according to weight and target anti-Xa level 4–6 h after dose 0.8–1.2 U/mL) should be considered in patients with a warfarin dose required of >5 mg/d (or phenprocoumon >3 mg/d or acenocoumarol >2 mg/d)	IIa	C
Discontinuation of OACs between weeks 6 and 12 and replacement by UFH or LMWH under strict dose control (as described above) may be considered on an individual basis in patients with warfarin dose required for therapeutic anticoagulation <5 mg/d (or phenprocoumon <3 mg/d or acenocoumarol <2 mg/d)	IIb	C
Continuation of OACs may be considered between weeks 6 and 12 in patients with a warfarin dose required for therapeutic anticoagulation >5 mg/d (or phenprocoumon >3 mg/d or acenocoumarol >2 mg/d)	IIb	C
LMWH should be avoided, unless anti-Xa levels are monitored	III	C

Abbreviation: OAC, oral anticoagulant.
[a] Level of evidence.
[b] Class of recommendation.
Adapted from Bax J, Auricchio A, Baumgartner H, et al. ESC Guidelines on the management of cardiovascular diseases during pregnancy: the Task Force on the management of cardiovascular diseases during Pregnancy of the European Society of Cardiology (ESC). Eur Heart J 2011;32(24):3147–97.

might suggest resistance to moderate doses of UFH in high-risk women with old-generation prosthetic heart valves. For this reason, if the decision is to use UFH, it should preferably be used as an intravenous continuous infusion and at high dose[16,39] and adjusted to achieve an aPTT ratio of greater than 2.5 times control value with careful maintenance of the central line to prevent infection and a risk of endocarditis. Because of high risk of valve thrombosis, subcutaneous administration of

UFH should be avoided if all possible. If no other choice is available in a woman who prefers not to use warfarin, a high dose (7500 to 20,000 U every 12 hours) should be used, aiming to achieve a mid-level (6 hours) of aPTT ratio of more than 2.5 control value.

Therapy with LMWH in pregnancy is an attractive and convenient alternative to VKAs and UFH. Substantial evidence shows the efficacy and safety of LMWH in prevention and treatment of

Table 2
Recommended approach for anticoagulation in women with MHV during pregnancy

	Higher Risk	Lower Risk
Definition	First-generation PHV (eg, Starr-Edwards, Bjork-Shiley) in the mitral position, MHV in the tricuspid position, AF, history of TE on anticoagulation	Second-generation PHV (eg, St Jude Medical, Medtronic-Hall) in the mitral position and any mechanical PHV in the aortic position
Treatment	Warfarin (INR 2.5–3.5) for 35–36 wk, followed by UFH[a] (aPTT ≥2.5) to parturition + ASA 80–100 mg every day or LMWH (trough anti-Xa ≥0.7, peak ≤ 1.5) or UFH[a] (aPTT ≥2.5) for 12 wk, followed by warfarin (INR 2.5–3.5) to 35–36 wk, then IV UFH[a] (aPTT >2.5) to parturition +ASA 80–100 mg every day	LMWH (trough anti-Xa ≥0.6, peak ≤ 1.5) to 35–36 wk then IV UFH (aPTT ≥2.0) to parturition or LMWH (trough anti-Xa ≥0.6, peak ≤1.5) for 12 wk, or UFH[a] (aPTT ≥2.0) followed by warfarin (INR 2.5–3.0) for 35–36 wk, then IV UFH (aPTT ≥2.0) to parturition

Abbreviations: ASA, acetylsalicylic acid; IV, intravenous; SC, subcutaneous; TE, thromboembolism.
[a] IV preferred.

thromboembolism during pregnancy in patients with evidence of deep vein thrombosis and thrombophilia,[38] and there is an increased experience with the use of this therapy in women with MHVs. Earlier published data on the use of LMWH in women with MHV during pregnancy were described by Elkayam and colleagues[47] and were limited to small groups of patients or to isolated reports; several of these cases were complicated by valve thrombosis and even death. However, a careful review of the reported cases indicated that most, if not all, were associated with an inadequate dose, lack of monitoring, or subtherapeutic anti-Xa levels.[23,48–54]

A more recent review by Oran and colleagues[52] comprising 81 pregnancies in women with MHV in whom LMWH was used reported 10 thromboembolic events in women with mechanical mitral valves, of which 9 occurred in the 30 pregnancies with a fixed LMWH dose and only 1 in the 51 pregnancies with adjusted LMWH dose. Rowan and colleagues[50] reported on their experience in 14 pregnancies in women with a mechanical prosthetic valve who were treated with LMWH; valve thrombosis was described in 1 patient, who had a new generation mechanical mitral valve and had stopped warfarin 3 months before conception. She presented at 8 weeks' gestation, on no anticoagulation treatment, with transient ischemic attacks and suspected thrombus on transesophageal echocardiography (TEE). The patient was started on enoxaparin, with apparent resolution of the thrombus on TEE, but she re-presented at 20 weeks' gestation after a further transient ischemic attack caused by subtherapeutic level of anticoagulation (peak anti-Xa level was 0.62 U/mL).

Yinon and colleagues[55] recently reported a series of 23 pregnancies in 17 women with MHVs treated with adjusted LMWH. There was a single maternal thromboembolic event in a patient with a new-generation mechanical aortic prosthesis despite peak anti-Xa levels described in the guidelines as therapeutic (ranging from 1.0 and 1.4 U/mL). This patient was treated with warfarin until 5 weeks of gestation and was then switched to LMWH and aspirin. At 24 weeks of gestation she presented with a transient ischemic event (peak anti-Xa level was 0.99 U/mL). Echocardiography showed an increased mean gradient across her aortic valve of 38 mm Hg (compared with her baseline mean gradient of 15 mm Hg). TEE was performed, and no thrombus was seen, but the aortic valve leaflets were not optimally visualized. The LMWH dose was increased, but at 26 weeks of gestation, the patient was admitted with cardiac arrest and died. The autopsy showed aortic valve thrombosis. This case shows the limitations of reliance on peak anti-Xa levels and the need to ensure a therapeutic trough level as well. Furthermore, because TEE may not allow adequate visualization of the aortic leaflets, significant change in gradients across the valve should alert physicians to the possibility of valve thrombosis, even when a thrombus cannot be seen, and patients should be hospitalized for further diagnosis and management. Abildgaard and colleagues[56] recently reported on 12 pregnancies with MHVs treated with LMWH, in which thromboembolism occurred in 2 women with aortic MHV. Both events were attributed to subtherapeutic doses of LMWH during the initial 3 weeks of pregnancy. Quinn and colleagues[57] conducted a prospective audit of the use of adjusted-dose LMWH in 12 pregnancies with MHV. LMWH ± low-dose aspirin was started at therapeutic dose with monitoring of anti-Xa levels to achieve a target level of 1.0 to 1.2 U/mL. This strategy necessitated a mean increase in the dose of LMWH of 54.4% over initial dose. One nonfatal valve thrombosis occurred at 26 weeks' gestation associated with subtherapeutic anti-Xa levels. Three patients experienced major bleeding.

More recently, McLintock and colleagues[58] reported thromboembolic complications in 7 of 47 pregnancies, of which 5 were believed to be associated with the use of enoxaparin therapy. Similar to other reports by other investigators described earlier, poor compliance with therapy and subtherapeutic peak anti-Xa levels were an issue in all cases. No thromboembolic complications occurred in the 20 pregnancies when enoxaparin was commenced before 6 weeks' gestation, a group that was compliant with medication and monitoring of peak anti-Xa levels.

There is increasing experience with the use of LMWH for anticoagulation in pregnant women with MHV. Most if not all the cases reported to have developed thromboembolic complications were related to poor compliance with therapy, inadequate monitoring, and subtherapeutic levels of anticoagulation. The pharmacokinetics of LMWH have been shown to be altered during pregnancy with lower plasma concentrations, probably related to higher clearance and volume of distribution.[34] Therefore, administration of LMWH by weight alone is inadequate, and peak anti-Xa levels may not reflect adequacy of anticoagulation around the clock.[47] The potential importance of measurement of trough anti-Xa levels was suggested by Barbour and colleagues,[59] who evaluated 138 peak and 112 troughs anti-Xa levels in 13 pregnancies in 12 patients. With peak levels of 0.63, 0.70, and 0.69 U/m, respectively, at the first, second, and third trimesters, mean trough level were 0.21, 0.30, and 0.40 U/mL, with only 9% of the measurements greater than 0.5 U/mL. Even when peak levels were between 0.75 and 1.0 U/mL, only 15% of trough levels were greater than 0.5 U/mL.[59] Similarly, in a recent series of 15 pregnant women at different gestational ages, a subtherapeutic anti-Xa level was reported in 20% of the peak levels and 73% of the trough levels, despite therapeutic enoxaparin administration 1 mg/kg twice a day.[60]

In our unpublished study of 26 pregnant women who received anticoagulation with LMWH for various indications, including 9 patients with MHV subcutaneously every 12 hours, we analyzed both through and peak anti-Xa levels throughout pregnancy for a total of 177 determinations.[61] Adjusted-dose LMWH achieving a peak anti-Xa between 0.7 U/mL and 1.2 U/mL, as recommended by guidelines, were associated with subtherapeutic trough anti-Xa levels in about 50% of cases. On the other hand, therapeutic trough anti-Xa levels 0.6 U/mL to 0.8 U/mL were rarely associated with excessive peak anti-Xa levels. These data, in addition to the documented risk of valve thrombosis with subtherapeutic predose anti-Xa levels, suggest the importance of routine measurement and maintenance of trough levels at therapeutic range as recommended by Elkayam and Bitar (anti-Xa ≥0.6 in low-risk patients and ≥0.7 U/mL in high-risk patients) (see **Table 2**). Because of possible bleeding complications,[16] peak levels should also be monitored to prevent excessive anticoagulation (anti-Xa levels >1.5 U/mL), in which case, an 8-hourly rather than a 12-hourly dosage should be used. To ensure patient compliance and adequate prophylaxis, anti-Xa activity should be measured once weekly for the first 4 weeks and later at least once every 2 weeks. Catheter placement for epidural anesthesia is not advisable within 10 to 12 hours of the last dose, because of the longer half-life of LMWH.[47] For this reason, and to prevent spinal or epidural hematoma, LMWH should be withdrawn 18 to 24 hours before an elective delivery and substituted with intravenous UFH. Because of the potential added benefit, a small dose of aspirin (75–100 mg/d), which is safe during pregnancy,[39,47] might be added in high-risk patients to further reduce the incidence of thromboembolism.

OTHER CARDIAC DISORDERS REQUIRING ANTICOAGULATION IN PREGNANCY
Mitral Stenosis

Mitral stenosis (MS) is the most common valvular heart disease in pregnancy, with a significant impact on both maternal and fetal outcome, and it is a disease that carries a significant risk of thromboembolism.[39,62,63] Prophylactic anticoagulation is indicated in MS patients who have the highest risk for thromboembolic events (ie, patients with atrial fibrillation [AF] or a previous history of an embolic event).[39] According to the ACC/AHA guidelines, anticoagulation may be considered for asymptomatic patients with severe MS and left atrial dimension greater than or equal to 55 mm by echocardiography. The hypercoagulable state of pregnancy appears as another risk factor for thromboembolism in pregnant patients with MS, and the investigators suggest considering anticoagulation therapy in pregnant patients with MS, even in the absence of AF. These recommendations are supported by a recently published case series that reported left atrial thrombus formation and ensuing clinical events in 3 pregnant patients with MS in the absence of AF.[64] Strong consideration should therefore be given to prophylactic full-dose anticoagulation in patients with severe MS, especially those with an enlarged left atrium, throughout pregnancy, even in the absence of AF or a history of thromboembolism.

Peripartum Cardiomyopathy and Pre-existent Dilated Cardiomyopathy

Peripartum cardiomyopathy (PPCM) is a cardiomyopathy of unknown cause presenting with heart failure secondary to left ventricle (LV) systolic dysfunction toward the end of pregnancy or in the months after delivery.[65] This condition is associated with important and lasting complications, including thromboembolic events, which can lead to severe morbidity and mortality. LV thrombus has been found on initial echocardiography in 10% to 17% of patients,[65,66] and several reports have described severe thromboembolic events as a result of embolization to the coronary, pulmonary, peripheral, and cerebral arteries.[65–74] Goland and colleagues[68] recently described 4 patients with severe embolic complications, all of them with left ventricular thrombus: 3 presented as a cerebrovascular accident with residual brain damage (plus pulmonary embolism in one), and 2 with leg ischemia (requiring amputation in one). The increased incidence of thromboembolism in women with PPCM is related to the hypercoagulable state of pregnancy,[7,10] cardiac dilatation and dysfunction, endothelial injury, venous stasis, and prolonged bed rest. Embolic events usually occur during the period of LV dysfunction until LV function recovers and anticoagulation is therefore strongly advisable.[75] Anticoagulation seems particularly important during pregnancy and the first 6 to 8 weeks post partum because of the persistent hypercoagulable state.[6] As mentioned earlier, because of warfarin-related risk to the fetus, either UFH or LMWH is favored in pregnancy, because (unlike warfarin) they do not cross the placenta.[76] Neither warfarin nor heparin is secreted into breast milk, and both drugs are therefore compatible with breastfeeding.[76]

There is an increased risk of thromboembolism in all types of dilated cardiomyopathy. The risk of thromboembolism in nonpregnant patients may be particularly high in women with concomitant AF, a history of venous thromboembolism, and LV thrombus who require chronic anticoagulation. Because of the increased risk of thromboembolic events during pregnancy[77] all patients with dilated cardiomyopathies and left ventricular ejection fraction 40% or less should be anticoagulated even in the absence of the other risk factors for TE events mentioned earlier.[77–81] LMWH are the preferred drugs for this population, and the dose has to be adjusted to achieve therapeutic trough anti-Xa levels ($\geq$0.6 U/mL).

Pregnant Women with AF

Increased frequency of arrhythmia has been reported during pregnancy in healthy women or in women with structural heart disease, especially when cardiac output increases 30% to 50%.[82–84] However, the incidence of AF during pregnancy is low and is usually secondary to congenital or rheumatic valvular disease, hypertrophic cardiomyopathy, thyroid disease, or a pre-excitation syndrome.[85–87] However, it can represent a benign, episode of lone AF in a pregnant woman with a normal heart.[88] In pregnant women who develop AF, the role of anticoagulation to prevent systemic arterial embolism has not been systematically studied in pregnant patients with nonvalvular AF.

Anticoagulation therapy is not required in pregnant women with a short lone episode of AF. If spontaneous conversion to normal sinus rhythm does not occur, cardioversion should be considered within 48 hours of the onset of AF to avoid the need for anticoagulation. Procainamide or quinidine are recommended for chemical cardioversion, whereas other medications, including flecainide, have also been used successfully in pregnancy.[89] However, some antiarrhythmic drugs such as amiodarone are contraindicated, because of their teratogenic effect. Synchronized cardioversion is safe and can quickly restore hemodynamic stability and perfusion of vital organs of the mother and the fetus, and can be used in the emergency situation or when chemical cardioversion failed.[89] Beta-blockers, calcium channel blockers, and digoxin are recommended for rate control in pregnant women with AF rapid ventricular response. However, precardioversion and postcardioversion anticoagulation with LMWH is recommended. If the arrhythmia or symptom onset began more than 48 hours before presentation in a stable patient, then anticoagulation should be given for 3 to 4 weeks before and after cardioversion.[89] TEE may be performed to rule out thrombus in a pregnant woman in whom cardioversion is considered earlier than 3 to 4 weeks or in those at high risk for bleeding complications with anticoagulation.

Patients with chronic AF, who are considered to be at increased risk for embolic stroke, should be anticoagulated during pregnancy. Although the risk of embolic events in a pregnant patient with loan AF is not clear, we have been anticoagulating such women because of the hypercoagulable state of pregnancy.

REFERENCES

1. Bremme KA. Haemostatic changes in pregnancy. Best Pract Res Clin Haematol 2003;16:153–68.
2. Franchini M. Haemostasis and pregnancy. Thromb Haemost 2006;95:401–13.
3. Rosenkranz A, Hiden M, Leschnik B, et al. Calibrated automated thrombin generation in normal uncomplicated pregnancy. Thromb Haemost 2008;99:331–7.
4. Clark P, Walker I. The phenomenon known as acquired activated protein C resistance. Br J Haematol 2001;114:767–73.
5. Kjellberg U, Anderson NE, Rosen S, et al. APC resistance and other haemostatic variables during pregnancy and puerperium. Thromb Haemost 1999;81:527–31.
6. James AH. Pregnancy-associated thrombosis. Hematology Am Soc Hematol Edu Program 2009;277–85.
7. Heit JA, Kobbervig CE, James AH, et al. Trends in the incidence of venous thromboembolism during pregnancy or postpartum: a 30-year population-based study. Ann Intern Med 2005;143:697–706.
8. James AH, Bushnell CD, Jamison MG, et al. Incidence and risk factors for stroke in pregnancy and the puerperium. Obstet Gynecol 2005;106:509–16.
9. James AH, Jamison MG, Biswas MS, et al. Acute myocardial infarction in pregnancy: a United States population-based study. Circulation 2006;113:1564–71.
10. James AH, Jamison MG, Brancazio LR, et al. Venous thromboembolism during pregnancy and the postpartum period: incidence, risk factors, and mortality. Am J Obstet Gynecol 2006;194:1311–5.
11. Brenner B. Haemostatic changes in pregnancy. Thromb Res 2004;114:409–14.
12. McGehee W. Anticoagulation in pregnancy. In: Elkayam U, Gleicher N, editors. Cardiac problems in pregnancy. 3rd edition. New York: Wiley-Liss; 1998. p. 407–17.
13. Bom D, Martinez EE, Almeida PA, et al. Pregnancy in patients with prosthetic heart valves: the effects of anticoagulation on mother, fetus and neonate. Am Heart J 1992;124:413–7.
14. Sbarouni E, Oakley CM. Outcome of pregnancy in women with valve prostheses. Br Heart J 1994;71:196–201.
15. Chan WS, Anand S, Ginsberg JS. Anticoagulation of pregnant women with mechanical heart valves: a systematic review of the literature. Arch Intern Med 2000;160:191–6.
16. Elkayam U, Bitar F. Valvular heart disease and pregnancy: prosthetic valves part II. J Am Coll Cardiol 2005;46:403–10.
17. Blickstein D, Blickstein I. The risk of fetal loss associated with warfarin anticoagulation. Int J Gynaecol Obstet 2002;78:221–5.
18. Srivastava AK, Gupta AK, Singh AV, et al. Effect of oral anticoagulant during pregnancy with prosthetic heart valve. Asian Cardiovasc Thorac Ann 2002;10:306–9.
19. Meschengieser SS, Fondevila CG, Santarelli MT, et al. Anticoagulation in pregnant women with mechanical heart valve prostheses. Heart 1999;82:23–6.
20. Chen WW, Chan CS, Lee PK, et al. Pregnancy in patients with prosthetic heart valves: an experience with 45 pregnancies. Q J Med 1982;51:358–65.
21. Cotrufo M, De Feo M, De Santo LS, et al. Risk of warfarin during pregnancy with mechanical valve prostheses. Obstet Gynecol 2002;99:35–40.
22. Wesseling J, Van Driel D, Heymans HS, et al. Coumarins during pregnancy: long-term effects on growth and development of school-age children. Thromb Haemost 2001;85:609–13.
23. Bates SM, Greer IA, Pabinger I, et al. Venous thromboembolism, thrombophilia, antithrombotic therapy and pregnancy: American College of Chest Physicians Evidence-Based Clinical Practice Guidelines (8th edition). Chest 2008;133(Suppl 6):844S–86S.
24. Vitale N, De Eeo M, De Santo LS, et al. Dose-dependent fetal complications of warfarin in pregnant women with mechanical heart valves. J Am Coll Cardiol 1999;33:1637–41.
25. Sadler L, MeCowan L, White H, et al. Pregnancy outcomes and cardiac complications in women with mechanical, bioprosthetic and homograft valves. Br J Obstet Gynecol 2000;107:245–53.
26. Flessa HC, Kapstrom AB, Glueck HI, et al. Placental transport of heparin. Am J Obstet Gynecol 1965;93:570–3.
27. Schneider D, Heilmann L, Harenberg J. Placental transfer of low-molecular weight heparin. Geburtshilfe Frauenheilkd 1995;55:93–8.
28. Barbour LA, Pickard J. Controversies in thromboembolic disease during pregnancy: a critical review. Obstet Gynecol 1995;86:621–33.
29. Dahlman TC. Osteoporotic fractures and the recurrence of thromboembolism during pregnancy and the puerperium in 184 women undergoing thromboprophylaxis with heparin. Am J Obstet Gynecol 1999;168:1265–70.
30. Gordon M, Gabbe S, Niebyl J, et al, editors. Maternal physiology in pregnancy. Normal and problem pregnancies. 4th edition. New York: Churchill Livingstone; 2002. p. 63–92.
31. Brancazio LR, Roperti KA, Stierer R, et al. Pharmacokinetics and pharmacodynamics of subcutaneous heparin during the early third trimester of pregnancy. Am J Obstet Gynecol 1995;173:1240–5.

32. Mazzolai L, Hohlfeld P, Spertini F, et al. Fondaparinux is a safe alternative in case of heparin intolerance during pregnancy. Blood 2006;108:1569–70.

33. Evans W, Laifer SA, McNanley TJ, et al. Management of thromboembolic disease associated with pregnancy. J Matern Fetal Med 1997;6:21–7.

34. Casele HL, Laifer SA, Woelkers DA, et al. Changes in the pharmacokinetics of the low-molecular-weight heparin enoxaparin sodium during pregnancy. Am J Obstet Gynecol 1999;181:1113–7.

35. Sanson BJ, Lensing AW, Prins MH, et al. Safety of low-molecular-weight heparin in pregnancy: a systematic review. Thromb Haemost 1999;81:668–72.

36. Greer IA, Nelson-Piercy C. Low-molecular-weight heparins for thromboprophylaxis and treatment of venous thromboembolism in pregnancy: a systematic review of safety and efficacy. Blood 2005;106:401–7.

37. Casele H, Haney EI, James A, et al. Bone density changes in women who receive thromboprophylaxis in pregnancy. Am J Obstet Gynecol 2006;195:1109–13.

38. James AH. Venous thromboembolism in pregnancy. Arterioscler Thromb Vasc Biol 2009;29(3):326–31.

39. Bonow RO, Carabello BA, Chatterjee K, et al, American College of Cardiology/American Heart Association Task Force on Practice Guidelines. 2008 focused update incorporated into the ACC/AHA 2006 guidelines for the management of patients with valvular heart disease: a report of the American College of Cardiology/American Heart Association Task Force on Practice Guidelines (Writing Committee to revise the 1998 guidelines for the management of patients with valvular heart disease). Endorsed by the Society of Cardiovascular Anesthesiologists, Society for Cardiovascular Angiography and Interventions, and Society of Thoracic Surgeons. J Am Coll Cardiol 2008;52(13):e1–142.

40. Bax J, Auricchio A, Baumgartner H, et al. ESC Guidelines on the management of cardiovascular diseases during pregnancy: the Task Force on the Management of Cardiovascular Diseases during Pregnancy of the European Society of Cardiology (ESC). Eur Heart J 2011. [Epub ahead of print].

41. Geelani MA, Singh S, Verma A, et al. Anticoagulation in patients with mechanical valves during pregnancy. Asian Cardiovasc Thorac Ann 2005;13(1):30–3.

42. Al-Lawati AA, Venkitraman M, Al-Delaime T, et al. Pregnancy and mechanical heart valves replacement: dilemma of anticoagulation. Eur J Cardiothorac Surg 2002;22(2):223–7.

43. Iturbe-Alessio I, Fonseca MC, Mutchinik O, et al. Risks of anticoagulant therapy in pregnant women with artificial heart valves. N Engl J Med 1986;315(22):1390–3.

44. Khan AO. Optic nerve dysfunction in a child following low-dose maternal warfarin exposure. Ophthalmic Genet 2007;28(3):183–4.

45. Finkelstein Y, Chitayat D, Schechter T, et al. Motherisk rounds. Warfarin embryopathy following low-dose maternal exposure. J Obstet Gynaecol Can 2005;27(7):702–6.

46. Sillesen M, Hjortdal V, Vejlstrup N, et al. Pregnancy with prosthetic heart valves: 30 years' nationwide experience in Denmark. Eur J Cardiothorac Surg 2011;40(2):448–54.

47. Elkayam U, Singh H, Irani A, et al. Anticoagulation in pregnant women with prosthetic heart valve. J Cardiovasc Pharmacol Ther 2004;9:107–15.

48. Lev-Ran O, Kramer A, Gurevitch J, et al. Low-molecular-weight heparin for prosthetic heart valves: treatment failure. Ann Thorac Surg 2000;69:264–5.

49. Berndt N, Khan I, Gallo R. A complication in anticoagulation using low-molecular weight heparin in a patient with mechanical valve prosthesis: a case report. J Heart Valve Dis 2000;9:844–6.

50. Rowan JA, McCowan LM, Raudkivi PJ, et al. Enoxaparin treatment in women with mechanical heart valves during pregnancy. Am J Obstet Gynecol 2001;185:633–7.

51. Arnaout MS, Kazma H, Khalil A, et al. Is there a safe anticoagulation protocol for pregnant women with prosthetic valves. Clin Exp Obstet Gynecol 1998;25:101–4.

52. Oran B, Lee-Parritz A, Ansell J. Low molecular weight heparin for the prophylaxis of thromboembolism in women with prosthetic mechanical heart valves during pregnancy. Thromb Haemost 2004;92:747–51.

53. Anticoagulation and enoxaparin use in patients with prosthetic heart valves and/or pregnancy. In: Clinical cardiology consensus reports, vol. 3. Atlanta (GA): American Health Consultants; 2002. p. 1–20.

54. Lovenox Injection [packet insert]. Bridgewater (NJ): Aventis Pharmaceuticals; 2004.

55. Yinon Y, Siu SC, Warshafsky C, et al. Use of low molecular weight heparin in pregnant women with mechanical heart valves. Am J Cardiol 2009;104(9):1259–63.

56. Abildgaard U, Sandset PM, Hammerstrom J, et al. Management of pregnant women with mechanical heart valve prosthesis: thromboprophylaxis with low molecular weight heparin. Thromb Res 2009;124:262–7.

57. Quinn J, Von Klemperer K, Brooks R, et al. Use of high intensity adjusted dose low molecular weight heparin in women with mechanical heart valves during pregnancy: a single-center experience. Haematologica 2009;94(11):1608–12.

58. McLintock C, McCowan LM, North RA. Maternal complications and pregnancy outcome in women with mechanical prosthetic heart valves treated with enoxaparin. BJOG 2009;116(12):1585–92.

59. Barbour LA, Oja JL, Schultz LK. A prospective trial that demonstrates that dalteparin requirements

increase in pregnancy to maintain therapeutic levels of anticoagulation. Am J Obstet Gynecol 2004;191: 1024–9.

60. Friedrich E, Hameed AB. Fluctuations in anti-factor Xa levels with therapeutic enoxaparin anticoagulation in pregnancy. J Perinatol 2010;30(4):253–7.

61. Fan J, Goland S, Khatri N, et al. Monitoring of anti Xa in pregnant patients with mechanical prosthetic valves receiving low molecular weight heparin: peak or trough levels? [abstract]. Circulation 2011;122:A18219.

62. Reimold SC, Rutherford JD. Valvular heart disease in pregnancy: clinical practice. N Engl J Med 2003; 349:52–9.

63. Hameed A, Karaalp IS, Tummala PP, et al. The effect of valvular heart disease on maternal and fetal outcome of pregnancy. J Am Coll Cardiol 2001;37:893–9.

64. Hameed A, Akhter MW, Bitar F, et al. Left atrial thrombosis in pregnant women with mitral stenosis and sinus rhythm. Am J Obstet Gynecol 2005;193: 501–4.

65. Sliwa K, Hilfiker-Kleiner D, Petrie MC, et al. Current state of knowledge on aetiology, diagnosis, management, and therapy of peripartum cardiomyopathy: a position statement from the Heart Failure Association of the European Society of Cardiology Working Group on peripartum cardiomyopathy. Eur J Heart Fail 2010;12:767–78.

66. Amos A, Jaber WA, Russell SD. Improved outcomes in peripartum cardiomyopathy with contemporary. Am Heart J 2006;152:509–13.

67. Napporn AG, Kane A, Damorou JM, et al. Intraventricular thrombosis complicating peripartum idiopathic-myocardiopathy. Ann Cardiol Angeiol 2000; 49:309–14.

68. Goland S, Modi K, Bitar F, et al. Clinical profile and predictors of complications in peripartum cardiomyopathy. J Card Fail 2009;15:645–65.

69. Agunanne E. Peripartum cardiomyopathy presenting with a pulmonary embolism: an unusual case. South Med J 2008;101:646–7.

70. Box LC, Hanak V, Arciniegas JG. Dual coronary emboli in peripartum cardiomyopathy. Tex Heart Inst J 2004;31:442–4.

71. Ibebuogu UN, Thornton JW, Reed GL. An unusual case of peripartum cardiomyopathy manifesting with multiple thrombo-embolic phenomena. Thromb J 2007;5:18.

72. Jha P, Jha S, Millane TA. Peripartum cardiomyopathy complicated by pulmonary embolism and pulmonary hypertension. Eur J Obstet Gynecol Reprod Biol 2005;123:121–3.

73. Quinn B, Doyle B, McInerney J. Postnatal pre-cordial pain, Pulmonary embolism or peripartum cardiomyopathy. Emerg Med J 2004;21:746–7.

74. Shimamoto T, Marui A, Oda M, et al. A case of peripartum cardiomyopathy with recurrent left ventricular apical thrombus. Circ J 2008;72:853–4.

75. Elkayam U. Clinical characteristics of peripartum cardiomyopathy in the United States: diagnosis, prognosis, and management. J Am Coll Cardiol 2011;58(7):659–70.

76. Briggs GG, Freeman RK, Yatte SJ. Drugs in pregnancy and lactation. 8th edition. Philadelphia: Wolters Kluwer; 2008.

77. Chan F, Ngan Kee WD. Idiopathic dilated cardiomyopathy presenting in pregnancy. Can J Anaesth 1999;46(12):1146–9.

78. Stergiopoulos K, Shiang E, Bench T. Pregnancy in patients with pre-existing cardiomyopathies. J Am Coll Cardiol 2011;58(4):337–50.

79. Siu SC, Sermer M, Colman JM, et al. Prospective multicenter study of pregnancy outcomes in women with heart disease. Circulation 2001;104:515–52.

80. Siu SC, Sermer M, Harrison DA, et al. Risk and predictors for pregnancy-related complications in women with heart disease. Circulation 1997;96: 2789–94.

81. Grewal J, Siu SC, Ross H, et al. Pregnancy outcomes in women with dilated cardiomyopathy. J Am Coll Cardiol 2009;55:45–52.

82. Shotan A, Ostrzega E, Mehra A, et al. Incidence of arrhythmias in normal pregnancy and relation to palpitations, dizziness, and syncope. Am J Cardiol 1997;79:1061–4.

83. Yarnoz MJ, Curtis AB. More reasons why men and women are not the same (gender differences in electrophysiology and arrythmias). Am J Cardiol 2008;101:1291–6.

84. Gowda RM, Punukollu G, Khan IA, et al. Lone atrial fibrillation during pregnancy. Int J Cardiol 2003;88: 123–4.

85. Bryg RJ, Gordon PR, Kudesia VS, et al. Effect of pregnancy on pressure gradient in mitral stenosis. Am J Cardiol 1989;63:384–6.

86. Whittemore R, Hobbins JC, Engle MA. Pregnancy and its outcome in women with and without surgical treatment of congenital heart disease. Am J Cardiol 1982;50:641–51.

87. Forfar JC, Miller HC, Toft AD. Occult thyrotoxicosis: a correctable cause of "idiopathic" atrial fibrillation. Am J Cardiol 1979;44:9–12.

88. DiCarlo-Meacham A, Dahlke J. Atrial fibrillation in pregnancy. Obstet Gynecol 2011;117(2 Pt 2): 489–92.

89. Fuster V, Rydén LE, Cannom DS, et al. ACC/AHA/ ESC 2006 Guide for the management of patients with atrial fibrillation: a report of the American College of Cardiology/American Heart Association task force on practice guidelines and European Society of Cardiology committee for practice guidelines: developed in collaboration with the European Heart Rhythm Association and the Heart Rhythm Society. Circulation 2006; 114:257–354.

Hypertension in Pregnancy

Amanda R. Vest, MBBS, MRCP[a], Leslie S. Cho, MD[b],*

KEYWORDS

- Pregnancy • Hypertension • Gestational • Preeclampsia • Eclampsia • Placenta • Angiogenic
- Antiangiogenic

KEY POINTS

- Preeclampsia can result in fetal growth restriction and preterm delivery.
- Hypertensive disease during pregnancy increases the risk of hypertension and cardiovascular diseases later in the woman's life.
- Little evidence exists as to optimal treatment thresholds, blood pressure targets, and antihypertensive agents in pregnancy; blood pressures of 150 to 160 mm Hg systolic and/or 100 to 110 mm Hg diastolic and greater should be treated to minimize maternal end-organ damage.
- Oral methyldopa, labetalol, hydralazine, and nifedipine have relative merits and risks.
- Intravenous labetalol, hydralazine, or sodium nitroprusside may be used in hypertensive emergencies, but with minimal data regarding fetal outcomes.
- Angiotensin-converting enzyme inhibitors and angiotensin receptor antagonists are contraindicated in pregnancy.
- Women with preeclampsia should be closely monitored and receive intravenous magnesium sulfate.
- The definitive treatment of preeclampsia or eclampsia is delivery of the fetus.

INTRODUCTION

Hypertensive disorders of pregnancy rank as the second most common cause of direct maternal death in the developed world.[1] Hypertension is also the most common medical complication encountered during pregnancy. The incidence in the United States is unknown, but hypertensive disorders are estimated to complicate 5% to 10% of pregnancies, depending on the population studied,[2,3] with the highest rates in black women, women more than 45 years old, and individuals with diabetes. Given the increasing prevalence of baseline hypertension, obesity, and diabetes in women of childbearing age in the United States, as well as the trend toward more advanced maternal age at childbirth, it is possible that the rates of hypertension in pregnancy established in the literature may be an underestimate of contemporary incidence.

There is significant maternal and neonatal morbidity associated with hypertension in pregnancy, with increased rates of intracerebral hemorrhage, placental abruption, intrauterine growth retardation, prematurity, and intrauterine death for expectant mothers with high blood pressure. The National High Blood Pressure Education Program (NHBPEP) Working Group on High Blood Pressure in Pregnancy published guidelines in 2000 that divided hypertensive disorders during pregnancy into 4 categories.[2]

- Chronic (or preexisting) hypertension
- Gestational hypertension (transient hypertension of pregnancy or chronic hypertension identified in the second half of pregnancy)
- Preeclampsia/eclampsia

Disclosures: None.
[a] Heart and Vascular Institute, Cleveland Clinic, 9500 Euclid Avenue, Cleveland, OH 44195, USA; [b] Preventive Cardiology and Rehabilitation, Robert and Suzanne Tomsich Department of Cardiovascular Medicine, Cleveland Clinic, 9500 Euclid Avenue, Cleveland, OH 44195, USA
* Corresponding author.
E-mail address: chol@ccf.org

Cardiol Clin 30 (2012) 407–423
doi:10.1016/j.ccl.2012.04.005
0733-8651/12/$ – see front matter © 2012 Elsevier Inc. All rights reserved.

cardiology.theclinics.com

- Preeclampsia superimposed on chronic hypertension.

The definitions for each of the 4 groups are presented in **Table 1**. The 2008 Canadian guidelines favor a simpler classification system with 2 categories, preexisting or gestational, plus the option to add "with preeclampsia" to either category. The 2011 European Society of Cardiology guidelines stipulate that gestational hypertension can be with or without significant proteinuria; when accompanied by proteinuria, it is then termed preeclampsia. The divergent and arbitrary classification systems highlight the incomplete understanding of the differing entities within this disease spectrum. However, each diagnostic system is intended to separate hypertensive cases that are similar to those seen outside pregnancy from the potentially life-threatening pregnancy-specific disease of preeclampsia. For the purposes of this article, the 2000 NHBPEP categories are used.

Diagnosis and Evaluation

The threshold for hypertension in pregnancy is based on absolute blood pressure measurements of greater than or equal to 140 mm Hg systolic and/or greater than or equal to 90 mm Hg diastolic. Most authorities distinguish mildly increased blood pressures from severe hypertension, which is generally agreed to be greater than or equal to 160 mm Hg systolic and/or greater than or equal to 110 mm Hg diastolic.[4–6] However, the NHBPEP refrained from using the terms mild or severe to emphasize that the degree of hypertension does not correlate with the likelihood of devastating outcomes such as eclamptic seizures. Increased readings should be confirmed on 2 occasions, with the patient seated or in the left lateral decubitus position and having rested for 10 minutes. The Korotkoff I sound, which is the onset of sounds, denotes the systolic pressure. The Korotkoff V sound, which is the silence encountered as the cuff pressure decreases to less than the diastolic blood pressure, should be used as the determinant of diastolic pressure in pregnant women. Ambulatory blood pressure monitoring has a role in pregnancy and has shown stronger outcome predictions than isolated clinic measurements.[7] Undiagnosed hypertension may not be evident in early pregnancy because of the physiologic

Table 1
Classification of hypertensive disorders in pregnancy

		Estimated Frequency
Chronic hypertension	Blood pressure ≥140/90 mm Hg present before pregnancy, before the 20th week of gestation, or persisting beyond the 42nd postpartum day	1%–5% of pregnancies
Gestational hypertension	Hypertension that (1) develops beyond 20 wk of gestation; (2) can be with or without proteinuria, but is not associated with other features of preeclampsia; and (3) usually resolves within 42 d postpartum	6%–7% of pregnancies
Preeclampsia/eclampsia	Hypertension presenting beyond 20 wk of gestation with >300 mg protein in a 24-h urine collection or >30 mg/mmol in a spot urine sample. Eclampsia is the occurrence of seizures in a pregnant woman with preeclampsia	5%–7% of pregnancies
Preeclampsia superimposed on chronic hypertension	The onset of features diagnostic of preeclampsia in a woman with chronic hypertension beyond 20 wk of gestation	20%–25% of chronic hypertension pregnancies

Data from Report of the National High Blood Pressure Education Program Working Group on High Blood Pressure in Pregnancy. Am J Obstet Gynecol 2000;183(1):S1–22; and Regitz-Zagrosek V, Blomstrom Lundqvist C, Borghi C, et al. ESC guidelines on the management of cardiovascular disease during pregnancy: the Task Force on the Management of Cardiovascular Diseases during Pregnancy of the European Society of Cardiology (ESC). Eur Heart J 2011;32(24):3147–97.

decrease in blood pressure that begins in the first trimester, thus causing confusion with gestational hypertension.

Evaluation of the Pregnant Patient with Hypertension

Evaluation of the pregnant patient with hypertension should also encompass a thorough history for the symptoms associated with preeclampsia (described later), a review of the risk factors listed in **Table 2**, and evaluation for rare secondary causes of hypertension such as Cushing syndrome or aortic coarctation. Although a third heart sound is a normal finding in pregnancy, a fourth heart sound is not and suggests either long-standing hypertension with left ventricular hypertrophy, or more acute diastolic dysfunction during a rapid increase in afterload as seen with the vasospasm of preeclampsia. Physical examination in suspected preeclampsia should include palpation of the right upper quadrant, fundoscopy for retinal vasospasm or edema, assessment of mental status, examination for exaggerated reflexes or clonus, cardiorespiratory examination for a volume-overloaded state, quantification of edema (especially in nondependent regions), and inspection for petechiae or ecchymoses.

Investigations for risk-stratification of the pregnant woman with hypertension include urinalysis, 24-hour urine collection, complete blood count, serum creatinine, serum uric acid, and liver enzymes. Close obstetric monitoring of the fetus is essential in pregnancies with a suspected or confirmed diagnosis of preeclampsia. Techniques may include biophysical profiles and fetal nonstress tests. Fetal heart rate monitoring can serve as a surrogate for uteroplacental perfusion, and fetal ultrasounds are used to confirm gestation and document fetal weight, growth velocity, and amniotic fluid volume. Doppler ultrasound of the uterine arteries may be performed beyond 16 weeks' gestation. Umbilical artery Doppler velocimetry may also be useful to determine a placental origin of intrauterine fetal growth restriction.[8]

Diagnosis of Preeclampsia

As displayed in **Table 1**, the diagnosis of preeclampsia is made when there is hypertension beyond 20 weeks' gestation that is accompanied by greater than 300 mg protein in a 24-hour urine collection or greater than 30 mg/mmol in a spot urine sample. Some guidelines permit 1+ or more protein by urinary dipstick as a diagnostic criterion, although a dipstick result requires confirmation and quantification by either a random or 24-hour urine protein/creatinine ratio. Note that false-negatives can also occur with urine dipsticks. The 24-hour collection is the most accurate method.[9] Preeclampsia can

---

Table 2
Maternal, medical, fetal, and paternal risk factors for preeclampsia

Maternal	Maternal age >40 y Black ethnicity, compared with other groups Interpregnancy interval less than 2 y or longer than 10 y Mother born small for gestational age Nulliparity
Medical	Preeclampsia or gestational hypertension in a prior pregnancy Chronic hypertension Obesity and/or insulin resistance[97,98] Prepregnancy diabetes (especially with microvascular complications) Chronic kidney disease Thrombophilia Systemic lupus erythematosus History of migraine[99] Use of SSRIs beyond the first trimester[100] Maternal infections (eg, periodontal)[101]
Fetal	Multiparity Gestational trophoblastic disease Hydrops fetalis Triploidy
Paternal	First pregnancy with partner Pregnancies following donor insemination or limited paternal sperm exposure Partner who fathered a preeclamptic pregnancy in another woman[102]

Abbreviation: SSRI, selective serotonin reuptake inhibitor.

occur in the absence of proteinuria (14% were without proteinuria in one series[10]), and should be suspected when hypertension is associated with headache, blurred vision, right upper quadrant or epigastric pain, hyperreflexia or clonus, thrombocytopenia, or transaminitis. Edema is no longer a diagnostic criterion because of its poor specificity within the pregnant population.

Particular vigilance is necessary to promptly identify superimposed preeclampsia in the patient with chronic hypertension. Diagnostic triggers include the new onset of proteinuria, the presence of hypertension and proteinuria before 20 weeks' gestation, a sudden increase in the degree of proteinuria, a loss of established blood pressure control, or a new thrombocytopenia or transaminitis. HELLP (hemolysis, elevated liver enzymes, and low platelets) syndrome is a laboratory diagnosis and represents a sector of the preeclampsia spectrum with poorer outcomes. Severe preeclampsia is a term used by some commentators to imply heavy proteinuria (≥5 g/d) or multiorgan involvement such as cerebral edema (a variation on the posterior reversible encephalopathy syndrome [PRES]), oliguria, pulmonary edema, or features of HELLP.[11]

Eclampsia, the life-threatening development of grand mal seizures in a woman with preeclampsia, is the most severe manifestation of the spectrum and is rare, with an estimated incidence of 4 to 5 cases per 10,000 live births.[12] Eclampsia may be preceded by a history of preeclampsia or may arise unexpectedly in a woman with minimally increased blood pressure and no proteinuria. There is significant risk of cardiorespiratory arrest during or after the seizure. Thirty-five percent of eclamptic seizures occur in the antepartum period, 9% are intrapartum, and 28% occur in the postpartum period. Late postpartum seizures, arising more than 48 hours after delivery, are increasingly recognized.[13]

Screening for Gestational Hypertension and Preeclampsia

Screening for gestational hypertension and preeclampsia is an area of active research. A group in the UK recently established a first-trimester screening protocol that moves beyond the traditional approach of reliance on the maternal history only.[14] Their prediction tool included mean arterial pressure, uterine artery pulsatility index, pregnancy-associated plasma protein-A (PAPP-A), and placental growth factor (PlGF). Of the 7797 singleton pregnancies prospectively studied, 2% developed preeclampsia and 1.7% developed gestational hypertension. Women who were subsequently affected by a hypertensive disorder in pregnancy had a higher mean arterial pressure and

uterine artery pulsatility index at 11 to 13 weeks, and decreased serum PAPP-A and PlGF concentrations. The algorithm combined baseline maternal data including maternal ethnicity, body mass index, and personal or family history of preeclampsia, and was able to identify approximately 90% of cases of early preeclampsia with 5% false-positives. This finding contrasts with an estimated 30% case detection for preeclampsia requiring delivery before 34 weeks that are identifiable by maternal history alone, with a false-positive rate of 5%.[15] However, PAPP-A and PlGF did not perform as well in predicting late preeclampsia or gestational hypertension. It remains to be seen whether uterine artery pulsatility index and biomarkers have a place in routine antenatal care and become incorporated into existing preeclampsia screening guidelines.[16,17]

An associated area of research is the identification and clinical implementation of biomarkers with a role in differentiation of gestational hypertension from the more concerning diagnosis of preeclampsia. Several recent publications have suggested that 2 antiangiogenic peptides of placental origin, soluble filmlike tyrosine kinase 1 (sFlt-1) and soluble endoglin (sEng), show increased serum levels in preeclampsia.[18–20] Serum sFlt-1 levels also seem to be high in women with preeclampsia superimposed on systemic lupus erythematosis[21] or glomerulonephritis,[22] and are higher during nulliparous than multiparous pregnancies.[23] Lupus, chronic kidney disease, and nulliparity are all preeclampsia risk factors. sEng levels decrease between the first and second trimesters of normal pregnancy, but there is blunting of this profile in individuals who subsequently develop preeclampsia.[24] Consistent with studies of sFlt-1, serum sEng is increased in preeclampsia, correlates with disease severity, and decreases postpartum.[25]

Placental protein 13 (PP-13) is another biomarker candidate. Maternal serum PP-13 levels normally increase during pregnancy, but lower levels at 9 to 12 weeks have been shown in women who progressed to preeclampsia, compared with controls.[26] Several investigators have found it useful to combine maternal serum PP-13 with uterine artery Doppler for early preeclampsia prediction, citing a 90% detecting rate with 6% false-positivity.[27] However, 1 group concluded that the use of first-trimester PP-13, PAPP-A, and uterine artery pulsatility index in combination did not offer enhanced predictive value compared with measurement of these parameters individually.[28] PP-13 has recently been credited with a pathophysiologic role in trophoblastic invasion and the development of preeclampsia (discussed further later). Additional proposed preeclampsia biomarkers being investigated include adiponectin, urine orosomucoid, inhibin A, and activin A.[29,30]

CAUSES AND CONTRIBUTORY FACTORS

Chronic hypertension occurs in approximately 20% of women of childbearing age, with the prevalence dependent on age, ethnicity, and comorbidities such as diabetes and obesity. The pathophysiology of gestational hypertension is unknown, but is probably the same as essential hypertension in the nonpregnant individual, because gestational hypertension increases future postpregnancy hypertension risk. Gestational hypertension and preeclampsia are separate disease processes with different mechanisms. Evidence supporting this theory includes that nulliparity is a strong preeclampsia risk factor, but not for gestational hypertension; there are specific histologic changes in the placenta and kidneys associated with preeclampsia; there are antiangiogenic peptides of placental origin that are increased in preeclampsia but not in gestational hypertension; and that the total circulating volume is lower in women with preeclampsia compared with gestational hypertension.[31] Furthermore, some authorities suggest that the pathophysiology of early preeclampsia (developing before 34 weeks) may differ from the preeclampsia seen nearer term, during labor, or postpartum.[32]

Preeclampsia occurs in 2% to 5% of all pregnancies, 10% of first pregnancies, and in 20% to 25% of women with chronic hypertension.[33] **Table 2** summarizes the maternal, medical, and fetal factors that are currently considered to be preeclampsia risk factors. Extremes of maternal age (age <18 years or more than 35 years) were previously considered risk factors, but a recent large-scale analysis concluded that young maternal age was not an independent predictor of preeclampsia.[34] Of additional relevance to the cardiologist is the increased preeclampsia risk with aortic coarctation, pulmonary stenosis, pulmonary atresia with ventricular septal defect, and transposition of the great vessels.[2]

The pathophysiologic mechanisms of preeclampsia remain elusive, but it is widely accepted that the placenta is the inciting organ, leading to a syndrome of endothelial dysfunction and vasospasm. It has been observed that the extravillous trophoblastic cells of the placenta fail to invade the myometrium normally in preeclampsia, causing placental hypoperfusion. Placental development is closely regulated to balance sufficient nutrient delivery permitting normal fetal development against the maternal requirement for the fetus not to become so big that it cannot be supported by the maternal cardiac output or safely delivered through the birth canal. During early pregnancy, fetal chorionic villi that contact the uterine wall generate columns of cytotrophoblasts. An external layer of syncytiotrophoblasts actively penetrate into the uterine wall, disrupting the endothelium and tunica media of the spiral arteries, which are small branches of the uterine arteries. The spiral arteries are remodeled into the high-flow, low-resistance vessels necessary for nutrient delivery, with cytotrophoblasts identifiable in the endothelium of these arteries. Cytotrophoblastic invasion follows 2 stages: initial invasion of the decidual segments of the spiral arteries at 10 to 12 weeks' gestation, followed by deeper invasion of the myometrium at 15 to 16 weeks.[35] It is the invasion of the myometrial arteries that is aberrant in preeclampsia, with the spiral arteries remaining narrowed and resistive. Consequently, the uterine vasculature is unable to meet perfusion needs as pregnancy progresses, which may prompt placental release of antiangiogenic factors that cause the endothelial dysfunction characteristic of the diffuse endorgan disease manifestations.[30]

Investigators have recently evaluated the role of placental protein 13 (PP-13, also known as galectin 13) in the trophoblastic invasion sequence. Immunohistochemical analysis localized PP-13 to the syncytiotrophoblasts lining the chorionic villi and in the zones of necrosis around decidual veins. **Table 3** this group hypothesized that PP-13 is secreted into the intervillus space, drains through the decidua basalis veins, and facilitates conversion of the maternal spiral arterioles.[36] Women who develop severe preeclampsia are

---

Table 3
Angiogenic and antiangiogenic placental factors

Angiogenic: Underexpressed in Preeclampsia	Antiangiogenic: Oversecreted in Preeclampsia
VEGF	sFlt-1 (soluble receptor for VEGF and PlGF)
Placental growth factor	sEng (coreceptor for transforming growth factor β1)
PP-13	—
PAPP-A	

Abbreviations: PAPP-A, pregnancy-associated plasma protein-A; VEGF, vascular endothelial growth factor.

more likely to have low levels of serum PP-13 between gestational weeks 6 and 13,[37] suggesting a possible mechanistic role. Other placental factors being investigated as biomarkers may also have causal roles. Simultaneous inoculation of adenoviruses encoding both sFlt-1 and sEng into pregnant rats produces severe hypertension, heavy proteinuria, increased liver enzymes, and circulating schistocytes, mirroring the human manifestations of severe preeclampsia.[38]

The reason for placental hypersecretion of these proteins remains unknown. Parallel lines of investigation in preeclampsia research include immunologic mechanisms, oxidative stress, and inflammation.[39] The questions surrounding the immunologic privilege of the fetus and placenta that enables their nonmaternal cells to evade host immune destruction have been entertained for decades.[40] It has long been recognized that a 4-fold to 5-fold excess of preeclampsia occurs in first pregnancies, and that parous women with a new partner in a subsequent pregnancy seem to lose the protective effect of a prior birth.[41,42] A more recent study reported that the protective effect of a prior abortion operated only among women who conceived again with the same partner.[43] A longer period of unprotected intercourse with the father of the subsequent fetus was also protective for preeclampsia in several epidemiologic studies, suggesting that maternal sensitization to paternal antigens may attenuate an immune process instrumental in the disease.[44,45] An allied observation is that artificial donor insemination results in a substantial increase in preeclamptic pregnancies in a 584-patient cohort.[46,47] These findings all point toward a contribution of immunologic intolerance between maternal and fetal tissues in the pathogenesis of preeclampsia. Links are increasingly being established between the immune mechanisms and endothelial dysfunction, with natural killer cells playing a bridging role. Natural killer cells aggregate around the invading cytotrophoblasts until approximately 20 weeks, when placentation is complete, and secrete cytokines such as vascular endothelial growth factor (VEGF) and PlGF (both potently antagonized by sFlt) as well as proinflammatory interferon-γ.[48] Despite these causal pathways, preeclampsia does not ensue in all women with high sFlt-1 and low PlGF levels, and does develop in some women with low sFlt-1 and high PlGF levels.[18] These recent pathophysiologic insights are reviewed in greater depth elsewhere.[32,49]

COMPLICATIONS AND PROGNOSIS

Chronic and gestational hypertension is usually associated with good maternal and fetal outcomes, although severe hypertension confers risks of maternal intracerebral hemorrhage and poorer fetal outcomes. As many as a quarter of women with chronic hypertension progress to preeclampsia during pregnancy, with the risk of superimposed preeclampsia increasing with greater duration of hypertension.[50] Even without preeclampsia development, the likelihood of preterm birth is increased 5-fold, and there is a 50% excess risk of a small-for-gestational-age neonate for women with chronic hypertension.[51] In addition, just as gestational diabetes may predict future diabetes, gestational hypertension may be a precursor to hypertension and an increased cardiovascular risk profile in later life.[52] The presence of hypertension before pregnancy or in the first 20 weeks of gestation is also associated with an increased risk in development of gestational diabetes mellitus during the pregnancy. A case-control study of singleton pregnancies showed a small increased risk of gestational diabetes with blood pressures in the 120 to 139/80 to 89 mm Hg range early in pregnancy, and an odds ratio of 2.04 (95% confidence interval, 1.14–3.65) for gestational diabetes with blood pressures in the greater than or equal to 140 and/or greater than or equal to 90 mm Hg range, compared with women with normal pressures and after adjustment for age, race/ethnicity, gestational week of blood pressure, body mass index, and parity.[53]

Preeclampsia can manifest as a maternal syndrome, a fetal syndrome, or a disease in which both the mother and fetus are adversely affected. There is significant potential for fetal and maternal morbidity and mortality, with the specific risks depending on the gestational age at the time of disease onset, the severity of the condition, and the presence of maternal comorbidities. Preeclamptic conditions represent a third of cases of severe obstetric morbidity[54] and are a major identifiable risk factor in pregnancies resulting in stillbirth of an otherwise viable neonate.[55] There are also strong associations between preeclampsia and intrauterine growth restriction, low birth weight, preterm delivery, neonatal respiratory distress syndrome, and admission to a neonatal intensive care unit.

The mortality associated with preeclampsia and eclampsia remains significant; in the 2006 to 2008 period, the mortality in the United Kingdom was 0.83 per 100,000 maternities, which amounted to 22 deaths.[1] Fourteen of the 22 women died of cerebral pathologies, of which 9 were intracranial hemorrhage, and 5 were anoxic brain injury following cardiac arrest during eclamptic seizures. A further 3 women died of liver necrosis or hemorrhage, and 2 died of multiorgan failure. Two deaths in this category were the result of acute fatty liver of pregnancy, and 1 death was caused by intra-abdominal hemorrhage of uncertain cause. None of the preeclampsia-eclampsia deaths in this time period were the result of pulmonary edema.

Of these 22 deaths, 14 (64%) were judged to have involved a major degree of substandard care, and a further 6 (27%) involved a minor degree of substandard care. A particular area of weakness was the failure to appropriately refer to specialist services, often because of underappreciation of the significance of symptoms or signs of preeclampsia. The report also identified several cases in which the timely involvement of a senior obstetric clinician did not occur. Combining the United Kingdom Obstetric Surveillance System (UKOSS) data[56] and data from the Eighth Report of the Confidential Enquiries, the case fatality rate from eclampsia is estimated at 3.1%. The UKOSS data show that the incidence of eclamptic seizures halved in the United Kingdom since 1992, presumably as a result of the widespread adoption of magnesium sulfate prophylaxis.

Hypertension caused by preeclampsia typically improves within a few days of delivery and should return to baseline by 12 weeks following delivery. Counseling the postpartum woman regarding the risk for future pregnancies depends on the diagnosis of the hypertensive disorder during the index pregnancy. For women who were diagnosed with preeclampsia, there is a low rate of preeclampsia recurrence, although this is higher if the onset of disease was early in the pregnancy, or if HELLP or eclampsia were diagnosed. Overall, the rate of recurrence is 16% in a future pregnancy, but increases to 25% with severe preeclampsia requiring delivery before 34 weeks, and to 55% if delivery had to occur before 28 weeks.[57,58] There is no additional risk of recurrence with an interpregnancy interval of up to 10 years. Previously affected women should be advised to maintain a healthy weight before the next pregnancy, because obesity increases their risk. Women with a preeclampsia diagnosis have a 13% to 53% risk of gestational hypertension in a future pregnancy. For women who had gestational hypertension, the risk of recurrence for a future pregnancy is 16% to 47%. A 2% to 7% risk of preeclampsia is expected in future pregnancies.[5]

Hypertensive diseases during pregnancy seem to increase the risk of hypertension and stroke later in life,[59,60] and even the risk of stroke in the adult offspring of preeclamptic pregnancies.[61] Severe hypertensive disease in pregnancy has a stronger association with the later development of ischemic heart disease than mild hypertensive disease, and recurrent hypertensive disease in pregnancy is more strongly associated with future

heart disease than nonrecurrent disease.[62] It is plausible that the positive association with future cardiovascular events is largely caused by shared risk factors rather than a direct influence of the disease in pregnancy on the heart or vasculature.[63-65] Cardiologists should be aware of these associations to better evaluate the cardiovascular risk of female patients who have previously been pregnant.[52,66]

MANAGEMENT GOALS AND GUIDELINES

Significant uncertainty remains regarding optimal management of chronic and gestational hypertension in the absence of preeclamptic features. There is general agreement, reflected in the NHBPEP and American College of Obstetricians and Gynecologists guidelines, that blood pressures in the range of 150 to 160 mm Hg systolic and/or 100 to 110 mm Hg diastolic and greater should be treated. Treatment is designed to minimize maternal end-organ damage, for which systolic (rather than diastolic) pressure is now judged to be the strongest predictor.[67]

Mild-to-moderate chronic or gestational hypertension is less likely to produce end-organ disorders, and treatment has been shown to neither improve neonatal outcomes nor prevent superimposed preeclampsia. A Cochrane review of 46 trials, encompassing 4282 patients with modest blood pressure increases, showed no benefits of treatment in terms of stillbirth, preterm birth, or small-for-gestational-age neonates.[68] Excessive blood pressure lowering in such patients may even prove detrimental to fetal growth via placental hypoperfusion.[69] Many physicians think that, in the absence of preeclampsia, a short period of mild-to-moderate hypertension in a young woman has little impact on maternal organ function or long-term cardiovascular risk. However, baseline blood pressures in women of childbearing age are often significantly lower than those of the general population.

When making decisions regarding blood pressure management for pregnant women, the physician should be aware of several issues specific to this patient group. There are few randomized trials with adequate sample sizes to determine optimal treatment of hypertension in pregnancy. The meta-analyses currently available provide useful guidance, but most incorporate heterogeneous studies with varying diagnostic criteria and small numbers of patients. Furthermore, there are no standardized requirements for rigorous animal testing before human studies, and hence childbearing potential without reliable contraception is an exclusion criterion from almost all trials of new cardiovascular medications.[70] There is little incentive for drug companies to develop medications specific to the pregnant cohort, or to test existing medications in this high-risk population. The US Food and Drug Administration (FDA) has a system of grading the risk of specific medications in pregnancy that relies mainly on available animal studies, postmarketing surveillance, and case reports. An understanding of the FDA grades is also essential for physicians who care for women of childbearing age, so that appropriate prepregnancy counseling and prescription decisions can be made.

Focused, large-scale studies to determine both the optimal blood pressure targets and drug regimens for pregnant women with hypertension are urgently needed. A pilot study that begins to address this knowledge deficit was recently published.[71] The Control of Hypertension in Pregnancy Study (CHIPS; ClinicalTrials.gov number NCT01192412) is a large, prospective, randomized, multicenter trial evaluating the impact of a diastolic blood pressure target of 100 versus 85 mm Hg on maternal and neonatal outcomes.[72] However, at the current time there is no consensus regarding the treatment thresholds or targets for blood pressure during pregnancy, with considerable variations in practice existing between, as well as within, countries. The major society thresholds and targets are outlined in **Table 4**.

PHARMACOLOGIC STRATEGIES IN CHRONIC AND GESTATIONAL HYPERTENSION

Blood pressure typically decreases by 10 mm Hg by the end of the second trimester compared with before conception, because of decreased systemic vascular resistance induced by hormonal changes and the low-resistance vessels of the uteroplacental bed **Table 5**. The 2000 NHBPEP report therefore supports stopping antihypertensive medications in women with preexisting hypertension and no target organ involvement, with plans for reinstating appropriate medications should the blood pressure increase to more than 150 to 160/100 to 110mm Hg. The NHBPEP report also endorses the use of the central adrenergic inhibitor methyldopa as the first-line medication, based on 3 decades of postmarketing surveillance and 7.5 years of neonatal follow-up.[73] Oral methyldopa carries a category B designation from the FDA, meaning either that animal reproduction studies have not shown a fetal risk but there are no controlled studies in pregnant women, or animal reproduction studies have shown an adverse effect that was not confirmed in controlled studies in women in the first trimester. However, the National Institute for Health and Clinical Excellence (NICE) guidelines from the United Kingdom raise concerns regarding the precipitation of maternal depression with this medication, and specifically advise against the continuation of

Table 4
Summary of society guidelines regarding blood pressure treatment thresholds and targets

Guideline	Treatment Threshold (mm Hg)	Target (mm Hg)
NHBPEP Working Group Report 2000	150–160 systolic or 100–110 diastolic	—
ACOG Practice Bulletin 2001	150–160 systolic or 100–110 diastolic 160 systolic or 105–110 diastolic in preeclampsia	—
European Society of Cardiology 2011	140/90 if higher risk, otherwise 150/95	—
Society of Obstetricians and Gynaecologists of Canada 2008	160/110	130–155/80–105 130–139/80–89 if comorbidities
Society of Obstetric Medicine of Australia and New Zealand 2008[103]	170/110 in all cases 160/100 in chronic HTN 140–160/90–100 reasonable to consider treatment	<160/100 in eclampsia
NICE 2010	150–159/100–109 (140/90 if end-organ damage in chronic HTN)	<150/80–100, 140/90 if end-organ damage

Abbreviations: ACOG, American College of Obstetricians and Gynecologists; HTN, hypertension; NICE, National Institute for Health and Clinical Excellence.

Table 5
Oral antihypertensive drugs in pregnancy

Drugs	Fetal Risk	Breastfeeding	Risk Class[a]
Methyldopa	Most commonly used agent Longest fetal outcome data Avoid in women at risk of depression	Safe	B oral C intravenous
Labetalol	Associated with intrauterine growth restriction and neonatal bradycardia	Safe, but observe neonate for bradycardia	C
Atenolol, metoprolol	Associated with intrauterine growth restriction, preterm delivery, neonatal hypoglycemia, and bradycardia; avoid atenolol	Safe, but observe neonate for bradycardia	D atenolol C metoprolol
Nifedipine	Avoid sublingual preparation Good safety data for slow-release preparation	Safe	C
Amlodipine	Has been used effectively, but safety data lacking Calcium channel blockers are tocolytics	No data, avoid	C
Hydralazine	Potential associations include hypospadias, neonatal thrombocytopenia, lupuslike syndrome	Safe	C
Hydrochlorothiazide	Neonatal hypoglycemia, thrombocytopenia, hemolytic anemia, and maternal electrolyte disturbances	Safe, but may reduce milk volume	B
Medications to Avoid During Pregnancy			
Captopril, lisinopril	Oligohydramnios, intrauterine growth restriction, hypocalvaria, renal dysplasia, anuria, neonatal hypotension, limb contractures, death	No data, avoid	D (C first trimester)
Losartan, valsartan	No human data, but potential renal and skull defects, neonatal hypotension, anuria	No data, avoid	D (losartan C first trimester)
Aliskiren (direct renin inhibitor)	Teratogenicity extrapolated from ACE and ARB data, but has not been shown by existing animal studies	No data, avoid	D (C first trimester)

Abbreviations: ACE, angiotensin-converting enzyme; ARB, angiotensin receptor blocker.

[a] Risk class B: either animal reproduction studies have not shown a fetal risk but there are no controlled studies in pregnant women, or animal reproduction studies have shown an adverse effect that was not confirmed in controlled studies in women in the first trimester (and there is no evidence of risk in later trimesters). Risk class C: either studies in animals have revealed adverse effects on the fetus and there are no controlled studies in women, or studies in women are not available. Drug should be given only if the potential benefit justifies the potential risk to the fetus. Risk class D: there is positive evidence of human fetal risk, but the benefits from use in pregnant women may be acceptable despite the risk.

Data retrieved from Micromedex 2.0, correct as of October 1 2011; *and Adapted from* Vest AR, Maroo A, Raymond RE. Pregnancy and heart disease. In: Brian PG, Samir RK, Curtis MR, editors. Cleveland Clinic cardiology board review, 2nd edition. Philadelphia: Lippincott Williams & Wilkins; 2012; with permission.

methyldopa beyond the second day postpartum. Other commonly used oral medications such as labetalol, hydralazine, and nifedipine are all category C agents, implying either that animal studies have revealed adverse effects on the fetus and there are no controlled studies in women, or that studies in women are not available. The FDA advises that category C drugs should only be given if the potential benefits justify the potential fetal risks.

Labetalol, a combined α-blocker and β-blocker, has gained popularity in pregnancy and is first line for gestational or preeclamptic hypertension in the 2010 NICE guidelines, based on expert opinion. The 2001 American College of Obstetricians and Gynecologists (ACOG) Practice Bulletin supports labetalol or methyldopa as first line,[74] and the 2008 Society of Obstetricians and Gynaecologists of Canada guidelines favor labetalol, nifedipine, or hydralazine.[4] Alternate β-blockers are generally considered safe during pregnancy, although there are case reports of adverse fetal events. Atenolol carries a category D classification because of its association with low birth weight, preterm delivery, and neonatal hypoglycemia and bradycardia. Metoprolol received a class C designation based primarily on studies in rats. One small human study in the 1970s compared metoprolol alone or in combination with hydralazine in 101 pregnant women with the outcomes for 97 hypertensive pregnant women receiving hydralazine. In both groups, a small dose of a thiazide was added. Perinatal mortality was lower in the metoprolol group (2.0%) than in the hydralazine group (8.0%), and the rate of fetal growth restriction was also lower in the metoprolol group (11.7 vs 16.3%).[75]

Successful long-term therapy with oral hydralazine usually requires combination therapy (typically with a sympatholytic agent such as methyldopa or a β-blocker), which prevents reflex tachycardia.[76] There are possible associations between first-trimester hydralazine use and hypospadias, third-trimester use and neonatal thrombocytopenia, and maternal or neonatal lupuslike syndrome. The 3 to 4 times daily dosing schedule of hydralazine is also a disadvantage.

Experience with calcium channel blockers in the first and second trimester is limited. Slow-release nifedipine is the most commonly used agent. Animal studies have raised concerns of teratogenicity, but postmarketing data have not revealed any association with congenital abnormalities. Concurrent administration of calcium channel blockers and magnesium sulfate has traditionally been avoided because of the potentially synergistic blood pressure effects, although the 2008 SOGC guidelines support contemporaneous use. Calcium channel blockers also have potential tocolytic effects.

The prescription of diuretics for blood pressure control during pregnancy remains controversial, even though hydrochlorothiazide is FDA category B. The total body volume is reduced in preeclampsia, and hence diuresis can precipitate clinically significant hypovolemia and placental hypoperfusion. Diuretics may reduce milk volume, although the American Academy of Pediatrics considers their use compatible with breastfeeding. There are also associations with maternal electrolyte disturbances and, rarely, with neonatal thrombocytopenia and hemolytic anemia.

Hypertensive emergencies during pregnancy necessitate the use of medications with more rapid onset of action. In an individual with severely increased blood pressure or evidence of maternal or fetal compromise, the systolic blood pressure should be lowered by approximately 25% over the first few minutes to hours. Common strategies are intravenous labetalol, hydralazine, or sodium nitroprusside. Rapidly acting oral nifedipine is also an option, but has never been FDA approved for hypertensive emergencies, and carries a substantial risk of precipitating severe hypotension and cerebral infarction. Intravenous nitroglycerin is a good choice in the setting of pulmonary edema.[77] Intravenous labetalol and hydralazine showed similar pressure lowering in a Cochrane review, with insufficient evidence to make practice recommendations.[78] In the presence of suspected PRES, labetalol may be a sensible choice because it does not cerebrally vasodilate. Heart failure, bradycardia, and asthma are contraindications to labetalol, and neonatal bradycardia has been reported. The role of intravenous hydralazine was questioned by a meta-analysis that reported poorer maternal and perinatal outcomes for hydralazine compared with other antihypertensives, particularly labetalol and nifedipine. Hydralazine was also found to be a less effective antihypertensive than nifedipine and did not clearly differ from labetalol. Hydralazine showed association with an excess of maternal hypotension, placental abruption, caesarean section, maternal oliguria, and low Apgar scores at 1 minute.[79] Sodium nitroprusside can be used, but with caution, especially in women with renal impairment who require frequent monitoring of thiocyanate levels (or cyanide levels if there is hepatic failure) to avoid cyanide toxicity.[80]

Angiotensin-converting enzyme (ACE) inhibitors and angiotensin receptor blockers are contraindicated throughout pregnancy. Observed fetal effects of drugs in these classes include oligohydramnios, intrauterine growth restriction, hypocalvaria, renal dysplasia, anuria, and death.[81] The newer direct renin inhibitors have a related mechanism of action and are therefore contraindicated in pregnancy. However, existing animal studies have not supported teratogenicity, and aliskiren has been assigned to FDA pregnancy categories C (first trimester) and D (second and third trimesters). The following antihypertensives are judged to have little or no effects for neonates receiving breast milk: labetalol, nifedipine, enalapril, captopril, metoprolol. Angiotensin receptor blockers, amlodipine, and ACE inhibitors other than enalapril and captopril should not be prescribed during lactation[5]; atenolol should also be avoided if possible.[82]

Ongoing hypertension control with oral agents may be required after delivery, especially for women who were hypertensive before the pregnancy. The NHBPEP recommends that, for women with normal or unknown prepregnancy blood pressure, it is reasonable to discontinue the antihypertensives after 3 to 4 weeks and observe the blood pressure at intervals of 1 to 2 weeks for 1 month, and then at intervals of 3 to 6 months for a year. If there is a recurrence of hypertension, it should be treated.

Novel therapies currently being investigated for hypertension in pregnancy include heme oxygenase 1, marinobufagenin, placental leucine aminopeptidase, and aminopeptidase A.[77]

PHARMACOLOGIC STRATEGIES SPECIFIC TO PREECLAMPSIA AND ECLAMPSIA

Preeclampsia and eclampsia necessitate more complex management decision than blood pressure control alone. Guidelines regarding delivery are outlined later. Intravenous magnesium sulfate has a crucial role in the prevention of seizures in preeclamptic women by slowing neuromuscular conduction and raising the seizure threshold. About a quarter of women experience minor side effects such as flushing. The high magnesium doses used in this setting can cause loss of deep tendon reflexes, mental status changes, and respiratory depression. Careful monitoring is essential with serum levels in patients with impaired renal function. A loading dose of 4 to 6 g is usually diluted in 100 mL of normal saline and infused over 15 to 20 minutes, followed by a continuous infusion of 2 g per hour. The therapeutic range for serum magnesium is 4 to 7 mg/dL.[83] The antidote is intravenous calcium gluconate. Seizure prophylaxis with magnesium should continue for 12 to 24 hours postpartum.

The Magpie Trial showed the benefits of magnesium in the preeclamptic patient.[84] This study recruited 10,141 pregnant women with blood pressures greater than 140/90 mm Hg and proteinuria greater than or equal to 1+ (30 mg/dL). Subjects were randomized to receive magnesium sulfate versus placebo. Primary outcomes were eclamptic seizures and, for women randomized before

delivery, perinatal death. Magnesium was found to half the risk of eclampsia without significant adverse maternal or fetal effects. In a patient already having eclamptic seizures, magnesium has shown superiority in prevention of recurrent seizures compared with phenytoin.[85]

As highlighted in the Eighth Report of the Confidential Enquiries, the combination of oxytocin and ergometrine (trade name Syntometrine) should not be used to precipitate delivery of the placenta and prevent postpartum hemorrhage in women with hypertension. Ergometrine is a powerful vasoconstrictor and has been implicated in cases of hypertensive morbidity in the immediate postpartum phase. Intramuscular oxytocin without ergometrine is an acceptable uterotonic.[86] Neither the routine use of intravenous fluids nor routine administration of diuretics is an appropriate response to maternal oliguria.[4]

Several therapies have been proposed and studied for their potential to prevent the development of preeclampsia in high-risk women when taken early in pregnancy. Aspirin may address an imbalance between prostacyclin and thromboxane arising early in the preeclampsia process. A Cochrane review of 36,500 women in 59 trials revealed a 17% risk reduction for preeclampsia, with a number needed to treat of 72.[87] Patients with high-risk maternal histories are advised to take 75 to 100 mg of aspirin daily by the NHBPEP, NICE, and Society of Obstetricians and Gynecologists of Canada guidelines.

Studies of calcium supplementation suggest that its benefit lies with women who have a high preeclampsia risk and a low dietary calcium intake.[88,89] A few preliminary trials showed benefit from vitamins C and E,[90] but an adequately powered study did not support this hypothesis.[91,92] Trials of magnesium and zinc supplements, fish oils, garlic, a low-salt diet, and folic acid have failed to show an impact on the risk of preeclampsia. Other agents specifically recommended against by the guidelines are nitric oxide donors, progesterone, and low-molecular-weight heparin.[5] Women who smoke during pregnancy have an increased rate of various negative obstetric outcomes, but smoking may be protective for hypertensive complications of pregnancy.[93] However, a substudy of one of the large calcium trials showed that smokers who quit before becoming pregnant did not have a risk reduction for gestational hypertension or preeclampsia.[94]

NONPHARMACOLOGIC STRATEGIES

The definitive treatment of preeclampsia or eclampsia is delivery of the fetus. Delivery greatly reduces the risk of complications such as seizures, cerebral edema, placental abruption, pulmonary edema, and dissemination intravascular coagulopathy. However, despite the potential for intrauterine growth restriction and still birth during this disease process, delivery may not be the right choice for the fetus, especially earlier in gestation. Therefore, management of the preeclamptic patient is a complex balance between competing maternal and fetal risks, and should be orchestrated by an obstetrician and/or fetal-maternal medicine subspecialist. **Fig. 1** shows an algorithm for recommended management of mild gestational hypertension or preeclampsia. **Fig. 2** shows an algorithm for recommended management of severe preeclampsia.

Expectant management, with adequate monitoring for uteroplacental insufficiency, is appropriate in mild preeclampsia. In such patients, delivery is generally not indicated until at least 27 to 28 weeks, but should occur by 40 weeks.[2] In more severe forms of preeclampsia, hospital

admission for prophylaxis of seizures and tight blood pressure control is essential. Expedited delivery will be coordinated if the disease arises after 34 weeks, or if features of severe preeclampsia are detected before 34 weeks.[95] Expert opinion supports delivery within 24 hours for women with treatment-resistant hypertension or maternal or fetal compromise, regardless of gestational age or fetal lung maturity. Beyond 34 weeks' gestation, or in cases in which fetal lung maturity has been achieved, delivery should occur without delay.[11]

The other nonpharmacologic intervention is bed rest, which is widely recommended for hypertension of any cause in pregnancy. Four small trials, involving 449 subjects, were evaluated by a Cochrane review.[96] One trial associated bed rest with reduced risks of severe hypertension and prematurity, but none of the studies evaluated the potential for deep vein thrombosis, or potential social and economic implications. The reviewers concluded that current evidence is insufficient to provide clinical

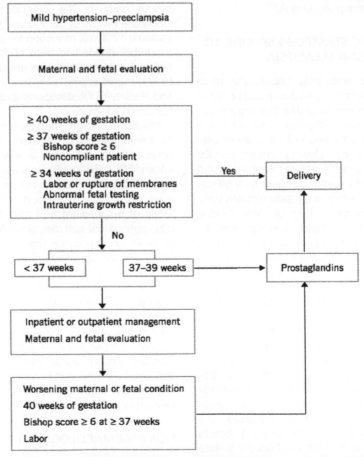

Fig. 1. Recommended management of mild gestational hypertension or preeclampsia. (*From* Sibai BM. Diagnosis and management of gestational hypertension and preeclampsia. Obstet Gynecol 2003;102(1):181–92; with permission.)

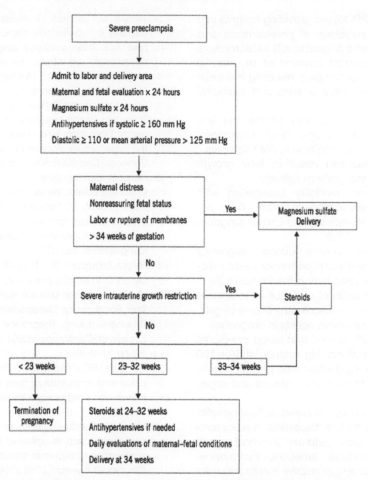

Fig. 2. Recommended management of severe preeclampsia. Maternal distress: thrombocytopenia, imminent eclampsia, pulmonary edema, and hemolysis plus increased liver enzyme levels. (*From* Sibai BM. Diagnosis and management of gestational hypertension and preeclampsia. Obstet Gynecol 2003;102(1):181–92; with permission.)

guidance, and therefore bed rest should not be routinely recommended.

SUMMARY

- 5% to 10% of women are diagnosed with hypertension during pregnancy, based on a systolic blood pressure greater than or equal to 140 mm Hg and/or diastolic greater than or equal to 90 mm Hg
- The National High Blood Pressure Education Program Working Group on High Blood Pressure in Pregnancy 2000 guidelines divide hypertensive disorders into chronic hypertension, gestational hypertension, preeclampsia/eclampsia, and preeclampsia superimposed on chronic hypertension
- Preeclampsia occurs in 2% to 5% of all pregnancies, 10% of first pregnancies, and 20% to 25% of women with chronic hypertension

- Diagnostic flags for preeclampsia include proteinuria greater than 300 mg per 24 hours (or >30 mg/mmol in a spot urine sample), an increase in proteinuria or loss of blood pressure control in a woman with preexisting hypertension, onset of headache, blurred vision, abdominal pain, transaminitis, or thrombocytopenia
- HELLP syndrome is a laboratory diagnosis and represents preeclampsia cases with poorer outcomes
- Eclampsia is the development of grand mal seizures in a woman with preeclampsia, but occasionally occurs with minimal blood pressure increase and no proteinuria
- Risk factors for preeclampsia include advanced maternal age, black ethnicity, nulliparity, and maternal diabetes or renal disease
- Angiogenic and antiangiogenic placental peptides (including PAPP-A, PlGF, sFlt-1,

sEng, and PP-13) are providing insights into the pathophysiology of preeclampsia and may establish a diagnostic role as biomarkers
- There is aberrant invasion of myometrial arteries in preeclampsia, resulting in unusually resistive spiral arteries and placental hypoperfusion
- Natural killer cells may bridge the link between immunologic and endothelial dysfunction mechanisms in preeclampsia
- Preeclampsia can result in fetal growth restriction and preterm delivery
- The maternal mortality associated with preeclampsia/eclampsia was 0.8 per 100,000 maternities in the United Kingdom from 2006 to 2008
- Hypertensive disease during pregnancy increases the risk of hypertension and cardiovascular diseases later in the woman's life
- There is a paucity of evidence as to optimal treatment thresholds, blood pressure targets, and antihypertensive agents in pregnancy
- It is generally agreed that blood pressures of 150 to 160 mm Hg systolic and/or 100 to 110 mm Hg diastolic and greater should be treated to minimize maternal end-organ damage
- A Cochrane review showed no fetal benefits of blood pressure treatment; medications could even prove detrimental to fetal growth
- Oral methyldopa, labetalol, hydralazine, and nifedipine have relative merits and risks
- Intravenous labetalol, hydralazine, or sodium nitroprusside may be used in hypertensive emergencies, but with minimal data regarding fetal outcomes
- ACE inhibitors and angiotensin receptor antagonists are contraindicated in pregnancy
- Women with preeclampsia should be closely monitored and receive intravenous magnesium sulfate at 4 to 6 g over 15 to 20 minutes, followed by a 2 g/h infusion
- The definitive treatment of preeclampsia or eclampsia is delivery of the fetus.

REFERENCES

1. Centre for Maternal and Child Enquiries (CMACE). Saving mothers' lives: reviewing maternal deaths to make motherhood safer: 2006–08. The Eighth Report on Confidential Enquiries into Maternal Deaths in the United Kingdom. BJOG 2011; 118(Suppl 1):1–203.
2. Report of the National High Blood Pressure Education Program. Working group report on high blood pressure in pregnancy. Am J Obstet Gynecol 2000;183:S1–22.
3. Tanaka M, Jaamaa G, Kaiser M, et al. Racial disparity in hypertensive disorders of pregnancy in New York State: a 10-year longitudinal population-based study. Am J Public Health 2007;97:163–70.
4. Magee LA, Helewa M, Moutquin JM, et al, for the Hypertension Guideline Committee, Society of Obstetricians and Gynaecologists of Canada, Treatment of the hypertensive disorders of pregnancy. Diagnosis, evaluation, and management of the hypertensive disorders of pregnancy. J Obstet Gynaecol Can 2008;30(3 Suppl 1):S24–36.
5. National Collaborating Centre for Women's and Children's Health. Hypertension in pregnancy. The management of hypertensive disorders during pregnancy. London: National Institute for Health and Clinical Excellence (NICE); 2010. p. 46. (Clinical guideline; no. 107).
6. Regitz-Zagrosek V, Blomstrom Lundqvist C, Borghi C, et al. ESC guidelines on the management of cardiovascular disease during pregnancy: the Task Force on the Management of Cardiovascular Diseases during Pregnancy of the European Society of Cardiology (ESC). Eur Heart J 2011; 32(24):3147–97.
7. Hermida RC, Ayala DE. Prognostic value of office and ambulatory blood pressure measurements in pregnancy. Hypertension 2002;40: 298–303.
8. Maulik D, Mundy D, Heitmann E, et al. Evidence-based approach to umbilical artery Doppler fetal surveillance in high-risk pregnancies: an update. Clin Obstet Gynecol 2010;53(4):869–78.
9. Wheeler TL, Blackhurst DW, Dellinger EH, et al. Usage of spot urine protein to creatinine ratios in the evaluation of preeclampsia. Am J Obstet Gynecol 2007;196(5):465.e1–4.
10. Mattar F, Sibai BM. Eclampsia. VIII. Risk factors for maternal morbidity. Am J Obstet Gynecol 2000; 182:307–12.
11. Sibai BM. Diagnosis and management of gestational hypertension and preeclampsia. Obstet Gynecol 2003;102:181–92.
12. Douglas KA, Redman CW. Eclampsia in the United Kingdom. BMJ 1994;309:1395–400.
13. Hirshfeld-Cytron J, Lam C, Karumanchi SA, et al. Late postpartum eclampsia: examples and review. Obstet Gynecol Surv 2006;61(7):471–80.
14. Poon LC, Kametas NA, Maiz N, et al. First-trimester prediction of hypertensive disorders in pregnancy. Hypertension 2009;53(5):812–8.
15. Yu CK, Smith GC, Papageorghiou AT, et al. An integrated model for the prediction of preeclampsia using maternal factors and uterine artery Doppler velocimetry in unselected low-risk women. Am J Obstet Gynecol 2005;193:429–36.
16. Milne F, Redman C, Walker J, et al. The preeclampsia community guideline (PRECOG): how to screen for

and detect onset of preeclampsia in the community. BMJ 2005;330(7491):576–80.

17. Meads CA, Cnossen JS, Meher S, et al. Methods of prediction and prevention of pre-eclampsia: systematic reviews of accuracy and effectiveness literature with economic modelling. Health Technol Assess 2008;12(6):iii–iv.

18. Levine RJ, Maynard SE, Qian C, et al. Circulating angiogenic factors and the risk of preeclampsia. N Engl J Med 2004;350:672–83.

19. Levine RJ, Lam C, Qian C, et al. Soluble endoglin and other antiangiogenic factors in preeclampsia. N Engl J Med 2006;355:992–1005.

20. Salahuddin S, Lee Y, Vadnais M, et al. Diagnostic utility of soluble fms-like tyrosine kinase 1 and soluble endoglin in hypertensive diseases of pregnancy. Am J Obstet Gynecol 2007;197:28.e1–6.

21. Qazi U, Lam C, Karumanchi SA, et al. Soluble Fms-like tyrosine kinase associated with preeclampsia in pregnancy in systemic lupus erythematosus. J Rheumatol 2008;35:631–4.

22. Masuyama H, Suwaki N, Nakatsukasa H, et al. Circulating angiogenic factors in preeclampsia, gestational proteinuria, and preeclampsia superimposed on chronic glomerulo-nephritis. Am J Obstet Gynecol 2006;194:551–6.

23. Wolf M, Shah A, Lam C. Circulating levels of the antiangiogenic marker sFlt-1 are increased in first versus second pregnancies. Am J Obstet Gynecol 2005;193:16–22.

24. Rana S, Karumanchi SA, Levine RJ. Sequential changes in antiangiogenic factors in early pregnancy and risk of developing preeclampsia. Hypertension 2007;50:137–42.

25. Venkatesha S, Toporsian M, Lam C. Soluble endoglin contributes to the pathogenesis of preeclampsia. Nature Med 2006;12:642–9.

26. Chafetz I, Kuhnreich I, Sammar M. First-trimester placental protein 13 screening for preeclampsia and intrauterine growth restriction. Am J Obstet Gynecol 2007;197:35, e1–7.

27. Nicolaides KH, Bindra R, Turan OM. A novel approach to first-trimester screening for early pre-eclampsia combining serum PP-13 and Doppler ultrasound. Ultrasound Obstet Gynecol 2006;27:13–7.

28. Odibo AO, Zhong Y, Goetzinger KR, et al. First-trimester placental protein 13, PAPP-A, uterine artery Doppler and maternal characteristics in the prediction of pre-eclampsia. Placenta 2011;32(8): 598–602.

29. D'Anna R, Baviera G, Corrado F, et al. Plasma adiponectin concentration in early pregnancy and subsequent risk of hypertensive disorders. Obstet Gynecol 2005;106(2):340–4.

30. Carty DM, Delles C, Dominiczak AF. Novel biomarkers for predicting preeclampsia. Trends Cardiovasc Med 2008;18(5–24):186–94.

31. Silver HM, Seebeck M, Carlson R. Comparison of total blood volume in normal, preeclamptic, and nonproteinuric gestational hypertensive pregnancy by simultaneous measurement of red blood cell and plasma volumes. Am J Obstet Gynecol 1998; 179:87.

32. Sibai B, Dekker G, Kupferminc M. Pre-eclampsia. Lancet 2005;365:785–99.

33. Seely EW, Ecker J. Chronic hypertension in pregnancy. N Engl J Med 2011;365:439–46.

34. Duckitt K, Harrington D. Risk factors for pre-eclampsia at antenatal booking: systematic review of controlled studies. BMJ 2005;330:565.

35. Sargent IL, Smarason AK. Immunology of pre-eclampsia; current views and hypothesis. In: Kurpisz M, Fernandez N, editors. Immunology of human reproduction. Oxford (United Kingdom): BIOS Scientific Publishers; 1995. p. 355–70.

36. Kliman HJ, Sammar M, Grimpel YI, et al. Placental protein 13 and decidual zones of necrosis: an immunologic diversion that may be linked to preeclampsia. Reprod Sci 2011;19(1):16–30.

37. Gonen R, Shahar R, Grimpel YI, et al. Placental protein 13 as an early marker for preeclampsia: a prospective longitudinal study. BJOG 2008; 115(12):1465–72.

38. Li Z, Zhang Y, Ying Ma J, et al. Recombinant vascular endothelial growth factor 121 attenuates hypertension and improves kidney damage in a rat model of preeclampsia. Hypertension 2007; 50:686–92.

39. Adali E, Kurdoglu M, Adali F, et al. The relationship between brachial artery flow-mediated dilatation, high sensitivity C-reactive protein, and uterine artery Doppler velocimetry in women with pre-eclampsia. J Clin Ultrasound 2011;39:191–7.

40. Zhang J, Zeisler J, Hatch MC. Epidemiology of pregnancy-induced hypertension. Epidemiol Rev 1997;19(2):218–32.

41. Robillard PY, Hulsey TC, Alexander GR, et al. Paternity patterns and risk of preeclampsia in the last pregnancy in multiparae. J Reprod Immunol 1993;24:1–12.

42. Li DK, Wi S. Changing paternity and the risk of preeclampsia/eclampsia in the subsequent pregnancy. Am J Epidemiol 2000;151:57–62.

43. Saftlas AF, Levine RJ, Klebanoff MA, et al. Abortion, changed paternity, and risk of preeclampsia in nulliparous women. Am J Epidemiol 2003;157: 1108–14.

44. Robillard PY, Hulsey TC, Perianin J, et al. Association of pregnancy-induced hypertension with duration of sexual cohabitation before conception. Lancet 1994;344:973–5.

45. Klonoff-Cohen HS, Savitz DA, Cefalo RC, et al. An epidemiologic study of contraception and pre-eclampsia. JAMA 1989;262:3143–7.

46. Need JA, Bell B, Meffin F, et al. Pre-eclampsia in pregnancies from donor inseminations. J Reprod Immunol 1983;5:329–38.

47. Smith GN, Walker M, Tessier JL, et al. Increased incidence of preeclampsia in women conceiving by intrauterine insemination with donor versus partner sperm for treatment of primary infertility. Am J Obstet Gynecol 1997;177:455–8.

48. Croy BA, He H, Esadeg S, et al. Uterine natural killer cells; insight into their cellular and molecular biology from mouse modeling. Reproduction 2003;126:149–60.

49. Powe CE, Levine RJ, Karumanchi SA. Pre-eclampsia, a disease of the maternal endothelium. The role of antiangiogenic factors and implications for later cardiovascular disease. Circulation 2011; 123:2856–69.

50. Sibai BM, Lindheimer M, Hauth J, et al. Risk factors for preeclampsia, abruption placentae, and adverse neonatal outcomes among women with chronic hypertension. N Engl J Med 1998;339: 667–71.

51. Catov JM, Nohr EA, Olsen J, et al. Chronic hypertension related to risk for preterm and term small for gestational age births. Obstet Gynecol 2008;112: 290–6.

52. Mosca L, Benjamin EJ, Berra K, et al. Effectiveness-based guidelines for the prevention of cardiovascular disease in women. 2011 update: a guideline from the American Heart Association. J Am Coll Cardiol 2011;57:1404–23.

53. Hedderson MM, Ferrara A. High blood pressure before and during early pregnancy is associated with an increased risk of gestational diabetes mellitus. Diabetes Care 2008;31(12):2362–7.

54. Waterstone M, Bewley S, Wolfe C. Incidence and predictors of severe obstetric morbidity: case-control study. BMJ 2001;322:1089–94.

55. Maternal and Child Health Research Consortium. Confidential enquiry into stillbirths and deaths in infancy: 6th annual report, 1 January-31 December 1997. London: Maternal and Child Health Research Consortium; 1999.

56. Knight M. Eclampsia in the United Kingdom 2005. BJOG 2007;114:1072–8.

57. Chames MC, Haddad B, Barton JR, et al. Subsequent pregnancy outcome in women with a history of HELLP syndrome at < or = 28 weeks of gestation. Am J Obstet Gynecol 2003;188:1504–7.

58. Sibai BM, Mercer B, Sarinoglu C. Severe preeclampsia in the second trimester: recurrence risk and long-term prognosis. Am J Obstet Gynecol 1991;165:1408–12.

59. Manussen EB, Vatten LJ, Smith GD, et al. Hypertensive disorders in pregnancy and subsequently measured cardiovascular risk factors. Obstet Gynecol 2009;144:961.

60. Wilson BJ, Watson MS, Prescott GJ, et al. Hypertensive diseases of pregnancy and risk of hypertension and stroke in later life: results from cohort study. BMJ 2003;326:845.

61. Kajantie E, Eriksson JG, Osmond C, et al. Preeclampsia is associated with increased risk of stroke in the adult offspring: the Helsinki Birth Cohort Study. Stroke 2009;40:1176–80.

62. Wikstrom AK, Haglund B, Olovsson M, et al. The risk of maternal ischaemic heart disease after gestational hypertensive disease. BJOG 2005; 112:1486–91.

63. Parvin S, Samsuddin L, Ali A, et al. Lipoprotein (a) level in pre-eclampsia patients. Bangladesh Med Res Counc Bull 2010;36(3):97–9.

64. Ramsay JE, Stewart F, Green IA, et al. Microvascular dysfunction: a link between pre-eclampsia and maternal coronary heart disease. BJOG 2003;110:1029–31.

65. Romundstad PR, Magnussen EB, Smith GD, et al. Hypertension in pregnancy and later cardiovascular risk. Common antecedents? Circulation 2010;122:579–84.

66. Robbins CL, Dietz PM, Bombard J, et al. Gestational hypertension: a neglected cardiovascular disease risk marker. Am J Obstet Gynecol 2011; 204:336.e1–9.

67. Martin JN Jr, Thigpen BD, Moore RC, et al. Stroke and severe preeclampsia and eclampsia: a paradigm shift focusing on systolic blood pressure. Obstet Gynecol 2005;105(2):246–54.

68. Abalos E, Duley L, Steyn DW, et al. Antihypertensive drug therapy for mild to moderate hypertension during pregnancy. Cochrane Database Syst Rev 2007;1:CD002252.

69. von Dadelszen P, Magee LA. Fall in mean arterial pressure and fetal growth restriction in pregnancy hypertension: an updated metaregression analysis. J Obstet Gynaecol Can 2002;24:941–5.

70. Cifkova R. Why is the treatment of hypertension in pregnancy still so difficult? Expert Rev Cardiovasc Ther 2011;9(6):647–9.

71. Magee LA, von Dadelszen P, Chan S, et al, CHIPS Pilot Trial Collaborative Group. The control of hypertension in pregnancy Study pilot trial. BJOG 2007;114(6):770. e13–20.

72. Available at: http://www.controlled-trials.com/ISRCTN71416914. Accessed October 23, 2011.

73. Cockburn J, Moar VA, Ounsted M, et al. Final report of study on hypertension during pregnancy: the effects of specific treatment on the growth and development of the children. Lancet 1982; 1(8273):647–9.

74. ACOG practice bulletin no.29. Chronic hypertension in pregnancy. ACOG Committee on Practice Bulletins. Obstet Gynecol 2001;98(1):177–85.

75. Sandström B. Antihypertensive treatment with the adrenergic beta-receptor blocker metoprolol during pregnancy. Gynecol Invest 1978;9(4):195–204.

76. Magee LA. Treating hypertension in women of child-bearing age and during pregnancy. Drug Safety 2001;24(6):457–74.

77. Brown CM, Garovic VD. Mechanisms and management of hypertension in pregnant women. Curr Hypertens Rep 2011;13:338–46.

78. Duley L, Henderson-Smart DJ, Meher S. Drugs for treatment of very high blood pressure during pregnancy. Cochrane Database Syst Rev 2006;3:CD001449.

79. Magee LA, Cham C, Waterman EJ, et al. Hydralazine for treatment of severe hypertension in pregnancy: meta-analysis. BMJ 2003;327:955–60.

80. Sass N, Itamoto CH, Silva MP, et al. Does sodium nitroprusside kill babies? A systematic review. Sao Paulo Med J 2007;125:108–11.

81. Cooper WO, Hernandez-Diaz S, Arbogast PG, et al. Major congenital malformations after first-trimester exposure to ACE inhibitors. N Engl J Med 2006;354:2443–51.

82. Schimmel MS, Eidelman AI, Wilschanski MA, et al. Toxic effects of atenolol consumed during breast feeding. J Pediatr 1989;114:476.

83. ACOG Committee on Practice Bulletins—Obstetrics. ACOG practice bulletin no. 33, diagnosis and management of preeclampsia and eclampsia. Obstet Gynecol 2002;99(1):159–67.

84. Altman D, Carroli G, Duley L, et al. Do women with preeclampsia, and their babies, benefit from magnesium sulphate? The Magpie Trial: a randomised placebo-controlled trial. Lancet 2002;359:1877–90.

85. Duley L, Henderson-Smart D. Magnesium sulphate versus diazepam for eclampsia. Cochrane Database Syst Rev 2003;4:CD000127.

86. McDonald SJ, Abbott JN, Higgins SP. Prophylactic ergometrine-oxytocin versus oxytocin for the third stage of labour. Cochrane Database Syst Rev 2004;1:CD000201.

87. Duley L, Henderson-Smart DJ, Meher S, et al. Antiplatelet agents for preventing pre-eclampsia and its complications. Cochrane Database Syst Rev 2007;2:CD004659.

88. Hofmeyr GJ, Atallah AN, Duley L. Calcium supplementation during pregnancy for preventing hypertensive disorders and related problems. Cochrane Database Syst Rev 2006;3:CD001059.

89. Levine RJ, Hauth JC, Curet LB, et al. Trial of calcium to prevent preeclampsia. N Engl J Med 1997;337:69–76.

90. Rumiris D, Purwosunu Y, Wibowo N, et al. Lower rate of preeclampsia after antioxidant supplementation in pregnant women with low antioxidant status. Hypertens Pregnancy 2006;25:241–53.

91. Poston L, Briley AL, Seed PT, et al. Vitamin C and vitamin E in pregnant women at risk for pre-eclampsia (VIP trial): randomised placebo-controlled trial. Lancet 2006;367:1145–54.

92. Roberts JM, Myatt L, Spong CY, et al, for the Eunice Kennedy Shriver National Institute of Child Health and Human Development Maternal–Fetal Medicine Units Network. Vitamins C and E to prevent complications of pregnancy-associated hypertension. N Engl J Med 2010;362:1282–91.

93. Conde-Agudelo A, Althabe F, Belizan JM, et al. Cigarette smoking during pregnancy and risk of preeclampsia: a systematic review. Am J Obstet Gynecol 1999;181:1026–35.

94. England LJ, Levine RJ, Qian C, et al. Smoking before pregnancy and risk of gestational hypertension and preeclampsia. Am J Obstet Gynecol 2002;186:1035–40.

95. Friedman SA, Lubarsky S, Schiff E. Expectant management of severe preeclampsia remote from term. Clin Obstet Gynecol 1999;42:470–8.

96. Meher S, Abalos E, Carroli G. Bed rest with or without hospitalisation for hypertension during pregnancy. Cochrane Database Syst Rev 2005;4:CD003514.

97. O'Brien TE, Ray JG, Chan WS. Maternal body mass index and the risk of preeclampsia: a systematic overview. Epidemiology 2003;14:368–74.

98. Wolf M, Sandler L, Munoz K, et al. First trimester insulin resistance and subsequent preeclampsia: a prospective study. J Clin Endocrinol Metab 2002;87:1563–8.

99. Facchinetti F, Allais G, Nappi RE, et al. Migraine is a risk factor for hypertensive disorders in pregnancy: a prospective cohort study. Cephalalgia 2009;29(3):286–92.

100. Toh S, Mitchell AA, Louik C, et al. Selective serotonin reuptake inhibitor use and risk of gestational hypertension. Am J Psychiatry 2009;166(3):320–8.

101. Boggess KA, Lief S, Martha AP, et al. Maternal periodontal disease is associated with an increased risk for preeclampsia. Obstet Gynecol 2003;101:227–31.

102. Lie RT, Rasmussen S, Brunborg H, et al. Fetal and maternal contributions to risk of preeclampsia: a population based study. BMJ 1998;316:1343–7.

103. Lowe SA, Brown MA, Dekker GA, et al. Guidelines for the management of hypertensive disorders of pregnancy 2008. Aust N Z J Obstet Gynaecol 2009;49(3):242–6.

Arrhythmias in Pregnancy

John H. McAnulty, MD

KEYWORDS

- Arrhythmia • Pregnancy • Pacemakers • Defibrillators • Antiarrhythmic drugs

KEY POINTS

- Document the rhythm before treatment. The diagnostic criteria for arrhythmias are not changed by pregnancy.
- Treat hemodynamically significant rhythms early.
- Use necessary drugs.
- Avoid procedures requiring an X ray until after pregnancy. Fetal exposure to radiation can be teratogenic and may result in subsequent malignancies. If required during pregnancy for maternal safety, low-dose imaging with abdominal shielding should be used.
- Evaluate cardiac anatomy in those with sustained arrhythmias. An anatomic abnormality itself may require attention. Because the significance of rhythms varies depending on associated cardiac abnormalities, it would help dictate the need for the treatment of arrhythmias.
- Incorporate the expertise of a neonatologist in cases when a concern about fetal distress can influence treatment decisions.

INTRODUCTION

Which part of the elephant were they touching? As strange as it is to begin with that sentence, it could be asked of the scientists studying arrhythmias during pregnancy.

Literature on this subject comes from 3 broad sources: anecdotal reports, reports from referral centers with modestly large populations of pregnant women with structural heart disease, and reports from more general hospitals that have collected their experiences. Not surprisingly, this leads to differences in mechanisms, significance, and treatment recommendations. Although there is much we do not know, arrhythmias will not wait until we learn more. Available information does provide guidance.

Perhaps following 2 women through this article will allow the consideration of some key principles. With some concerns of entrapping the reader, they will be called our 2 women.

Two women

1. A 29-year-old woman, not pregnant, with sudden-onset racing heart; in emergency department: blood pressure, 80/50; heart rate, 190 beats per minute and regular
2. A 29-year-old woman, 7 months pregnant, with an identical presentation.

The arrhythmia is likely to be the same in these women. In most cases, the approach to an abnormal heart rhythm should also be the same. This article takes a particular interest in woman number 2. It is worth remembering, however, that woman number 1 could become woman number 2. The treatment decisions in women of childbearing age should always take that into consideration. A drug or procedure can affect a subsequent pregnancy. Although it could be argued that the treatment could be changed at the time a pregnancy occurs, many are unplanned and exposure to treatment or to untreated heart disease could occur when the fetus is most vulnerable.

KEY POINTS OF ARRHYTHMIA MANAGEMENT DURING PREGNANCY

- Document the rhythm before treatment. All treatments carry some risk to the mother

Disclosures: The author has no disclosures.
Legacy Good Samaritan Hospital and Medical Center, 1015 NW 22nd Avenue W-302, Portland, OR 97210, USA
E-mail address: jmcanult@lhs.org

Cardiol Clin 30 (2012) 425–434
doi:10.1016/j.ccl.2012.04.002
0733-8651/12/$ – see front matter © 2012 Elsevier Inc. All rights reserved.

and fetus, thus it is essential to know the reason for their use. The diagnostic criteria for arrhythmias are not changed by pregnancy.

- Treat hemodynamically significant rhythms early. During pregnancy, the mother's cardiovascular adaptations allow adequate blood flow to both the fetus and herself, with the uterus receiving 17% of the cardiac output at term (compared with the usual 2%) along with increased flow to the kidneys, breast, and skin. If the mother's own perfusion is compromised significantly, uterine vascular constriction will occur to allow vital maternal organ perfusion. Symptomatic rhythms in combination with the associated increased catecholamine levels and volume shifts may compromise uterine blood flow. Thus, pregnancy adds a sense of urgency to treat. Late in pregnancy, the uterus can obstruct the venous return through the inferior vena cava. The supine position should be discouraged during a symptomatic arrhythmia in favor of her lying on her left side.
- Evaluate for potential reversible causes. This point is important not only because it may be the optimal way to treat rhythms but also because the cause itself may require specific treatment for other reasons. Drugs, either those prescribed or those taken without prescription, are always suspect.
- Avoid drugs if possible. But, use drugs if necessary for maternal or fetal safety. All drugs used to treat an arrhythmia cross the placenta resulting in fetal exposure, and most are categorized as Food and Drug Administration (FDA) class C: "No adequate studies in humans. Teratogenicity has been shown in animals for some."[1] An implication of this is that there is not clear evidence for fetal harm. This point is generally interpreted to mean that the use of these drugs for maternal and fetal safety is justified. Expectant parents, like all patients, should be advised of both the purpose of the drug use and the potential concerns.
- Avoid procedures requiring an X ray until after the pregnancy. Fetal exposure to radiation can be teratogenic and may result in subsequent malignancies. If required during pregnancy for maternal safety, low-dose imaging with abdominal shielding should be used.
- Evaluate cardiac anatomy in those with sustained arrhythmias. An anatomic abnormality itself may require attention. Because the significance of rhythms varies depending on associated cardiac abnormalities, it would help dictate the need for the treatment of arrhythmias.
- Incorporate the expertise of a neonatologist in cases when a concern about fetal distress can influence treatment decisions. These colleagues can provide guidance.

The title of this section implies these key points relate to woman number 2. They are also reasonable recommendations for woman number 1.

ARRHYTHMIAS ARE COMMON IN PREGNANCY AND THE INCIDENCE IS INCREASING

Despite this being a time of improving care of heart disease, arrhythmias, and pregnancy, the incidence of arrhythmias is probably increasing. Two explanations are likely:

1. Increasing age: Pregnancy is increasingly common in women in their thirties and forties. Aging of the heart itself may increase arrhythmias but it also results in an increased chance of an associated disease process that is likely to increase the chance of heart disease and arrhythmias. The most obvious of these are hypertension, adult onset diabetes, atherosclerotic vascular disease, and chronic kidney disease.
2. Treatment success: Paradoxically, successful treatment of heart disease in infants and children has resulted in an increase in the prevalence of heart disease in women capable of having a successful pregnancy. Their children have a 5% to 50% chance of having a cardiac defect compared with 0.8% of all children born in the United States. These children, in turn, have an increased chance of reaching childbearing age, amplifying this phenomenon.

Arrhythmias are more common in women with heart disease. This fact is already apparent as evidenced in a population of women with congenital heart disease (**Fig. 1**).[2] Overall, 4.5% of women with congenital heart disease were determined to have arrhythmias compared with less than 1% of patients without recognized heart disease. If premature beats themselves are considered an arrhythmia, more than 50% of pregnant women have atrial or ventricular premature beats, which is a number that increases still further if there is any associated heart disease.[2–4]

> **Our 2 women**
>
> And so, it is not a great surprise to see women number 2. Since she is pregnant, her chance of having an arrhythmia exceeds that of woman number 1.

> **Our 2 women**
>
> It is important to avoid testing requiring radiation in woman number 2 if possible.
>
> This advice is not unreasonable for woman number 1 given the increasing concerns about serial studies, particularly computed tomography scans, and the accumulating adverse effects.
>
> In woman number 1, the possibility of an unknown pregnancy should be considered before any study.

DIAGNOSTIC TESTING DURING PREGNANCY

- *Rhythm detection*: The electrocardiogram, Holter monitoring, rhythm event monitor, and implantable loop recorder can be used as in nonpregnant patients. Standard exercise and tilt testing are appropriate if considered diagnostically useful.
- *Imaging*: Occasionally, imaging is important for understanding prognosis and guiding therapy. Echocardiography carries no risks to the fetus or the mother; the only concerns are general overuse, expense, and the potential misinterpretation of the changes of a normal pregnancy. On occasion, cardiac magnetic resonance imaging may be indicated (for example, in an assessment for an arrhythmogenic right ventricular dysplasia [ARVD]). It is safe during pregnancy, although gadolinium should not be used. If possible, procedures requiring radiation should be avoided. If they are required for maternal safety, efforts to minimize radiation dose and to use abdominal shielding are important.

TREATMENT OPTIONS
Eliminate Offending Causes

Drugs top the list, but metabolic and endocrine abnormalities (particularly hyperthyroidism given its prevalence of 0.5% in pregnancies) are additional potentially reversible causes.

Antiarrhythmic Drugs

All drugs used to treat arrhythmias cross the placenta and most are found in breast milk. There is insufficient evidence for each to be certain that they can be used safely. There is little enough information about drugs that have been available for many years that these old drugs are not clearly distinguishable from the newer drugs in regard to fetal safety. In this regard, the use of newer drugs seems justifiable if they have a significant

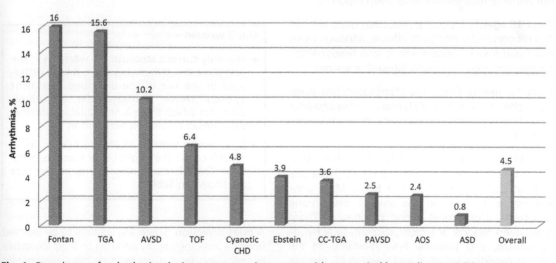

Fig. 1. Prevalence of arrhythmias during pregnancy in women with congenital heart disease. AOS, aortic stenosis; ASD, atrial septal defect, AVSD, atrioventricular septal defect; CC-TGA, congenital corrected transposition of the great arteries; CHD, congenital heart disease; Ebstein, Ebstein anomaly; Fontan, patients after Fontan repair; PAVSD, pulmonary atresia with ventricular septal defect; TGA, transposition of the great arteries; TOF, tetralogy of Fallot. (*Data from* Drenthen W, Pieper PG, Roos-Hesselink JW, et al. Outcome of pregnancy in women with congenital heart disease: a literature review. J Am Coll Cardiol 2007;49:2303–11.)

advantage over the old in protecting the mother. As always, the parents should understand the potential risks. As noted previously, most are considered FDA class C drugs. The current single most agreed on absolute regarding avoiding a drug relates to warfarin; it should not be used in the first trimester and preferably not at the time of labor and delivery.[5–10]

Atrioventricular node blocking agents

All beta-blockers have the potential for influencing fetal and newborn size, but only atenolol is singled out as being an FDA class D drug in this regard (ie, some evidence for harm to the fetus). The rest are FDA class B or C.

Digoxin (Lanoxin), verapamil (Calan), diltiazem (Cardizem, Dilacor), and adenosine (Adenocard) have their usual efficacy without adversely affecting the fetus.

Antiarrhythmia drugs (Vaughan-Williams classification)

Class IA drugs Modern arrhythmia treatment trends might make providers surprised to hear a discussion of these drugs. Experience during pregnancy is greater with quinidine (Quinaglute) than with all the other drugs. Probably many of you reading this article have never used this drug. It is difficult to recommend that you begin your experience with a pregnant woman, but it has been successful in treating both maternal and fetal arrhythmias. Procainamide (Pronestyl) and disopyramide (Norpace) use has been limited, but minimal fetal effects have been reported.

Class 1B agents Lidocaine has been used without any recognized teratogenic effects, although there has been some concern about fetal bradycardia. Experience with mexiletine (Mexitil) is sparse.

Class 1C agents Flecainide (Tambocor) has been used effectively to treat maternal rhythms and fetal arrhythmias. Less is known about propafenone (Rythmol).

Class III agents Sotalol (Betapace) has been effective in treating both fetal and maternal arrhythmias without apparent harm to the fetus. Most controversy exists around the use of amiodarone (Pacerone, Cordarone) during pregnancy. There have been reports of hypothyroidism, fetal hypothyroidism, and possible fetal mortality. In the largest reported series, it was used in 26 women to treat fetal arrhythmias without any recognized adverse fetal effects.[10] This finding has also been true when it has been used to treat maternal arrhythmias.[4] In balance, its use also seems reasonable if maternal safety is a concern. There

are isolated cases reports on the use of dofetilide (Tikosyn), dronedarone (Multaq), and ibutilide (Corvert).

Antithrombotic drugs

Given the potential thromboembolic complications of arrhythmias, antithrombotic drugs may be required. An increased recognition of atrial flutter (Aflutter) and atrial fibrillation (AFib) during pregnancy (often associated with heart disease and previous heart surgery) makes this discussion increasingly relevant. Aspirin (ASA) has potential detrimental effects, such as premature closure of the ductus arteriosus, fetal bleeding, and growth retardation. All of this has earned aspirin a class D by the FDA. Others have given it a class C rating. Warfarin (Coumadin) should not be used in the first trimester because of its teratogenicity (arguably the only absolute drug prohibition rule) and at the time of delivery because of the bleeding risks. Heparin and the low molecular weight heparins (LMWH) (enoxaparin [Lovenox], dalteparin [Fragmin]) do not cross the placenta and can be used for the standard indications. Despite the need for parenteral administration, they are the medication of choice in the first trimester and at labor and delivery. The platelet inhibitors (clopidogrel [Plavix], prasugrel [Effient], and the 2b3a inhibitors) are all considered FDA class C with isolated reports of use without fetal harm. There is no information available about the direct thrombin inhibitor dabigatran (Pradaxa) or the factor 10A inhibitors, rivaroxaban (Xarelto) or apixaban (Eliquis).

> **Our 2 women**
>
> - The only current absolute: no warfarin in the first trimester. Otherwise, there is little difference in the use of the described treatment options. Newer cardiovascular arrhythmic drugs for which there is no available information should be chosen with this in mind.
>
> - Drug use in woman #1 should take in mind consideration she might be, or become, pregnant. Overall, the author's drug preferences are shown in **Table 1**.

A brief diversion There are lessons to be learned from neonatologists. In addition to their expertise in assessing fetal distress, they have experience in treating fetal arrhythmias by administering antiarrhythmic drugs to the mother. Between 1% and 3% of all fetuses have an arrhythmia; most have atrial or ventricular ectopy. About 10% of fetal arrhythmias are sustained and increase the risk of fetal hydrops

Table 1
Antiarrhythmic drugs during pregnancy: author's preference

	IV	Oral
AV node blocking agents	adenosine metoprolol verapamil	metoprolol verapamil digoxin
Antiarrhythmic agents	lidocaine amiodarone	flecainide sotalol quinidine
Antithrombotic agents	LMWH heparin	Aspirin[a] warfarin (second & third trimester)

Abbreviations: AV, atrioventricular; IV, intravenous.
[a] Dose of 325 mg daily for prevention of thrombo-emboli.

and fetal death. The most common of these rhythms seems to be paroxysmal supraventricular tachycardia (PSVT) or Aflutter. Sustained fetal arrhythmias are associated with a 2% to 30% incidence of fetal mortality.[11,12]

Success in treating fetal arrhythmias has been achieved by treating mothers with both intravenous and oral medications. Digoxin, quinidine, flecainide, sotalol, and amiodarone have been used most often. This fact offers some comfort regarding fetal safety when using the drugs to treat a maternal arrhythmia. Although fetal mortality is thought to be related to its arrhythmia or the associated heart disease, because drugs have been used, their role cannot be excluded.

Cardioversion has been used in pregnancy without any reported adverse fetal effects.[13]

Ablation Procedures

There are few reports about the efficacy and safety of ablation procedures during pregnancy. They can be performed and be effective.[13] Potential fetal risks are radiation exposure and anesthetic drugs. Increased reliance on echocardiography to guide the procedure can decrease irradiation. In balance, if medication can achieve reasonable rhythm control, it is preferable to defer ablation until the pregnancy is completed.

Device Insertion

Again, it is the use of radiation that would seem to be the greatest risk of inserting either a pacemaker or defibrillator during pregnancy. If it is essential for maternal safety, either can be inserted while attempting to minimize the radiation used. Neither cardiac pacing nor defibrillator discharge has been reported to adversely affect the fetus.[14]

ARRHYTHMIAS
Tachyarrhythmias

Sinus tachycardia

This most common of tachycardias by at least 10^{10} (author's estimate) is a common cause of tachycardia-related hospital admission during pregnancy (**Fig. 2**).[15]

The resting sinus node rate increases gradually through pregnancy by about 20 beats per minute. It rarely exceeds 100 beats per minutes. Rates faster than this are a reason to assess the electrocardiogram carefully to be certain that the rhythm is originating in the sinus node. If it is sinus tachycardia, there may be an explainable cause; again, drugs should be considered. It may signal hyperthyroidism, which occurs in 1 in 200 pregnancies. As in nonpregnant women, it may go unexplained and is labeled inappropriate sinus tachycardia. The postural orthostatic tachycardia syndrome is one variant of this. (The rate increases by greater than 30 beats per minute when going from the supine to standing position). It is common in young women (5:1 female-to-male ratio) but does not adversely affect a pregnancy.[16,17] Unless associated with unacceptable symptoms, treatment of sinus tachycardia is not appropriate. If symptoms are not acceptable, treatment with a beta-blocker is occasionally successful.

Ectopy

Atrial and ventricular premature beats are common, occurring in more than 50% of pregnancies. As in nonpregnant individuals, premature beats are often described as a skipped beat. Shotan and colleagues[3] found that palpitations do not always correlate well with these beats (**Table 2**). Only 10% of episodes of palpitations were associated with an arrhythmia. This evaluation also revealed ectopic beats in more than 50% of pregnancies with a decrease in frequency postpartum.

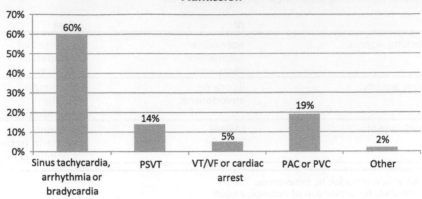

Fig. 2. Distribution of various arrhythmias in women hospitalized because of an arrhythmia during pregnancy. PAC, premature atrial complex; PVC, premature ventricular complex; VF, ventricular fibrillation; VT, ventricular tachycardia. (*Data from* Li JM, Nguyen C, Joglar JA, et al. Frequency and outcome of arrhythmias complicating admission during pregnancy: experience from a high-volume and ethnically diverse obstetric service. Clin Cardiol 2008;31:538–41.)

Neither atrial nor ventricular ectopy has been associated with increased morbidity or mortality during pregnancy. Although not required for protection, beta-blockers or an antiarrhythmic drug can be used if symptoms are intolerable.

Paroxysmal supraventricular tachycardia

This is the most common non-sinus tachycardia tachycardia in women of childbearing age. (That awkward sentence is left in as a reminder to consider sinus tachycardia in the differential diagnosis of any regular tachycardia.) In their series of 207 young women with PSVT, Lee and colleagues[18] confirmed dual atrioventricular (AV) node physiology as the mechanism in 48% (AV node reentry tachycardia [AVNRT]). In the other 52% of these women, the PSVT resulted from

accessory atrial ventricular pathways (atrial ventricular reentry tachycardia [AVRT]). In this latter group with 127 accessory pathways, only 32% had evidence of preexcitation on the resting electrocardiogram (ECG) (a short PR interval with the delta wave, ie, the Wolff Parkinson White syndrome [WPW]). Both mechanisms are a form of congenital heart disease with not fully defined transmission patterns. Accessory pathways can be associated with structural heart disease, the two most common being Ebstein anomaly and hypertrophic obstructive cardiomyopathy.

Eighty-four percent of the 207 women had at least one pregnancy. The PSVT was noted for the first time during pregnancy in 7/107 (6%) of those with AVRT and in only 1/100 (1%) of those with AVNRT. Although this would suggest that pregnancy will not necessarily cause PSVT if a woman has not had it, others have noted PSVT presenting for the first time in pregnancy in up to 90%.[15] There is more agreement that women with PSVT before pregnancy are likely to have a recurrence during pregnancy.[4,18]

The treatment of PSVT in pregnancy should be the same as in nonpregnant women, although with a heightened sense of urgency. Because a sympathetic tone is a little higher during pregnancy, valsalva maneuvers and carotid massage may be less successful. Adenosine (12 mg) (or intravenous verapamil or metoprolol) is highly effective in terminating the rhythm. If the PSVT is a recurrence, daily oral verapamil (240 mg) or metoprolol (50–100 mg) may prevent further episodes. If not, an antiarrhythmic drug may be

Table 2 Pregnant women with no heart disease[a]	
With Palpitations	**No Palpitations**
PACs 56%	58%
>100/hour 7%	4%
PVCs 59%	50%
>50/hour 22%	2%

Abbreviations: PAC, premature atrial complex; PVC, premature ventricular complex.

[a] No known heart disease.

Data from Shotan A, Ostrzega E, Mehra A, et al. Incidence of arrhythmias in normal pregnancy and relation to palpitations, dizziness, and syncope. Am J Cardiol 1997;79(8):1061–4.

successful. Ablations can and have been performed successfully; radiation exposure should be minimized.

There are consequences of having PSVT before or during pregnancy: (1) recurrence is likely, (2) rhythms are more symptomatic,[3] and (3) the rhythms are associated with an increased risk of fetal complications.[4] Although successful ablations before pregnancy have not been proven to change these, they are a reason to consider that treatment before pregnancy in women with PSVT or preexcitation on the ECG.

Our 2 women

- Given the presentation, the implied good health, the young age and the documented heart rate, PSVT is the most likely explanation for the tachycardia in both of our women. Acute management should be the same except for a somewhat greater sense of urgency in women number 2.

- If there is a recurrence in women number 2, treatment with verapamil or metoprolol is appropriate. If women number 1 is considering pregnancy , an ablation procedure is reasonable given the consequences of the rhythm during pregnancy as just mentioned in the above text.

Atrial tachycardia/ectopic atrial tachycardia
This arrhythmia is noted only occasionally during pregnancy. The reports have focused on the incessant nature of the rhythms. Maintaining reasonable hemodynamics with rate control or antiarrhythmic drug suppression of the ectopic focus will allow completion of a successful pregnancy.

AFib and Aflutter
Why are these rhythms being discussed? They are uncommon in women of childbearing age. Yes, but they are occurring more frequently. This result is another of the seemingly paradoxic results of successful heart treatment. Women who have had previous surgical or catheter treatment of structural heart disease are more prone to developing these rhythms.[4]

If AFib or Aflutter results in a rapid ventricular response, urgent treatment is required. Intravenous verapamil (or metoprolol or diltiazem) will likely slow the ventricular rate by at least a third. If this is not achieved, cardioversion proceeded by moderate sedation should be performed. Once the rate is controlled, chronic treatment decisions can be considered.

AFib and Aflutter are associated with an increased risk of a thromboembolic stroke. Women of childbearing age, pregnant or not, have not been included in studies evaluating prophylactic antithrombotic treatment. Still, these studies can be used as guides. Women with AFib or Aflutter (paroxysmal or persistent) who have had a stroke (or who have a mechanical valve) should be on an anticoagulant: LMWH in the first trimester and the last weeks of the third trimester and warfarin in the second and early third trimester. Given the hypercoagulable state of pregnancy, all others should be on daily aspirin (325 mg). There is no evidence that a lesser dose provides stroke prevention.

Regarding the rhythm itself, if rate control is easily achieved and the woman becomes asymptomatic, oral metoprolol or verapamil can be continued throughout pregnancy. If neither of these is true, cardioversion can be performed and a decision made about the institution of an antiarrhythmic drug. Again, flecainide or sotalol are the optimal choices.

In general, treatment of Aflutter should be the same as for AFib. But if recurrent Aflutter is a problem despite drug treatment and by the ECG, it is likely to be a tricuspid annulus/inferior vena cava isthmus-dependent rhythm; ablation can be a consideration given the relative efficacy and safety of that procedure.

Wide QRS tachycardias
Diagnosis of the regular QRS tachycardias is as difficult during pregnancy as at other times. Clues suggestive (although not diagnostic) of ventricular tachycardia (VT) include a QRS greater than 0.14 seconds with a slurred initial vector (ugly wide). Precordial QRS concordance is near diagnostic of VT.[19] A response to a vagal maneuver or adenosine would make a supraventricular rhythm most likely.

VT does occur in pregnancy. Centers reporting on structural heart disease in pregnancy report on many different mechanisms[4] with some presumably scar-based from previous surgery. Acute treatment should include the drugs or cardioversion needed to protect the mother.[20] Reports from outside the large referral centers include more women without structural heart disease and with more benign VTs.[21] These conditions are frequently compatible with a right ventricular outflow tract (RVOT) tachycardia (left bundle branch block and vertical axis morphology). These conditions are often effectively suppressed with beta-blockers or verapamil. Ablation can be considered after the pregnancy if the rhythm does not respond to chronic treatment with drugs.

If the ventricular pattern is chaotically irregular, AFib is the likely mechanism no matter what the

Our 2 women

If not PSVT/AT, the other rhythm most likely in this presenting woman would be VT given the presentation and the rate and regularity of the rhythm. If the ECG reveals a wide QRS, treatment as discussed in this article is appropriate for both women. From the brief histories, it is not implied that either has structural heart disease or previous heart surgery. This factor makes an RVOT tachycardia somewhat more likely.

QRS morphology. Although examples of ECGs could be shown for any of the rhythms discussed in this article, that shown in **Fig. 3** is the chosen one because of the importance of considering accessory pathway conduction as a possible cause of the wide QRS and treating accordingly. In this young population, the wide QRS complex should increase suspicion of antegrade accessory pathway conduction (although normal pathway conduction with bundle branch block is possible). Initial treatment with metoprolol may be ineffective (verapamil and digoxin should not be used). Intravenous procainamide or lidocaine may block or slow pathway conduction. Cardioversion may be required.

Bradycardia

Sinus node dysfunction resulting in bradycardia is rare in pregnancy, although its incidence may increase in those with complex congenital heart disease. Symptomatic sinoatrial arrest should optimally be treated before pregnancy. Temporary and permanent pacing can be performed during pregnancy if required (minimizing irradiation) for maternal safety or fetal distress. Here an evaluation of the fetus by a neonatologist may be helpful.

A common bradycardia situation in young people relates to the vasovagal or neurocardiogenic syndrome. Despite the volume, hormonal and possibly neurologic changes of pregnancy, there is no reported consistent improvement or exacerbation of symptom in patients with this syndrome. The supine hypotension syndrome of pregnancy (syncope when supine, relief from lateral position) may involve an abnormal parasympathetic response along with the inferior vena caval obstruction, but a bradycardia has not been identified as a significant component.

Although 1° AV block or Mobitz type I, 2° AV block are reasons to assess for a cause, treatment is rarely indicated. Acquired Mobitz type II, 2° AV block or complete heart block require permanent

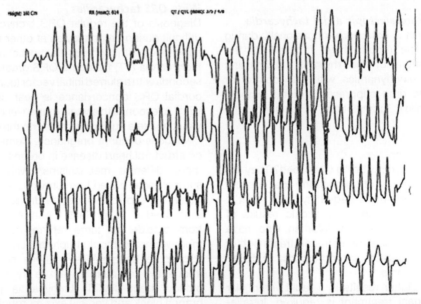

Fig. 3. This rhythm tracing is the one chosen in this article because of its potential consequence and the need to consider treatment limitations. It shows a variable QRS width and an irregular tachycardia. It is from a woman with WPW when she developed syncopal atrial fibrillation. Because of likely accessory pathway conduction, AV node blocking agents could not be relied on to slow the ventricular rate, which approaches 300 beats per minute. Calcium blockers and digoxin should not be used because they might actually accelerate pathway conduction. The irregularity makes it atrial fibrillation. She was sedated and cardioverted successfully and subsequently underwent pathway ablation. She was not pregnant but she was planning a pregnancy.

pacemaker treatment. Controversy exists about congenital complete heart block unrelated to pregnancy.[22] Increasingly, permanent pacing is the preferred approach, even when the rhythm is first recognized in pregnancy. Again, by assessing fetal distress, the neonatologist may help define the need for a pacemaker.

REPOLARIZATION ABNORMALITIES ASSOCIATED WITH VENTRICULAR TACHYCARDIA
Long QT Syndrome

This syndrome is the most common arrhythmogenic repolarization abnormality syndrome in women of childbearing age.[23–26] Drugs are a common and potentially reversible cause. A specific genetic mutation can be defined as a cause in up to 70% of those with a congenital long QTc. Although there are at least 10 known mutations, $LQTC_1$ occurs in about 50%, $LQTC_2$ in about 45%, and $LQTC_3$ in 5% with very small numbers with the other mutation. In the patients with LQT_1 and LQT_2, adverse cardiac events are not clearly increased during pregnancy but are increased in the first 9 postpartum months. Women with LQT_3 may have a higher incidence of arrhythmia during pregnancy. Beta-blocker drugs have a protective effect and are recommended during and after pregnancy. A woman with a long QTc presenting with syncope or VT during pregnancy presents a dilemma. Beta-blocker therapy should be started. If it is late in pregnancy, some have advised hospitalization with rhythm monitoring until the baby is delivered.

ARVD, Brugada Syndrome, Catecholaminergic VT

As might be expected in rhythm syndromes that are so uncommon, there are only anecdotal reports of their association with pregnancy and there are no patterns that can guide treatment recommendations.[25]

Our 2 women

- Assessing the ECG during and after the arrhythmia is important in defining the mechanism of the rhythm.
- An ECG looking for repolarization abnormalities would have been important if either woman had presented with syncope, palpitations, or a family history of early sudden death.

CARDIAC ARREST

Whatever the arrhythmia or nonarrhythmic cause, cardiopulmonary resuscitation should be performed. If it occurs in late pregnancy, tilting the abdomen/pelvis up on the left side may enhance the venous return by decreasing uterine compression of the inferior vena cava. If the pregnancy is greater than 28 weeks, an emergency cesarean section should be considered and has been performed.[27]

SUMMARY

Finally, it seems the approach to our 2 women should not be all that different. Some final reminders in relation to pregnancy itself:

1. Treat hemodynamically significant arrhythmias with more urgency.
2. Consider risks to the fetus when choosing treatment.
3. Defer radiation procedures to after delivery if possible.

REFERENCES

1. Federal Register. 2008; vol. 73: p. 104.
2. Drenthen W, Pieper PG, Roos-Hesselink JW, et al. Outcome of pregnancy in women with congenital heart disease: a literature review. J Am Coll Cardiol 2007;49:2303–11.
3. Shotan A, Ostrzega E, Mehra A, et al. Incidence of arrhythmias in normal pregnancy and relation to palpitations, dizziness, and syncope. Am J Cardiol 1997;79(8):1061–4.
4. Silversides CK, Harris L, Haberer K, et al. Recurrence rates of arrhythmias during pregnancy in women with previous tachyarrhythmia and impact on fetal and neonatal outcomes. Am J Cardiol 2006;97(8):1206–12.
5. Mitani GM, Steinberg I, Lien EJ, et al. The pharmacokinetics of antiarrhythmic agents in pregnancy and lactation. Clin Pharmacokinet 1987; 12(4):253–91.
6. Qasqas SA, McPherson C, Frishman WH, et al. Cardiovascular pharmacotherapeutic considerations during pregnancy and lactation. Cardiol Rev 2004; 12:201–21.
7. Adamson DL, Nelson-Piercy C. Managing palpitations and arrhythmias during pregnancy. Heart 2007;93:1630–6.
8. Burkart TA, Conti JB. Cardiac arrhythmias during pregnancy. Curr Treat Options Cardiovasc Med 2010;12(5):457–71.
9. Elkayam U, Goodwin TM. Adenosine therapy for supraventricular tachycardia during pregnancy. Am J Cardiol 1995;75(7):521–3.

10. Strasburger JF, Cuneo BF, Michon MM, et al. Amiodarone therapy for drug-refractory fetal tachycardia. Circulation 2004;109(3):375–9.

11. Strasburger JF, Cheulkar B, Wichman HJ. Perinatal arrhythmias: diagnosis and management. Clin Perinatol 2007;34(4):627–52.

12. Srinivasan S, Strasburger J. Overview of fetal arrhythmias. Curr Opin Pediatr 2008;20(5):522–31.

13. Trappe HJ. Emergency therapy of maternal and fetal arrhythmias during pregnancy. J Emerg Trauma Shock 2010;3(2):153–9.

14. Natale A, Davidson T, Geiger MJ, et al. Implantable cardioverter-defibrillators and pregnancy. A safe combination? Circulation 1997;96:2808–12.

15. Li JM, Nguyen C, Joglar JA, et al. Frequency and outcome of arrhythmias complicating admission during pregnancy: experience from a high-volume and ethnically diverse obstetric service. Clin Cardiol 2008;31:538–41.

16. Kanjwal K, Karabin B, Kanjwal Y, et al. Outcomes of pregnancy in patients with preexisting postural tachycardia syndrome. Pacing Clin Electrophysiol 2009;32(8):1000–3.

17. Kimpinski K, Iodice V, Sandroni P, et al. Effect of pregnancy on postural tachycardia syndrome. Mayo Clin Proc 2010;85(7):639–94.

18. Lee SH, Chen SA, Wu TJ, et al. Effects of pregnancy on first onset and symptoms of paroxysmal supraventricular tachycardia. Am J Cardiol 1995;76:675–8.

19. Wellens HJ. Electrophysiology: ventricular tachycardia: diagnosis of broad QRS complex tachycardia. Heart 2001;86(5):579–85.

20. Kron J, Conti JB. Arrhythmias in the pregnant patient: current concepts in evaluation and management. J Interv Card Electrophysiol 2007;19(2):95–107.

21. Nakagawa M, Katou S, Ichinose M, et al. Characteristics of new-onset ventricular arrhythmias in pregnancy. J Electrocardiol 2004;37(1):47–53.

22. Epstein AE, DiMarco JP, Ellenbogen KA, et al. ACC/AHA/HRS 2008 guidelines for device-based therapy of cardiac rhythm abnormalities: a report of the American College of Cardiology/American Heart Association Task Force on Practice Guidelines (Writing Committee to Revise the ACC/AHA/NASPE 2002 Guideline Update for Implantation of Cardiac Pacemakers and Antiarrhythmia Devices): developed in collaboration with the American Association for Thoracic Surgery and Society of Thoracic Surgeons. Circulation 2008;117:e350.

23. Rashba EJ, Zareba W, Moss AJ, et al. Influence of pregnancy on the risk of cardiac events in patients with hereditary long QT syndrome. Circulation 1998;97(5):451–6.

24. Khositseth A, Tester DJ, Will ML, et al. Identification of a common genetic substrate underlying postpartum cardiac events in congenital long QT syndrome. Heart Rhythm 2004;1(1):60–4.

25. Heradien MJ, Goosen A, Crotti L, et al. Does pregnancy increase cardiac risk for LQT1 patients with the KCNQ1-A341V mutation? J Am Coll Cardiol 2006;48(7):1410–5.

26. Seth R, Moss AJ, McNitt S, et al. Long QT syndrome and pregnancy. J Am Coll Cardiol 2007;49:1092–8.

27. American Heart Association and the International Liason Committee on Resuscitation. Guidelines 2000 for cardiopulmonary resuscitation and emergency cardiovascular care. Part 8: advanced challenges in resuscitation. Section 3: special challenges in ECC. 3F: cardiac arrest associated with pregnancy. Circulation 2000;102(Suppl 8):1247–9.

Peripartum Cardiomyopathy

Uri Elkayam, MD[a,b,*], Sawan Jalnapurkar, MD[a,b],
Mohamad Barakat, MD[a,b]

KEYWORDS

- Pregnancy • Peripartum cardiomyopathy • Bromocriptine • Pentoxifylline • BNP • Heart failure
- Cardiac transplantation

KEY POINTS

- Peripartum cardiomyopathy (PPCM) has a higher incidence in women older than 30 years, in patients with a history of hypertension and preeclampsia, in multifetal pregnancies, and in African American women in the United States.
- PPCM can be associated with severe complications, including pulmonary edema, cardiogenic shock, arrhythmias, thromboembolic events, and mortality.
- Treatment of heart failure in patients with PPCM should follow recent guideline recommendations; drug therapy may need to be changed during pregnancy and lactation to prevent side effects to the fetus or lactating infant.
- In patients who are diagnosed during pregnancy and can be stabilized with therapy, continuation of pregnancy to allow fetal maturity may be possible under close monitoring. Termination of pregnancy often results in improvement of both symptoms and cardiac function and should be considered in patients with deteriorating symptoms or cardiac function.

DEFINITION

In 1971, Demakis and colleagues[1] established the term peripartum cardiomyopathy (PPCM) and defined it by the following criteria based on the clinical profile of their patients:

1. Development of heart failure (HF) in the last month of pregnancy or within 5 months of delivery
2. Absence of a determinable cause for HF
3. Absence of demonstrable heart disease before the last month of pregnancy
4. Left ventricular (LV) systolic dysfunction demonstrated by echocardiography with LV ejection fraction (EF) less than 45%, fractional shortening less than 30% or both is an additional criterion added in 1997 by a National Heart, Lung, and Blood Institute workshop on PPCM[2]; the criterion had been previously proposed by Hibbard and colleagues.[3]

Realizing that these criteria are arbitrary and that PPCM often presents earlier in pregnancy,[4–6] the definition of PPCM has been recently updated by a working group on PPCM of the European Society of Cardiology: "idiopathic cardiomyopathy presenting with HF secondary to LV systolic dysfunction toward the end of pregnancy or in the months following delivery where no other cause of HF is found. The left ventricle (LV) may not be dilated but the ejection fraction (EF) is nearly always reduced below 45%".[7]

INCIDENCE

The incidence of PPCM in the United States has ranged in different publications between 1:1149 and 1:4350 live births,[8–11] with an average of 1:3186. A significantly higher incidence[12,13] has been reported in South Africa (1:1000) and Haiti

a Division of Cardiology, Department of Medicine, University of Southern California Keck School of Medicine, Los Angeles, CA, USA; b Department of Obstetrics and Gynecology, University of Southern California Keck School of Medicine, Los Angeles, CA, USA
* Corresponding author. LAC/USC Medical Center, 2020 Zonal Avenue, Los Angeles, CA 90033.
E-mail address: elkayam@usc.edu

Cardiol Clin 30 (2012) 435–440
doi:10.1016/j.ccl.2012.04.009
0733-8651/12/$ – see front matter © 2012 Elsevier Inc. All rights reserved.

cardiology.theclinics.com

(1:300). No information is available regarding the incidence of this condition in Europe.

CAUSE

The cause of PPCM is still unknown and many potential theories have been proposed and discussed in details in a recent review.[14] The most recent hypothesis is based on experimental work that has demonstrated the development of PPCM in female mice with a cardiomyocyte-specific deletion of signal transducer and activator of transcription 3.[15] This study suggested that an unprotected increase in oxidative stress leads to increased expression and proteolytic activity of cardiac cathepsin D, which results in conversion of the nursing hormone prolactin into an antiangiogenic and proapoptotic 16-kDa form with a detrimental effect on coronary microvasculature resulting in a myocardial insult caused by hypoxemia and apoptosis.

RISK FACTORS

The incidence of PPCM has been found to be higher in women older than 30 years, in patients with a history of hypertension and preeclampsia, multifetal pregnancies, and in African American women in the United States.[4] In addition, recent studies have demonstrated a high incidence of PPCM in families with dilated cardiomyopathies[16,17] suggesting that in a proportion of patients, PPCM may have a genetic cause.[6]

CLINICAL PRESENTATION

Many of the signs and symptoms of PPCM are similar to those of HF caused by other factors. Because normal pregnancy is often associated with signs and symptoms that can mimic those of HF, the diagnosis of PPCM is often missed or delayed.[18]

Biomarkers

B-type natriuretic peptide (BNP) levels remain grossly unchanged during normal pregnancy and are only mildly elevated in women with preeclampsia.[19] Similar to other forms of HF, BNP levels increase significantly in symptomatic patients with PPCM.[20] Troponin can be slightly elevated, especially in patients with a substantial myocardial insult at the time of the diagnosis.[21]

Laboratory Evaluation

An electrocardiogram usually shows sinus tachycardia and nonspecific ST-segment and T-wave changes. LV hypertrophy and conduction abnormalities can also be seen. A chest radiograph commonly demonstrates cardiomegaly, pulmonary venous congestion, and occasionally pulmonary edema and pleural effusion. An echocardiogram shows a dilated LV size in most patients but can also be within normal range; dilation of the other cardiac chambers is also commonly found. LV systolic dysfunction is the rule, with moderate to severe depression of LVEF and a small pericardial effusion. Doppler evaluation usually shows moderate to sever mitral and tricuspid valve regurgitation, mild to moderate pulmonic regurgitation, and pulmonary hypertension.[4,7]

PROGNOSIS

PPCM can be associated with severe complications, including pulmonary edema, cardiogenic shock, arrhythmias, thromboembolic events, and mortality.[18]

Mortality

PPCM continues to be an important cause of pregnancy-related death in the United States and other countries.[22,23] The rate of mortality, however, seems to vary geographically and is considerably higher in South Africa (28%–40%), Haiti (15%–30%), and Turkey (30%) compared with the United States where the reported mortality rate from PPCM has been lower than from other forms of cardiomyopathies and has varied between 0% and 19%.[9-11,24-30] The risk of death increases with older age, severe myocardial insult (LVEF <25%), multiparity, African American ethnicity, and when the diagnosis is delayed.[18,22]

Recovery of Cardiac Function

The most recent publications in the United States have demonstrated improvement of LV function in at least 50% of patients with PPCM, mostly occurring within 2 to 6 months after the diagnosis.[5,28,31] An exception to these findings was reported in 1 US study[30] that found recovery of LV function in only 35% of 40 indigent, mostly African Americans women, with a median time to recovery of 54 months. These data are similar to a low recovery rate of 21% to 43% reported in South Africa, Haiti, and Turkey[7] and suggest that race, ethnicity, and environmental differences as well as access to medical care may be responsible for poorer outcomes.

Outcome of Subsequent Pregnancy

A retrospective study published in 2001 reported on the outcome of 60 subsequent pregnancies in 44 women, 28 with normal LV function (group 1) and 16 with persistent LV dysfunction (group 2).[32]

Subsequent pregnancies were associated with a significant reduction in mean LVEF in both groups. A substantial (>20%) reduction in LVEF was seen in 21% of group 1 and 44% of group 2 patients, there was 0% mortality in group 1 women and 19% in group 2. When aborted pregnancies were excluded, rate of unfavorable maternal and fetal outcome was even higher, especially in women with persistent LV dysfunction, suggesting the rational for early termination of pregnancy in women with severely depressed LV function. A recent publication by Fett and colleagues[33] based on data mostly obtained from an Internet support group in the United States reported on 61 post-PPCM pregnancies, with a relapse of PPCM in 29% of the group and a significantly higher rate (46%) in women with LVEF of less than 55%.

TREATMENT

Standard drug therapy for acute and chronic HF includes the potential use of several drugs, including diuretics, angiotensin converting enzyme (ACE) inhibitors, or angiotensin receptor blockers (ARB) as well as beta-blockers, spironolactone, digoxin, intravenous (IV) and oral vasodilators, and IV inotropes.[34] In general, the treatment of HF in patients with PPCM should follow recent guideline recommendations, although drug therapy may need to be changed during pregnancy and lactation to prevent side effects to the fetus or the lactating infant. The safety of HF therapy in pregnancy and lactation is shown in **Table 1**.

Experimental Therapy

A successful effect of IV immune globulin was reported in a small number of women with PPCM compared with 11 historical control patients who received conventional therapy alone.[35] The study was limited by an open design and a small number of patients. Sliwa and colleagues[36] reported a significant improvement in a combined end point of death, persistent LV dysfunction, or NYHA functional class III to IV at the last follow-up in a group of South African women with PPCM treated with pentoxifylline. However, no further studies have been performed to confirm these results. More recently, Sliwa and colleagues[25] have used bromocriptine, a prolactin blocker in the treatment of 10 South African patients with PPCM. The treatment was associated with a significantly larger rate of LV recovery and decreased rate of mortality and symptomatic HF at 6 months compared with a control group of 10 patients with PPCM treated with standard therapy alone. Because of the small number of patients reported and known side

effects of bromocriptine, more information is needed to clearly establish the safety and efficacy of this therapy for the treatment of PPCM.

Implantable Cardioverter-Defibrillators

Because improvement of LV function is common and failure to improve can not be predicted early after diagnosis, the use of a wearable external defibrillator[37] or an entirely subcutaneous implantable cardioverter–defibrillator[38] rather than implantable cardioverter-defibrillators (ICD) should be considered in high-risk patients as a bridge to recovery or to implantable ICD in cases with persistent LV dysfunction despite appropriate trial of medical therapy.

Cardiac Assist Devices

An intra-aortic balloon pump, extracorporeal membrane oxygenation, and LV assist devices have been used successfully as a bridge for recovery or transplantation in patients with PPCM and should be considered in rapidly deteriorating patients who are not responding to medical therapy, including vasoactive medications.[39–42]

Cardiac Transplantation

This procedure has been performed successfully in patients with PPCM. A recent publication by Rasmusson and colleagues[43] reported on 485 women who had PPCM as an indication for cardiac transplantation. Compared with patients with other causes of transplantation, patients with PPCM had more posttransplant rejection during the index transplant hospitalization and during the first year. In addition, graft survival was inferior and age-adjusted survival was lower in patients with PPCM.

LABOR AND DELIVERY

In patients who are diagnosed during pregnancy, the continuation of pregnancy to allow fetal maturity may be possible under close monitoring in a woman who can be stabilized with therapy. The termination of pregnancy often results in the improvement of both symptoms and cardiac function and should be considered in patients with deteriorating symptoms or cardiac function.

The mode of delivery in stable patients with PPCM should be decided jointly by the obstetrician and the cardiologist. In general, vaginal delivery is preferred in stable patients. Cesarean section should be performed for obstetric reasons or because of maternal instability. In cases of vaginal delivery, instrumental delivery is recommended to reduce maternal efforts and shorten labor. Hemodynamic monitoring for labor and

Table 1
Drug safety during pregnancy and lactation

Drug	Risk Category	Information in Humans	Potential Complications	Safety for Breast Feeding
Furosemide	C	Limited	Hypotension and decreased uterine perfusion	Compatible
Intravenous nitroglycerin	B	Modest	Hypotension and decreased uterine perfusion	Unknown
Intravenous nitroprusside	C	Limited	Thiocyanate toxicity	Unknown
Nesiritide	N/A	None	Hypotension and decreased uterine perfusion; effect on the fetus unknown	Unknown
Dopamine	C	Limited	Unknown	Unknown
Dobutamine	B	Limited	Unknown	Unknown
Milrinone	C	Limited	Unknown	Unknown
ACE inhibitors/ ARBs	C	Limited	Renal insufficiency, oligohydramnios, IUGR, prematurity, bony malformation, limb contractures, PDA, pulmonary hypoplasia, RDS, hypotension, anemia, and neonatal death	Compatible
Carvedilol	C	Not available	Unknown, beta 2 receptor blocking may cause premature uterine contractions	Unknown
Bisoprolol	C	Not available	Unknown	Unknown
Metoprolol succinate	C	Not available	Unknown	Unknown
Metoprolol tartrate	C	Modest	Relatively safe	Compatible, monitoring of infants for signs of beta blockade recommended
Digoxin	C	Modest used for both maternal and fetal indications	None reported	Compatible
Spironolactone	C	Limited	Possible antiandrogenic effect and feminization	Compatible
Warfarin	D	Modest	Teratogenic effect in first trimester (warfarin embryopathy), increased maternal and fetal bleeding	Compatible
Heparins	C	Extensive	Do not cross the placenta	Compatible

Abbreviations: IUGR, intrauterine growth retardation; N/A, not available; PDA, patient ductus arteriosus; RDS, respiratory distress syndrome.

delivery is advisable in patients who are diagnosed during pregnancy for hemodynamic optimization before delivery and monitoring during and after the delivery.

REFERENCES

1. Demakis JG, Rahimtoola SH, Sutton GC, et al. Natural course of peripartum cardiomyopathy. Circulation 1971;44:1053–61.
2. Pearson GD, Veille JC, Rahimtoola SH, et al. Peripartum cardiomyopathy: National Heart, Lung, and Blood Institute and Office of Rare Diseases (National Institutes of Health) workshop recommendations and review. JAMA 2000;283:1183–8.
3. Hibbard JU, Lindheimer M, Lang R. A modified definition for peripartum cardiomyopathy and prognosis based on echocardiography. Obstet Gynecol 1999;94:311–6.
4. Lang RM, Lampert MB, Poppas A, et al. Peripartal cardiomyopathy. In: Elkayam U, Gleicher N, editors. Cardiac problems in pregnancy. 3rd edition. New York: Wiley-Liss Inc; 1998. p. 87–100.
5. Elkayam U, Akhter MW, Singh H, et al. Pregnancy-associated cardiomyopathy: clinical characteristics and a comparison between early and late presentation. Circulation 2005;11:2050–5.
6. Anderson JL, Horne BD. Birthing the genetics of peripartum cardiomyopathy. Circulation 2010;121:2157–9.
7. Sliwa K, Hilfiker -Kleiner D, Petrie MC, et al. Current state of knowledge on aetiology, diagnosis, management, and therapy of peripartum cardiomyopathy: a position statement from the Heart Failure Association of European Society of Cardiology Working Group on peripartum cardiomyopathy. Eur J Heart Fail 2010;12:767–78.
8. Witlin AG, Mabie WC, Sibai BM. Peripartum cardiomyopathy: an ominous diagnosis. Am J Obstet Gynecol 1997;176:182–8.
9. Chapa JB, Heiberger HB, Weinert L, et al. Prognostic value of echocardiography in peripartum cardiomyopathy. Obstet Gynecol 2005;105:1303–8.
10. Mielniczuk LM, Williams L, Davis DR, et al. Frequency of peripartum cardiomyopathy. Am J Cardiol 2006;97:1765–8.
11. Brar SS, Khan SS, Sandha GK, et al. Incidence, mortality, and racial differences in peripartum cardiomyopathy. Am J Cardiol 2007;100:302–4.
12. Desai D, Moodley J, Naidoo D. Peripartum cardiomyopathy: experience at King Edward VIII Hospital, Durban, South Africa and review of the literature. Trop Doct 1995;25:118–23.
13. Fett JD, Christie LG, Caraway RD, et al. Five year prospective study of the incidence and properties of peripartum cardiomyopathy at a single institution. Mayo Clin Proc 2005;80:1602–6.
14. Ntusi NB, Mayosi BM. Aetiology and risk factors of peripartum cardiomyopathy a systematic review. Int J Cardiol 2009;131:168–79.
15. Hilfiker-Kleiner D, Kaminski K, Podewski E, et al. A cathepsin D-cleaved 16 kDa form of prolactin mediates postpartum cardiomyopathy. Cell 2007;128:589–600.
16. Morales A, Painter T, Li R, et al. Rare variant mutations in pregnancy-associated or peripartum cardiomyopathy. Circulation 2010;121:2176–82.
17. Van Spaendonck-Zwarts KY, van Tintelen JP, van Veldhuisen DJ, et al. Peripartum cardiomyopathy as a part of familial dilated cardiomyopathy. Circulation 2010;121:2169–75.
18. Goland S, Modi K, Bitar F, et al. Clinical profile and predictors of complications in peripartum cardiomyopathy. J Card Fail 2009;15:645–50.
19. Resnik JL, Hong C, Resnik R, et al. Evaluation of B-type natriuretic peptide (BNP) levels in normal and preeclamptic women. Am J Obstet Gynecol 2005;193:450–4.
20. Forster O, Hilfiker-Kleiner D, Ansari AA, et al. Reversal of IFN-gamma, oxLDL and prolactin serum levels correlate with clinical improvement in patients with peripartum cardiomyopathy. Eur J Heart Fail 2008;10:861–8.
21. Hu CL, Li YB, Fang JH, et al. Troponin T measurement can predict persistent left ventricular dysfunction in peripartum cardiomyopathy. Heart 2007;93:488–90.
22. Whitehead SJ, Berg CJ, Chang J. Pregnancy-related mortality due to cardiomyopathy; United States, 1991-1997. Obstet Gynecol 2003;102:1326–31.
23. Lang CT, King JC. Maternal mortality in the United States. Best Pract Res Clin Obstet Gynaecol 2008;22:517–31.
24. Sliwa K, Forster O, Tibarazwa K, et al. Long term outcome of peripartum cardiomyopathy in a population with high seropositivity for human immunodeficiency virus. Int J Cardiol 2011;147:202–8.
25. Sliwa K, Blauwet Tibazarwa K, et al. Evaluation of bromocriptine in the pilot study. Circulation 2010;121:1465–73.
26. Fett J, Carraway RD, Dowell DL, et al. Peripartum cardiomyopathy in the Hospital Albert Schweitzer District of Haiti. Am J Obstet Gynecol 2009;201:171e1–5.
27. Duran N, Gunes H, Duran I, et al. Predictors of prognosis in patients with peripartum cardiomyopathy. Int J Obstet Gynecol 2008;111:2050–5.
28. Amos A, Jaber WA, Russel SD. Improved outcomes in peripartum cardiomyopathy with contemporary. Am Heart J 2006;152:509–13.
29. Felker GM, Thompson RE, Hare J, et al. Underlying causes and long-term survival in patients with initially unexplained cardiomyopathy. N Engl J Med 2000;342:1077–84.

30. Modi KA, Illum S, Jariatul K, et al. Poor outcome of indigent patients with peripartum cardiomyopathy in the United States. Am J Obstet Gynecol 2009; 201:171–2.

31. Safirstein JG, Ro AS, Grandhi S, et al. Predictors of left ventricular recovery in a cohort of peripartum cardiomyopathy patients recruited via the Internet. Int J Cardiol 2012;154:27–31.

32. Elkayam U, Tummala PP, Rao K, et al. Maternal and fetal outcomes of subsequent pregnancies in women with peripartum cardiomyopathy. N Engl J Med 2001;334:1567–71.

33. Fett JD, Fristoe KL, Welsh SN. Risk of heart failure relapse in subsequent pregnancy among peripartum cardiomyopathy mothers. Int J Gynaecol Obstet 2010;109:34–6.

34. Lindenfeld J, Albert NM, Boehmer JA, et al. Executive summary; HFSA 21006 comprehensive heart failure practice guidelines. J Card Fail 2006;12:10–38.

35. Bozkurt B, Villaneuva FS, Holubkov R, et al. Intravenous immune globulin in the therapy of peripartum cardiomyopathy. J Am Coll Cardiol 1999;34: 177–80.

36. Sliwa K, Skudicky D, Candy G, et al. The addition of pentoxifylline to conventional therapy improves outcome in patients with peripartum cardiomyopathy. Eur J Heart Fail 2002;4:305–9.

37. Reck S, Geller JC, Meltendorf U, et al. Clinical efficacy of wearable defibrillator in acutely terminating episodes of ventricular fibrillation using biphasic shocks. Pacing Clin Electrophysiol 2003;26: 2016–22.

38. Bardy GH, Smith WM, Hood MA, et al. An entirely subcutaneous implantable cardioverter – defibrillator. N Engl J Med 2010;363:36–44.

39. Yang HS, Hong YS, Rim SJ, et al. Extracorporeal membrane oxygenation in a patient with peripartum cardiomyopathy. Ann Thorac Surg 2007;84:262–4.

40. Oosterom L, de Jonge N, Kirkels JH, et al. Left ventricular assist device as a bridge for recovery in a young woman admitted with peripartum cardiomyopathy. Neth Heart J 2008;16:426–8.

41. Zimmerman H, Bose R, Smith R, et al. Treatment of peripartum cardiomyopathy with mechanical assist devices and cardiac transplantation. Ann Thorac Surg 2010;89:1211–7.

42. Zimmerman H, Coelho- Anderson R, Smith R, et al. Bridge to recovery with a thoracic biventricular assist device for postpartum cardiomyopathy. ASAIO J 2010;50:479–80.

43. Rasmusson K, Braunisholz K, Budge D, et al. Peripartum cardiomyopathy: post transplant outcome from the United Network for Organ Sharing database. J Heart Lung Transplant 2012;31:180–6.

Pregnancy After Cardiac Transplantation

Scott W. Cowan, MD[a], John M. Davison, MD[b],
Cataldo Doria, MD, PhD,[a], Michael J. Moritz, MD[c],
Vincent T. Armenti, MD, PhD[a],*

KEYWORDS

- Pregnancy • Heart transplantation • Immunosuppression • Outcomes complications

KEY POINTS

- Successful pregnancy is possible following heart transplantation.
- Prepregnancy counseling, including an assessment of immunosuppression medications, should take place.
- Stable maternal cardiac function, with no recent rejection, and overall good maternal health is recommended.
- Long-term maternal survival should be discussed prepregnancy.
- Genetic counseling is recommended in some cases, depending on the original diagnosis in the mother.
- Follow-up of children born to cardiac transplant recipients is positive and ongoing studies continue.

INTRODUCTION

The first successful pregnancy after transplantation occurred in 1958 in a kidney recipient, although it was not reported until 1963.[1] This recipient was from the early series of identical twin transplants performed by Dr Joseph Murray and his team in Boston, Massachusetts, USA. Within 2 years of her transplant, the recipient approached her caretakers because she wanted to have a child. As well as discussing issues regarding pregnancy safety, a major concern at this time was the potential compressive effect of the expanding uterus on a kidney transplanted in the pelvis. Because she was an identical twin recipient, there were no concerns of immunosuppression. The patient became pregnant and she safely delivered a healthy boy by cesarean delivery on March 10, 1958. This heralded the beginning of an era in which the success of transplantation subsequently resulted in thousands of pregnancies.[2,3]

The first successful pregnancy after heart transplantation was reported in 1988, the woman having been transplanted at 18 years of age for dilated cardiomyopathy and conceiving less than 2 years posttransplant.[4] She was maintained on immunosuppression, including cyclosporine and prednisone during the pregnancy. A healthy girl was delivered at 31 weeks and weighed 1450 g with no malformations reported. The recipient and infant were both healthy 7 months postpartum.

Since 1988, approximately 12,900 heart transplants have been performed in women, with a 5-year graft and patient survival of approximately 67.4% and 69%, respectively.[5] Fertility and pregnancy in this patient population raise complex

The NTPR is supported by grants from Novartis Pharmaceuticals Corporation, Astellas Pharma US, Inc., Genentech, Inc, Pfizer Inc, Teva Pharmaceuticals USA, and Sandoz Pharmaceuticals.

[a] Department of Surgery, Thomas Jefferson University, 1025 Walnut Street, Suite 605, Philadelphia, PA 19107, USA; [b] Institute of Cellular Medicine, Newcastle University, Newcastle upon Tyne, UK; [c] Department of Surgery, Lehigh Valley Health Network, 1210 South Cedar Crest Boulevard, Suite 3300, Allentown, PA 18103, USA

* Corresponding author. Jefferson Medical College, 1025 Walnut Street, Suite 605, Philadelphia, PA 19107.
E-mail address: NTPR.registry@jefferson.edu

Cardiol Clin 30 (2012) 441–452
doi:10.1016/j.ccl.2012.05.001
0733-8651/12/$ – see front matter © 2012 Published by Elsevier Inc.

issues. Although successful outcomes have been reported, these pregnancies should be considered high risk for potential maternal and fetal complications. Issues that must be considered include overall maternal health, the effect of pregnancy on maternal graft function, and the effect of medications on the developing fetus. There are also longer term concerns about graft prognosis and any subtle effects on the growth and development of the offspring, including familial or genetic considerations. These longer term issues must also address the mother's survival prospects and the potential that a child could be without a parent. Data are more limited in this recipient population as compared with nonthoracic recipients.[3,6–18]

Advances in immunosuppression have led to increases in transplant recipient survival, allowing for more women to contemplate parenthood after cardiac transplantation. Data continue to accrue. Additionally, the face of heart transplantation is changing, because there are a proportion of younger patients being referred for evaluation that have complex congenital heart disease.[19] A shift toward younger recipients would dictate a greater need to assess the potential for parenthood in this population.

REGISTRIES AND SOURCES OF INFORMATION

Most data available regarding pregnancy following cardiac transplantation appears in the literature in the form of case reports, case series, and registry reports, including the National Transplantation Pregnancy Registry (NTPR)[3] and the United Kingdom Transplant Pregnancy Registry.[18] Currently, the NTPR is the only active ongoing pregnancy registry for transplant recipients. Recipients and pregnancies reported to the NTPR are shown in **Table 1**. Registries rely on patients self-reporting or caregivers contacting the registries and providing patient and outcome data. Continued patient accrual is paramount to determine and define potential risks to the mother, the transplanted graft, and the fetus amid the constant change in donors, recipients, and medications.

MANAGEMENT

Pregnancy in heart transplant recipients should be considered high risk for both the mother and the fetus. A tertiary center team composed of transplant cardiologists, maternal-fetal medicine specialists, and neonatologists should evaluate the recipient and, optimally, prepregnancy discussions between the recipient, her partner, and her doctors should take place.[20–23] Recommendations for prepregnancy counseling of kidney

Table 1
NTPR: pregnancies in female transplant recipients (December 2010)

Organ	Recipients	Pregnancies	Outcomes[a]
Kidney	886	1422	1466
Liver	166	292	298
Liver-Kidney	4	6	7
Small Bowel	1	1	1
Pancreas-Kidney	43	77	79
Pancreas Alone	1	4	5
Heart	58	103	107
Heart-Lung	5	5	5
Lung	21	30	32
Totals	1185	1940	2000

[a] Includes twins, triplets, and quadruplets.

transplant recipients were published in 1976 by Davison and colleagues. Based on a review of the literature at that time, along with their clinical experience, they formulated guidelines for counseling female kidney transplant recipients.[24] For the most part, these guidelines remain applicable today, and can be useful for other solid-organ recipients. The original recommendations consisted of the following eight guidelines: (1) good general health for at least 2 years since the transplant, (2) stature compatible with good obstetric outcome, (3) no proteinuria, (4) no significant hypertension, (5) no evidence of renal rejection, (6) no evidence of pelvicalyceal distention on a recent excretory urogram, (7) plasma creatinine of 2 mg/dL (180 μmol/L) or less, and (8) drug therapy: prednisone 15 mg/day or less, azathioprine 3 mg/kg/d or less.[22] In 2003, a Consensus Conference, organized by the Women's Health Committee of the American Society of Transplantation (AST), convened to address reproductive issues in transplant recipients.[22] The Consensus Summary is shown in **Box 1** and provides guidelines for clinicians caring for these high-risk patients. Consideration must be given to counseling recipients who may have a limited lifespan related to their disease process. Recipients should be encouraged to seek counseling regarding pregnancy risks before proceeding, although historically approximately 50% of pregnancies have been unplanned. Counseling should take into consideration the various risk

Box 1
Consensus summary

Basis on which to determine timing of pregnancy

- No rejection in the past year
- Adequate and stable graft function (eg, creatinine <1.5 mg/dL; true glomerular filtration rate [GFR] needs to be defined in prospective studies) or no or minimal proteinuria (level needs to defined)
- No acute infections that might affect fetus
- Maintenance immunosuppression at stable dosing

Special circumstances that affect recommendations

- Rejection within the first year (consider further graft assessment—biopsy and GFR)
- Maternal age
- Comorbid factors that may impact pregnancy and graft function
- Established medical noncompliance

Pregnancies outside the guidelines need to be evaluated on a case-by-case basis. In general these considerations could be met at 1 year posttransplant, based on individual circumstances.

Comorbid factors that may influence pregnancy outcome

- Cause of original disease (eg, risk of recurrent disease)
- Chronic allograft dysfunction
- Renal function and proteinuria
- Cardiovascular status and pulmonary status
- Diabetes mellitus (or history of)
- Hypertension
- Inherited diseases in mother and or father (genetic, vs chromosomal)
- Hepatitis B virus, hepatitis C virus, cytomegalovirus
- Obesity

Preconception counseling

- Should be introduced at least at the pretransplant evaluation
- Should be followed up throughout the posttransplant process
- Should be offered to both the patient and her partner
- Ideally patients should be vaccinated pretransplant; if not, should be vaccinated prepregnancy for influenza, pneumococcus, hepatitis B, and tetanus
- Must discuss consequences of preterm birth and long-term consequences of preterm birth for both the mother and child with *both* prospective parents

Obstetric management

- Management of all pregnant transplant patients should be by high-risk obstetrician (because of intrauterine growth retardation and preeclampsia) in conjunction with transplant physician
- Cesarean section indicated only for obstetric reasons
- Graft dysfunction during pregnancy warrants appropriate investigation (by biopsy if necessary)
- Immunosuppression must be maintained during pregnancy to avoid rejection
- Future studies need to address optimal selection and dosing of these agents
- Hyperemesis gravidarum may lead to decreased absorption or inadequate immunosuppression

Adapted from McKay DB, Josephson MA, Armenti VT, et al. Reproduction and transplantation: report on the AST Consensus Conference on Reproductive Issues and Transplantation. Am J Transplant 2005;5:1592–9.

factors related to each recipient, as well as the overall data, to give an assessment of the potential for childrearing issues that may arise. Avoidance of pregnancy is recommended for heart transplant female recipients who have allograft dysfunction or cardiac allograft vasculopathy (CAV). Recommendations on pregnancy after heart transplantation from the International Society for Heart and Lung Transplantation (ISHLT) guidelines include[25]: (1) that there be a multidisciplinary team involving specialists in maternal-fetal medicine, cardiology, transplant medicine, anesthesia, neonatology, psychology, genetics, and social services; (2) the management plan should be individualized according to the status of the mother and her transplanted heart, best achieved at the primary transplant institution, in collaboration with other referring physicians; (3) individual factors, including the risk of acute rejection and infection, and other therapies that are potentially toxic or teratogenic, should be reviewed; and (4) patients should be counseled on the risks of pregnancy and discouraged if graft function and significant CAV are expected to preclude a successful outcome. Typically, it is not recommended that pregnancy occur sooner than 1 year after transplant.

For a heart transplant recipient who wishes to become pregnant, there should be baseline tests including an EKG, ECG, and potentially coronary angiography, with the option of right heart catheterization and endomyocardial biopsy (EMB) if clinically indicated.[26] Baseline assessment of renal and liver function should be obtained. Frequent monitoring of blood pressure, urine cultures, and surveillance for preeclampsia and gestational diabetes are advised. Calcineurin inhibitors and steroids, if part of maintenance immunotherapy, should be continued. Blood levels of calcineurin inhibitors should be monitored during pregnancy with awareness that changes in plasma volume during pregnancy, gastrointestinal motility and absorption, and fetal metabolism must also be taken into account. The current recommendation includes discontinuation of mycophenolic acid products (MPA),[27,28] but alternatives to therapy must be evaluated, such as azathioprine. Surveillance for rejection is imperative and, if necessary, EMB under ECG guidance or fluoroscopy with leaded draping can be performed.[8,10]

TRANSPLANT TO CONCEPTION INTERVAL

Although the recommended transplant to conception interval for heart transplant patients has not been defined, it seems prudent to delay pregnancy for a year until graft function is proven stable. This recommendation is also supported in the ISHLT guidelines.[25] Factors to consider when counseling

transplant recipients about the timing of pregnancy should include infection risk, risk of acute or chronic rejection, and the use of medications that may have a deleterious effect on the fetus, as well as overall graft function and maternal health.[22] During the first year posttransplant, there is the greatest risk of rejection and infection.

CONTRACEPTION

The NTPR reported that at least 50% of all pregnancies in solid organ recipients are unplanned, emphasizing the need for early patient-caregiver discussions.[29] Recipients who choose to delay pregnancy should discuss contraception options with their doctors. There is a paucity of data regarding appropriate contraceptive options following solid organ transplantation. Barrier methods may be suboptimal owing to a need for consistent use.[30,31] Interactions between hormonal contraceptives and immunosuppressants have been observed,[32] whereas intrauterine devices have shown decreased effectiveness, with an increased risk of infection in the immunosuppressed patient.[25,33] Recently the Centers for Disease Control in conjunction with the World Health Organization published comprehensive recommendations for patients with medical conditions (**Box 2**).[34] Health care providers for patients with medical conditions are encouraged to become familiar with these guidelines.

PREGNANCY EFFECTS ON THE CARDIAC TRANSPLANT

Effects of pregnancy on the transplanted heart include increased cardiac workload, increased

---

Box 2
Categories for classifying hormonal contraceptives and intrauterine devices

1. A condition for which there is no restriction for the use of the contraceptive method

2. A condition for which the advantages of using the method generally outweigh the theoretical or proven risks

3. A condition for which the theoretical or proven risks usually outweigh the advantages of using the method

4. A condition that represents an unacceptable health risk if the contraceptive method is used

Data from Peterson HB, Curtis KM, Jamieson D, et al. U.S. Medical Eligibility Criteria for Contraceptive Use, 2010: adapted from the World Health Organization Medical Eligibility Criteria for Contraceptive Use, 4th edition. MMWR Recomm Rep 2010;59(RR-4):1–86.

cardiac output, and elevated maternal oxygen consumption.[11,35] The transplanted heart seems to adapt well to these changes when graft function is stable.[25,36]

COMORBID CONDITIONS DURING PREGNANCY
Hypertension and Diabetes

Comorbid conditions should be well controlled before pregnancy (**Table 2**).[3] Hypertension may contribute to a higher incidence of preterm delivery in this patient population.[37] In the NTPR, 39% of cardiac recipients reported taking medication for hypertension during pregnancy. Antihypertensive medications, including angiotensin-converting enzyme inhibitors and angiotensin receptor blockers should be avoided during pregnancy.[23] However, general management principles for treating hypertension during pregnancy should be applied to cardiac transplant recipients.[26] Although diabetes is common in adult heart transplant recipients with 1-year rates up to 30%, there is a lower incidence of diabetes treatment during pregnancy among cardiac transplant recipients reported to the NTPR (see **Table 2**).[3,25]

Preeclampsia

Preeclampsia can occur during pregnancy after cardiac transplantation. In the NTPR, the incidence of preeclampsia for cardiac recipients is 18% (see **Table 2**), lower than that seen in kidney transplant recipients,[3] but higher than the 2% to 7% in healthy nulliparous women.[38] Risk factors to take into consideration when assessing preeclampsia risk include increased maternal

age, chronic hypertension or renal disease, obesity with its associated insulin resistance, and prepregnancy diabetes mellitus. Preeclampsia can be difficult to diagnose in transplant recipients who may have baseline proteinuria and hypertension.[39] Also, because calcineurin inhibitors may increase uric acid levels, this test is not useful when diagnosing preeclampsia.[40] It is beneficial to have a baseline serum creatinine and urinalysis in nonrenal recipients before conception.[41] Delivery for preeclampsia should be based on obstetric algorithms.[38]

Infection

Infection in the mother and the fetus is a concern during pregnancy. Maternal immunosuppression in the cardiac transplant recipient leads to increased risk of viral, mycotic, and opportunistic infections.[6,7,42] Prepregnancy titers for rubella, varicella herpes simplex cytomegalovirus toxoplasmosis, HIV, and hepatitis B and C should be obtained.[21] As with all obstetric patients, female recipients not immune to cytomegalovirus should be counseled regarding preventive measures and those not immune to varicella zoster virus must avoid contact with chicken pox. If exposure does occur, then intervention with varicella zoster immune globulin should be considered. For patients at risk for recurrent herpes simplex, antiviral therapy may also be considered in the third trimester. Prophylactic antibiotics are indicated for cesarean delivery, and many physicians would advocate their use to cover vaginal delivery. However, antibiotic prophylaxis is not routinely recommended for vaginal delivery without specific indications with regard to prophylaxis against subacute endocarditis. No foci of infection and negative urine cultures should be confirmed before conception. In the NTPR, reported infections in heart transplant recipients during pregnancy include respiratory, urinary tract, and vaginal.[43,44] Infections reported to the NTPR have not been life-threatening and should be treated with the appropriate therapy.

Rejection

Monitoring for rejection in patients with a cardiac transplant may require endomyocardial biopsy. Graft rejection during pregnancy was reported in 11% of 103 pregnancies in 57 heart recipients reporting to the NTPR[3] with many of the episodes being low grade and without clinical consequence. Treatment of rejection was corticosteroids, cyclosporine dose increased, or with no change in several recipients with low grade rejection.[43] Noted in **Table 3** are the outcomes of pregnancies in heart

---

Table 2
NTPR: Comorbid conditions among 57 heart recipients reporting 103 pregnancies (106 outcomes, including twins and triplets)

Organ	Heart[3]
Maternal Factors (n = pregnancies)	**(103)**
Transplant-to-conception interval (mean)	6.0 ± 4.7 yrs
Range	0.1–18.9 yrs
Hypertension during pregnancy	39%
Diabetes during pregnancy	2%
Infection during pregnancy	13%
Rejection episode during pregnancy	11%
Preeclampsia	18%

Table 3
NTPR: rejection during pregnancy in female heart transplant recipients

Case	Rejection Grade	Treatment	Current Graft Status	Outcome
1 (2 biopsies)	1; 3	None; increase prednisone	Died 5.6 y postpartum	34 wk, 1814 gm
2 (pregnancy #1)	2	Prednisone	Died 5.5 y	8 wk termination
2 (pregnancy #2)	2; 2	None	postpartum	40 wk, 3813 gm
3 (2 biopsies)	2; 1A	None	Adequate	30 wk, 1191 gm
4	Moderate	Methylprednisolone	Adequate	33 wk, 2,240 gm
5 (pregnancy #1)	1A	None	Died 12.2 y	12 wk spontaneous
5 (pregnancy #2)	2	None	postpartum	abortion 30 wk, 1673 gm
6	2	Methylprednisolone	Died 10.8 y postpartum	34 wk, 2381 gm
7	Mild	Increase prednisone	Adequate	32 wk, 2523 gm
8	3A	Oral steroid pulse	Adequate	40 wk, 2495 gm
9 (2 biopsies)	1B; 1A	Increase cyclosporine, modified; none	Died 2.7 y postpartum	Stillbirth

transplant recipients in which rejection was reported to the NTPR. Some pregnancies resulted in viable and others in nonviable outcomes. To date, use of high-dose steroids or no therapy for rejections, depending on grade, have been reported to the registry; however, no antilymphocyte therapies have been noted. Postpartum rejection (within 3 months) was reported in 6% of patients. The ISHLT published guidelines on long-term care of heart transplant recipients regarding reproductive issues had the opinion that steroids are safe for antirejection therapy; however, the safety of antithymocyte sera and rituximab are unknown.[25] Reports of heart transplant recipients developing antibody-mediated rejection postpartum have occurred and recipients who develop features suggestive of rejection during or after pregnancy should be assessed for anti-HLA antibodies.[45]

SPECIAL CONSIDERATIONS

Among the cardiac recipients in the NTPR, it is worth noting that there are recipients who were transplanted for congenital heart disease who have gone on to have pregnancies. Additionally, many recipients have had more than one pregnancy, which does not seem to confer any increased incidence of pregnancy complications, graft rejection, or loss.[11,13] Such considerations need to be factored into counseling policy because a recipient that is doing well may want to have more than one baby.

For the patient with congenital heart disease, it is mandatory to consider the potential risk of

occurrence in the offspring, which depends on the type of maternal disease. For example, mitochondrial cardiomyopathy, a known genetic disorder as the cause for heart transplantation, further highlights the importance of preconception counseling. Interestingly, peripartum cardiomyopathy also has the theoretical risk of recurrence. However, a report of five cases by Morini and colleagues[12] did not report any recurrence, which is the experience of other investigators[9,13] as well as the NTPR.

PREGNANCY OUTCOMES

Pregnancy outcomes after cardiac transplant reported to the NTPR, compared with those reported to the UK Transplant Pregnancy Registry (up to 2000) are listed in **Table 4**[3,18]—most were live births. The rate of therapeutic abortion in cardiac transplant recipients seems similar to that of the general population.[12]

IMMUNOSUPPRESSION

Medication regimens to maintain transplant graft survival and prevent rejection have evolved, and can be divided into three categories. Induction regimens are used in the first week after transplantation and include agents such as antilymphocyte sera and interleukin-2 receptor blockade antibodies. Maintenance regimens are initiated soon after transplantation to prevent acute rejection episodes and provide long-term immunosuppression. Combination therapies are used to balance

Table 4
Pregnancy outcomes in cardiac transplant recipients

	NTPR[3]	UK Transplant Pregnancy Registry[18]
Recipients	57	17
Outcomes (n)	106[a]	18
Therapeutic abortions	5	0
Spontaneous abortions	32	1
Ectopic	2	1
Stillbirth	1	1
Live births	66	15
Live births (n)	(66)	(6[b])
Mean gestational age (wks)	36.8 ± 2.6	36.8 ± 1.5
Premature (<37 wks)	38%	33% (10[b])
Mean birthweight (g)	2600 ± 568	2458 ± 186
Low birthweight (<2500 g)	39%	80%
Cesarean section	40%	45%
Newborn complications	32%	NR
Neonatal deaths n (%) (within 30 days of birth)	0	NR

Abbreviation: NR, not reported.
[a] Includes twins and triplets.
[b] Number reported.

the benefits of these agents against the side effects and toxicities. Antirejection regimens are used to treat episodes and typically include high-dose short-term treatments such as corticosteroids and/or antilymphocyte sera.

The introduction of cyclosporine as the mainstay of therapy in the early 1980s was followed by significant improvement in the survival of heart transplant recipients. Since then, other agents have been introduced and ongoing studies continue to address questions such as the effectiveness of induction therapy, newer combinations of agents, and minimization or early elimination of steroids. Methods for managing acute rejection have also evolved, with strategies dependent on the histologic type of rejection (cellular vs antibody-mediated) and severity (by hemodynamic compromise or histologic grade). Although high-dose intravenous corticosteroids are used for symptomatic acute cellular rejection, cytolytic therapy with antilymphocyte sera, are considered in recipients with hemodynamically compromising rejection or high-grade cellular rejection.[46] Antibody-mediated rejection (AMR) therapies are evolving. If there is severe hemodynamic compromise, AMR is treated with high-dose corticosteroids, plasmapheresis, and other therapies such as intravenous immunoglobulin or rituximab. Ongoing studies are continuing to assess treatment strategies for antibody-mediated rejection.[46]

Most recipients with early rejection are asymptomatic; therefore, surveillance and myocardial biopsies are needed to detect then treat rejection before it results in transplant dysfunction. According to the ISHLT guidelines for the care of heart transplant recipients, there is no consensus on the optimal frequency of surveillance.[46] Typically, biopsies are more often undertaken in the first 3 months after transplant, and tapered thereafter up to one year. The schedule is based on the observation that the risk is highest in the first 6 months and then decreases after 12 months. The need to continue surveillance biopsies in recipients greater than 1 year after transplant is still being evaluated.

Immunosuppressive regimens used during pregnancy in the heart transplant recipient typically include a combination of corticosteroids, calcineurin inhibitors, antimetabolites, and/or macrolide antibiotics, and dose changes during pregnancy may be necessary.[43] The US Food and Drug Administration (FDA) pregnancy categories for immunosuppression are listed in **Table 5**. Adjustments in immunosuppressive medications and dosages should be anticipated before and during pregnancy due in part to increased volume of distribution and increased glomerular filtration rate. Slowed gastrointestinal motility with associated nausea and vomiting may result in altered drug levels requiring close

Table 5
FDA pregnancy categories for commonly used immunosuppressive drugs in transplantation

Drug	Pregnancy Category[a]
Corticosteroids (prednisone, methylprednisolone, others)	B
Azathioprine (Imuran)	D
Cyclosporine (Sandimmune, Neoral, et al)	C
Tacrolimus, FK506 (Prograf, et al)	C
Antithymocyte globulin (Atgam, ATG, Thymoglobulin)	C
Muromonab-CD3 (Orthoclone OKT3)	C
Mycophenolate mofetil (CellCept, others)	D
Enteric-coated mycophenolate sodium (Myfortic)	D
Basiliximab (Simulect)	B
Daclizumab (Zenapax)	C
Sirolimus (Rapamune)	C

[a] FDA categories briefly defined: B, no fetal risk, no controlled studies; C, fetal risk cannot be ruled out; D, evidence of fetal risk.

monitoring.[47,48] Although pregnancy is considered an immunosuppressed state, evidence shows that pregnant women do not have diminished systemic immunity and inappropriate reduction of immunosuppression will result in rejection.

Corticosteroids

Steroids have historically been a part of maintenance immunosuppression. Steroids cross the placenta and adrenal insufficiency and thymic hyperplasia have been reported but are uncommon when doses are <15 mg/d. In animal studies, a reproducible cleft palate has been shown with steroid exposure.[49] Although steroids have been implicated in premature rupture of membranes, their overall use is considered low teratogenic risk.[50] Currently some centers are using steroid minimization immunosuppression because of the long-term complications associated with steroid use.

Azathioprine

As new immunosuppressive medications have been developed, the use of azathioprine has decreased. The dose of azathioprine used originally was 1.5 to 3.0 mg/kg/d; doses used now are 0.5 to 1.5 mg/kg/d. A recent review of all births from Sweden with early exposure to azathioprine (most for inflammatory bowel disease), concluded that infants may be at a moderately increased risk of congenital malformations, specifically ventricular or atrial septal defects.[51] Although concern has always existed regarding azathioprine use during pregnancy, no pattern of birth defects has been observed in azathioprine-treated transplant recipients.[2,52,53]

Cyclosporine

Since the early 1980s, cyclosporine, a calcineurin inhibitor, has been widely used for maintenance therapy in transplantation. Cyclosporine is often used in conjunction with steroids, azathioprine, mycophenolic acid products, or sirolimus. Early on, fetal toxicities and abnormalities in animal studies had been published, although the concentration of cyclosporine used was much higher than clinically used.[54,55] Cyclosporine administered in pregnant patients can be associated with an increased risk of gestational diabetes, hypertension, preeclampsia, and low birthweight in the newborn.[23] From NTPR data, the incidence of malformations in those offspring exposed to cyclosporine has been approximately 4.9% and there has not been a specific pattern or increase in the incidence of malformations in recipient offspring.[56]

Tacrolimus

Tacrolimus is a macrolide antibiotic that is a more potent calcineurin inhibitor than cyclosporine. Initially approved for liver transplant recipients in the early 1990s, tacrolimus has slowly replaced cyclosporine over the ensuing years for maintenance immunosuppression. Tacrolimus is typically used in conjunction with other agents such as steroids, azathioprine, mycophenolic acid products, or sirolimus. In an earlier case report, thrombotic-dilated cardiomyopathy with degeneration of cardiac muscle was seen in a newborn born to a kidney recipient maintained on tacrolimus during pregnancy.[57] Tacrolimus has also been associated with transient neonatal hyperkalemia.[58] Similar to cyclosporine, no specific pattern or increase in malformation rate has been noted with tacrolimus exposure during pregnancy.

MPA

Two MPA preparations are available, mycophenolate mofetil (MMF) and enteric-coated mycophenolic acid (EC-MPA). MMF is a prodrug converted into MPA and used mostly in conjunction with calcineurin inhibitors. From reproductive animal studies, questions have been raised about safety in pregnancy because rats and rabbits exhibited malformations and intrauterine growth restriction, and fetal deaths also occurred at dosages that seemed to be in the clinical range based on body surface area. In 2007, the pregnancy category of MPA was changed from C to D based on NTPR and postmarketing data. Data collected by Roche Laboratories between 1995 and 2007, from the 77 women exposed to systemic MMF during pregnancy, revealed that 25 had spontaneous abortions and 14 had a malformed infant or fetus, six having ear abnormalities. Reports of newborn congenital malformations in transplant recipients treated with MMF and mycophenolate sodium have accumulated in the literature as well.[59–61] In cardiac recipients, the NTPR reported 21 pregnancies (23 outcomes) in patients exposed to MPA, 15 having spontaneous abortions, and 8 live births. Four of these were associated with birth defects that included facial defects, duodenal atresia, atrioventricular canal defect and Tetralogy of Fallot, laryngomalacia, and bicuspid aortic valve.[3] In 2002, the European Best Practice Group recommended eliminating MPA from immunosuppressive drug regimens at least 6 weeks before a planned conception.[62] The package inserts for MMF and EC-MPA recommend avoiding these medications for at least 6 weeks before pregnancy and complete avoidance during pregnancy.[27,28]

Sirolimus

This macrolide antibiotic was approved in the United States in 1999 and is used mostly in conjunction with a calcineurin inhibitor. In animal studies, sirolimus has been linked to decreased birthweight and delayed skeletal ossification.[63] Clinical outcomes have not shown sirolimus to be associated with any specific pattern of fetal malformation but data are limited.[59,64–67] In the NTPR, two cardiac recipients reported two pregnancies with exposure to sirolimus; one live birth with facial malformations (maternal immunosuppression also included MMF) and one spontaneous abortion. The package insert does recommend avoiding sirolimus during pregnancy and to discontinue the medication 12 weeks before conception.[63]

Statins

Statins are a common part of therapy in heart transplant recipients, but typically are not recommended during pregnancy owing to their potential teratogenic effects. A study from the Motherisk program suggested that the actual risks for an exposed pregnancy seem to be small and do not by itself warrant termination of pregnancy.[68] It is still advisable to avoid the use of these drugs to reduce fetal risks as much as possible. In the NTPR, 10 pregnancies have been evaluated in heart recipients with exposure to statins, with six live births and no structural birth defects in these newborn.[69]

DELIVERY

Vaginal delivery is the recommended method of delivery in heart transplant recipients.[22] Cesarean section should be performed for obstetric indications. In cardiac recipient pregnancies reported to the NTPR, 40% were cesarean deliveries. During labor, EKG monitoring is mandatory because of the increased risk of arrhythmias, with more invasive cardiovascular monitoring generally not necessary. Epidural anesthesia reduces pain-induced sympathetic responses and may reduce acute blood pressure fluctuations during labor.[21] Prophylactic antibiotics to prevent subacute bacterial endocarditis, are not routinely recommended. For heart recipients, the physician must be judicious when giving fluids during labor and delivery, and the health care provider must be aware that cardiac recipients may have an unpredictable response to vasoactive medications.[41] Immunosuppression must also be continued during labor and delivery. Some recommend a scheduled delivery to allow a more coordinated effort among the various specialists.[26]

PERINATAL OUTCOMES

The outcomes of newborns of cardiac recipients are listed in **Table 4**. Compared with kidney recipients, these babies are born closer to term and have higher birthweights, have a mean gestational age of 36.8 compared with 35 weeks, and have mean birthweights of 2600 g compared with 2500 g. A childhood follow-up for the 66 live births revealed that one had died a traumatic death, two had mitochondrial cardiomyopathy (same diagnosis as mother), and four had birth anomalies, including facial defects, duodenal atresia, atrioventricular canal defect, Tetralogy of Fallot, laryngomalacia, and bicuspid aortic valve (all maternal immunosuppression included MPA). The remaining 59 children were reported healthy and developing well.[3] Major structural malformations occur in 4% to 5% of pregnancies following solid organ transplantation, which is similar to the general population (3%–5%),[70] and no distinct pattern of malformations has been observed in patients treated with conventional immunosuppressants.[3] Discussions prepregnancy with heart transplant recipients should include genetic counseling, and they should be informed of the possibility of their offspring being subsequently diagnosed with the same condition. Although most children born to heart transplant recipients are healthy and developing normally, long-term follow-up of these children is necessary.[15,43]

BREASTFEEDING

Breastfeeding has typically been discouraged. Cyclosporine and tacrolimus have been detected in variable concentrations in infants breastfed by mothers maintained on these immunosuppressive medications.[23,58,71–75] The NTPR reported 89 women breastfeeding their children with no apparent adverse effects.[3] Six cardiac recipients reported breastfeeding their nine children from a few days to up to 3 years.

Breastfeeding has been shown to have beneficial health effects for the newborn that must be weighed carefully against the potential adverse effects of exposure to maternal immunosuppressive medications.[58,76] The conclusion of the AST Consensus Conference was that breastfeeding need not be viewed as absolutely contraindicated.[22] It is a topic that will surely remain controversial in this population.

CARDIAC FUNCTION POSTPARTUM

Most patients maintain adequate graft function following pregnancy.[3] In the NTPR, 40 recipients (70%) reported adequate transplant function postpartum and there were two recipients who had graft loss within 2 years of pregnancy. One recipient died 16.9 years after transplant. The second loss occurred 9 months after delivery, necessitating retransplant, and the recipient is currently healthy with adequate function.[3] Furthermore, maternal death was reported in 16 of the 57 female heart recipients by the NTPR, all occurring more than 2 years after pregnancy. Causes of death included vasculopathy, atherosclerosis, acute rejection, sepsis, and pneumonia. As emphasized previously, prepregnancy discussions must include the potentially limited lifespan of the heart transplant recipient.

SUMMARY

Although, in the past, pregnancy has often been discouraged for cardiac transplant recipients, most pregnancies reported result in a live birth and have positive graft outcomes for the recipient. In an ideal situation, there should be a planned pregnancy with coordinated efforts between the recipient and her health care team. Serious comorbidities reported during pregnancy include hypertension, preeclampsia, and infection. There are

also risks to the fetus, including preterm delivery and low birthweight. The cardiovascular changes that occur during pregnancy are usually tolerated by the recipient. Continued reporting via case, center, and registry reports will add to the body of knowledge regarding pregnancy after cardiac transplantation. The NTPR is an ongoing database initiated in 1991 for the study of pregnancy outcomes in transplant recipients. All centers are encouraged to report pregnancies to the NTPR to help to further modify and update guidelines for management of pregnancy in these high-risk recipient populations.

ACKNOWLEDGMENTS

The authors would like to thank Lisa A Coscia, RN, BSN, CCTC and Carolyn H. McGrory, MS, RN for their assistance in the preparation of the manuscript.

The NTPR acknowledges the cooperation of transplant recipients and the personnel in over 250 centers in North America who have contributed their time and information to the registry.

REFERENCES

1. Murray JE, Reid DE, Harrison JH, et al. Successful pregnancies after human renal transplantation. N Engl J Med 1963;269:341–3.
2. Registration Committee of the European Dialysis and Transplant Association. Successful pregnancies in women treated with dialysis and kidney transplantation. Report from the Registration Committee of the European Dialysis and Transplant Association. Br J Obstet Gynaecol 1980;87:839–45.
3. Coscia LA, Constantinescu S, Moritz MJ, et al. Report from the National Transplantation Pregnancy Registry (NTPR): outcomes of pregnancy after transplantation. In: Terasaki PI, Cecka JM, editors. Clinical Transplants 2010. Los Angeles (CA): Terasaki Foundation Laboratory; 2011. p. 65–85.
4. Lowenstein BR, Vain NW, Perrone SV, et al. Successful pregnancy and vaginal delivery after heart transplantation. Am J Obstet Gynecol 1988;158:589–90.
5. Organ Procurement Transplant Network Data. Available at: http://optn.transplant.hrsa.gov. Accessed October 11, 2011.
6. Camann WR, Goldman GA, Johnson MD, et al. Cesarean delivery in a patient with a transplanted heart. Anesthesiology 1989;71:618–20.
7. Key TC, Resnick R, Dittrich HC, et al. Successful pregnancy after heart transplantation. Am J Obstet Gynecol 1989;160:367–71.
8. Camann WR, Jarcho JA, Mintz KJ, et al. Uncomplicated vaginal delivery 14 months after cardiac transplantation. Am Heart J 1991;121:939–41.

9. Carvalho AC, Almeida D, Cohen M, et al. Successful pregnancy, delivery and puerperium in a heart transplant patient with previous peripartum cardiomyopathy. Eur Heart J 1992;13(11):1589–91.

10. Scott JR, Wagoner LE, Olsen SL, et al. Pregnancy in heart transplant recipients: management and outcome. Obstet Gynecol 1993;82:324–7.

11. Wagoner LE, Taylor DO, Olsen SL, et al. Immunosuppressive therapy, management and outcome of heart transplant recipients during pregnancy. J Heart Lung Transplant 1993;12:993–1000.

12. Morini A, Spina V, Aleandri V, et al. Pregnancy after heart transplant: update and case report. Hum Reprod 1998;13(3):749–57.

13. Branch KR, Wagoner LE, McGrory CH, et al. Risk of subsequent pregnancies on mother and newborn in female heart transplant recipients. J Heart Lung Transplant 1998;17:698–702.

14. Maglione A, Di Giorgio G. Successful outcome of pregnancy and vaginal delivery in a heart transplant recipient. Minerva Ginecol 2003;55:537–9 [in Italian].

15. Miniero R, Tardivo I, Centofanti P, et al. Pregnancy in heart transplant recipients. J Heart Lung Transplant 2004;23:898–901.

16. Wasywich CA, Ruygrok PN, Wilkinson L, et al. Planned pregnancy in a heart transplant recipient. Intern Med J 2004;34:206–9.

17. Ohler L, Coscia LA, McGrory CH, et al. National Transplantation Pregnancy Registry (NTPR): pregnancy outcomes in female thoracic transplant recipients. J Heart Lung Transplant 2007;2(Suppl 1): S158.

18. Sibanda N, Briggs JD, Davison JM, et al. Pregnancy after organ transplantation: a report from the U. K. Transplant Pregnancy Registry. Transplantation 2007;83:1301–7.

19. Hunt SA, Haddad F. The changing face of heart transplantation. J Am Coll Cardiol 2008;52(8):587–98.

20. Mastrobattista JM, Katz AR. Pregnancy after organ transplant. Obstet Gynecol Clin North Am 2004;31: 415–28.

21. Mastrobattista JM, Gomez-Lobo V. Pregnancy after solid organ transplantation. Obstet Gynecol 2008; 112:919–32.

22. McKay DB, Josephson MA, Armenti VT, et al. Reproduction and transplantation: report on the AST Consensus Conference on Reproductive Issues and Transplantation. Am J Transplant 2005;5:1592–9.

23. Wieglos M, Pietrzak B, Bobrowska K, et al. Pregnancy after organ transplantation. Neuroendocrinol Lett 2009;30(1):6–10.

24. Davison JM, Lind T, Uldall PR. Planned pregnancy in a renal transplant recipient. BJOG 1976;83:518–27.

25. Hunt S, Burch M, Bhat G, et al. The International society of Heart and Lung Transplantation guidelines for the care of heart transplant recipients Task force 3: Long-term care of heart transplant recipients. Available at: http://www.ishlt.org/publications/guidelines.asp. Accessed October 19, 2011.

26. Wu DW, Wilt J, Restaino S. Pregnancy after thoracic organ transplantation. Semin Perinatol 2007;31:354.

27. CellCept [package insert]. South San Francisco, CA: Genentech USA, Inc; 2010.

28. Myfortic [package insert]. East Hanover, NJ: Novartis Pharmaceuticals; 2009.

29. Armenti VT, Moritz MJ, Davison JM. Parenthood after transplantation: 50 years later. Transplantation 2008; 85:1389–90.

30. Riely CA. Contraception and pregnancy after liver transplantation. Liver Transpl 2001;7(1):S74–6.

31. Shlay JC, Mayhugh B, Foster M, et al. Initiating contraception in sexually transmitted disease clinic setting: a randomized trial. Am J Obstet Gynecol 2003;189:473–81.

32. Sucato GS, Murray PJ. Gynecologic health care for the adolescent solid organ transplant recipient. Pediatr Transplant 2005;9:346–56.

33. Zerner J, Doil KL, Drewry J, et al. Intrauterine contraceptive device failure in renal transplant patients. J Reprod Med 1981;26(2):99–102.

34. Peterson HB, Curtis KM, Jamieson D, et al. U.S. Medical Eligibility Criteria for Contraceptive Use, 2010: adapted from the World Health Organization Medical Eligibility Criteria for Contraceptive Use, 4th ed. MMWR Recomm Rep 2010;59(RR-4):1–86.

35. Metcalfe J, McAnulty JH, Ueland K. Cardiovascular physiology. Clin Obstet Gynecol 1981;24:693–710.

36. Hunt SA. Pregnancy in heart transplant recipients: a good idea? J Heart Lung Transplant 1991;10: 499–503.

37. McKay DB, Josephson MA. Pregnancy in recipients of solid organs—effects on mother and child. N Engl J Med 2006;354(12):1281–93.

38. Decker G. Hypertension. In: James DK, Steer PJ, Weiner CP, et al, editors. High risk pregnancy-management options. 4th edition. Philadelphia: Elsevier Science; 2011. p. 599–626.

39. Josephson MA, McKay DB. Considerations in the medical management of pregnancy in transplant recipients. Adv Chronic Kidney Dis 2007;14(2):156–67.

40. Morales JM, Hernández Poblete G, Andrés A, et al. Uric acid handling, pregnancy and cyclosporin in renal transplant women. Nephron 2005;37(9):3721–22.

41. Armenti VT, Moritz MJ, Davison JM. Pregnancy following transplantation. In: James DK, Steer PJ, Weiner CP, et al, editors. High risk pregnancy: management options. 4th edition. Philadelphia: Elsevier Science; 2011. p. 961–72.

42. Ahner R, Kiss H, Zuckermann A, et al. Pregnancy and spontaneous delivery 13 months after heart transplantation. Acta Obstet Gynecol Scand 1994;73(6):511–3.

43. Cowan SW, Coscia LA, Philips LZ, et al. Pregnancy outcomes in female heart and heart-lung transplant recipients. Transplant Proc 2002;34:1855–6.

44. Shen AY, Mansukhani PW. Is pregnancy contraindicated after cardiac transplantation? A case report and literature review. Int J Cardiol 1997;60:151–6.

45. O'Boyle PJ, Smith JD, Danskine AJ, et al. De novo HLA sensitization and antibody mediated rejection following pregnancy in a heart transplant recipient. Am J Transplant 2010;10:180–3.

46. Taylor D, Meiser B, Baran D, et al. The International society of Heart and Lung Transplantation guidelines for the care of heart transplant recipients. Task force 2: Immunosuppression and rejection. Available at: http://www.ishlt.org/publications/guidelines.asp. Accessed October 19, 2011.

47. Lindheimer MD, Katz AI. Gestation in women with kidney disease: prognosis and management. In: Lindheimer MD, Davison JM, editors. Baillieres Clin Obstet Gynaecol: renal disease in pregnancy. London: Baillere Tindall; 1994. p. 387–404.

48. Monga M. Maternal cardiovascular and renal adaptation to pregnancy. In: Creasy RK, Resnick R, editors. Maternal-fetal medicine. 4th edition. Philadelphia: WB Saunders; 1999. p. 783–92.

49. Fraser FC, Fainstat TD. Production of congenital defects in the offspring of pregnant mice treated with cortisone: a progress report. Pediatrics 1951; 8:527–33.

50. Armenti VT, Moritz MJ, Cardonick EH, et al. Immunosuppression in pregnancy: choices for infant and maternal health. Drugs 2002;62(16):2361–75.

51. Kallen B, Westgren M, Aberg A, et al. Pregnancy outcome after maternal organ transplantation in Sweden. BJOG 2005;112(7):904–9.

52. Davison JM. Dialysis, transplantation, and pregnancy. Am J Kidney Dis 1991;17:127–32.

53. Armenti VT, Ahlswede KM, Ahlswede BA, et al. National Transplantation Pregnancy Registry: outcomes of 154 pregnancies in cyclosporine-treated female kidney transplant recipients. Transplantation 1994;57:502–6.

54. Fein A, Vechoropoulos M, Nebel L. Cyclosporin-induced embryotoxicity in mice. Biol Neonate 1989;56:165–73.

55. Pickrell MD, Sawers R, Michael J. Pregnancy after renal transplantation: severe intrauterine growth retardation during treatment with cyclosporin A. Br Med J (Clin Res Ed) 1988;296:825.

56. Armenti VT, Radomski JS, Moritz MJ, et al. National Transplantation Pregnancy Registry (NTPR): Outcomes of pregnancy after transplantation. In: Cecka JM, Terasaki PI, editors. Clinical Transplants 2001. Los Angeles (CA): UCLA Immunogenetics Center; 2002. p. 97–105.

57. Vyas S, Kumar A, Piecuch S, et al. Outcome of twin pregnancy in a renal transplant recipient treated with tacrolimus. Transplantation 1999;67:490–2.

58. Jain A, Venkataramanan R, Fung JJ, et al. Pregnancy after liver transplantation under tacrolimus. Transplantation 1997;64(4):559–65.

59. Sifontis NM, Coscia LA, Constantinescu S, et al. Pregnancy outcomes in solid organ transplant recipients with exposure to mycophenolate mofetil or sirolimus. Transplantation 2006;82:1698–702.

60. Le Ray C, Coulomb A, Elefant E, et al. Mycophenolate mofetil in pregnancy after renal transplantation: a case of major fetal malformations. Obstet Gynecol 2004;103:1091–4.

61. Andrade Vila JH, da Silva JP, Guilhen CJ, et al. Even low dose of mycophenolate mofetil in a mother recipient of heart transplant can seriously damage the fetus. Transplantation 2008;86(2):369–70.

62. EPBG Expert Group on Renal Transplantation. European best practice guidelines for renal transplantation. Pregnancy in renal transplant recipients. Nephrol Dial Transplant 2002;17(4):50–5.

63. Rapamune package insert. Pfizer. Philadelphia, PA 2011.

64. Cardonick E, Moritz M, Armenti V. Pregnancy in patients with organ transplantation: a review. Obstet Gynecol Surv 2004;59:214–22.

65. Jankowska I, Oldakowska-Jednyak U, Jabiry-Zieniewicz Z, et al. Absence of teratogenicity of sirolimus used during early pregnancy in a liver transplant recipient. Transplant Proc 2004;36: 3232–3.

66. Guardia O, del Rial MC, Casadei D. Pregnancy under sirolimus-based immunosuppression. Transplantation 2006;81(4):636.

67. Chu SH, Liu KL, Chiang YJ, et al. Sirolimus used during pregnancy in a living related renal transplant recipient: a case report. Transplant Proc 2008;40(7):2446–8.

68. Kazmin A, Garcia-Bournissen F, Koren G. Risks of statin use during pregnancy: a systematic review. J Obstet Gynaecol Can 2007;29(11):906–8.

69. Sifontis NM, Constantinescu S, Coscia LA, et al. Long-term survival in female heart transplant recipients following pregnancy. Am J Transplant 2009;S2: 198A.

70. Finnell RH. Teratology: general considerations and principles. J Allergy Clin Immunol 1999;103:S337–42.

71. Muirhead N, Sabharwal AR, Rieder MJ, et al. The outcome of pregnancy following renal transplantation—the experience of a single center. Transplantation 1992;54:429–32.

72. Morton A. Cyclosporine and lactation. Nephrology (Carlton) 2011;16:249.

73. French AE, Soldin SJ, Soldin OP, et al. Milk transfer and neonatal safety of tacrolimus. Ann Pharmacother 2003;37:815–8.

74. Gardiner SJ, Begg EJ. Breastfeeding during tacrolimus therapy. Obstet Gynecol 2006;107:453–5.

75. Grimer M. Pregnancy, lactation and calcineurin inhibitors. Nephrology 2007;12:S98–105.

76. Flechner SM, Katz AR, Rogers AJ, et al. The presence of cyclosporine in body tissues and fluids during pregnancy. Am J Kidney Dis 1985;5:60–3.

Cardiopulmonary Resuscitation in Pregnancy

Christine K. Farinelli, MD*, Afshan B. Hameed, MD

KEYWORDS

- Pregnancy • Cardiopulmonary resuscitation • Sudden cardiac arrest
- Cardiopulmonary resuscitation

KEY POINTS

- Cardiac arrest in pregnancy requires timely identification, initiation of cardiopulmonary resuscitation (CPR), and expedited delivery of the infant to achieve optimal outcomes for mother and infant.
- The etiology of cardiac arrest varies, and it is imperative for treating physicians to be able to identify reversible causes in a timely fashion.
- The normal physiologic changes of pregnancy may have a profound effect on CPR, and require several modifications be made to the usual resuscitative algorithms.
- When determining whether to perform a perimortem cesarean, several factors must be accounted for: gestational age, features of the cardiac arrest, setting of the arrest.
- Clinical experience with the usual medications used for advanced cardiac life support is limited in pregnancy. Acutely, the benefits of restoring maternal circulation outweigh the potential risks.

INTRODUCTION

Cardiac arrest during pregnancy is a rare event complicating 1 in 30,000 pregnancies in the United States annually. Women increasingly are seeking pregnancy at a later age, as evidenced by recent statistics: approximately 1 in 12 first births in the United States in 2008 were to women aged 35 years and older compared with 1 in 100 in 1970.[1] Advances in medical care have improved survival and quality of life, leading to successful pregnancies in women with serious underlying medical conditions who are then predisposed to catastrophic outcomes requiring cardiopulmonary resuscitation (CPR). Cardiac arrest requires high-quality medical care consisting of timely identification, initiation of CPR, and expedited delivery of the infant within 4 to 5 minutes to achieve optimal outcomes for mother and infant. However, 2 recent publications[2,3] indicate that obstetricians, midwives, and anesthetists possess limited knowledge regarding the current recommendations for the treatment of maternal cardiac arrest. There is a need for the health care providers caring for pregnant women to raise their awareness of the recommendations for and training in CPR in pregnancy.

CASE PRESENTATION

A 34-year-old apparently healthy woman, 38 weeks pregnant, was admitted to labor and delivery for labor augmentation. On admission to the hospital, her vital signs were stable and the fetal heart tracing was normal. She had been having prodromal labor for several days and her cervical examination was 4 cm dilated, 50% effaced, at −2 station. Approximately 10 minutes after her membranes were artificially ruptured, she complained of sudden anxiety and developed witnessed cardiorespiratory arrest,

Disclosures: None.
Maternal Fetal Medicine, University of California, Irvine, 101 The City Drive South, Building 56, Suite 800, Orange, CA 92868, USA
* Corresponding author.
E-mail address: cfarinel@uci.edu

Cardiol Clin 30 (2012) 453–461
doi:10.1016/j.ccl.2012.04.006
0733-8651/12/$ – see front matter © 2012 Elsevier Inc. All rights reserved.

cardiology.theclinics.com

which was accompanied by severe fetal bradycardia. CPR was immediately started by the obstetrician and anesthesiologist, and the patient was rapidly transferred to the nearby operating room for an emergency cesarean delivery. Within 5 minutes of the cardiac arrest the infant was delivered, and resuscitation of the mother continued thereafter and was successful. The patient recovered slowly over many weeks in the intensive care setting, because of multisystem failure related to anaphylactoid syndrome of pregnancy and its complications, including disseminated intravascular coagulation, renal failure, and hepatic failure. She was discharged home with minor neurologic sequelae.

ETIOLOGY AND CONTRIBUTORY FACTORS

The etiology of cardiac arrest varies (**Box 1**), and it is imperative for treating physicians to be able to identify reversible causes in a timely fashion (**Box 2**). A typical gravid victim of cardiac arrest is younger with fewer underlying medical conditions than a nonpregnant victim; however, with the recent trends in delayed childbearing, this demographic may change. It is well known that

---

Box 1
Etiology of cardiac arrest in pregnancy

- Thromboembolism
- Pregnancy-induced hypertension (including preeclampsia, eclampsia)
- Sepsis/infection
- Trauma
- Hemorrhage
  - Placental abruption
  - Placenta previa
  - Uterine atony
  - Disseminated intravascular coagulation
- Cerebrovascular accident
- Asthma
- Iatrogenic
  - Medication allergy or error
  - Anesthestic complications
  - Hypermagnesemia
- Preexisting heart disease
  - Congenital
  - Acquired (cardiomyopathy)
- Anaphylactoid syndrome of pregnancy (previously amniotic fluid embolism)

Box 2
Possibly reversible causes of cardiac arrest

Hypovolemia

Hypoxia

Hydrogen ion acidosis

Hyperkalemia or hypokalemia, other metabolic

Hypothermia

Hypoglycemia

Trauma

Tamponade, cardiac

Tension pneumothorax

Thrombosis, coronary or pulmonary

Toxins (ie, amniotic fluid, preeclampsia)

Tablets (drug overdose)

---

pregnancy increases the risk of venous thromboembolic disease (VTE) because of hormonal stimulation of procoagulant proteins. Thromboembolic risk is enhanced by conditions necessitating bed rest (preterm labor, gestational hypertension), and is further amplified in the immediate postpartum period because of inactivity and tissue trauma.[4] Pregnancy also increases the risk of myocardial infarction by 3- to 4-fold over comparable nonpregnant women, especially in women older than 30 years.[5] Progesterone-mediated relaxation of smooth muscle may enhance the risk of coronary artery and aortic dissections seen in pregnant women in comparison with their nonpregnant counterparts.[6]

Pregnancy carries unique risks, including the anaphylactoid syndrome of pregnancy (previously termed amniotic fluid embolus) and gestational hypertension (GHTN). Anaphylactoid syndrome is characterized by cardiac depression, cardiopulmonary collapse, and coagulopathy. It is considered extremely morbid, with a 50% to 65% risk of cardiac arrest and maternal mortality.[7,8] This disorder is associated with profound vascular leaking, and resuscitation efforts may result in massive pulmonary edema; therefore, cardiovascular support and correction of coagulopathy is vital while avoiding fluid overresuscitation.

While the etiology of gestational hypertension remains to be fully elucidated, it is known that GHTN, including preeclampsia and eclampsia, results in maternal morbidity and even mortality, likely due to widespread endothelial injury and inflammation. Antihypertensive therapy along with magnesium as indicated for seizure prophylaxis may result in cardiopulmonary compromise, particularly with concomitant use of calcium-channel antagonists and magnesium. Magnesium sulfate toxicity may be reversed with typically 1 g of intravenous calcium carbonate.

PHYSIOLOGY AND TECHNIQUES OF CARDIOPULMONARY RESUSCITATION

In the event of a primary respiratory arrest the heart continues to pump for several minutes, providing oxygen to the lungs and bloodstream to support life for up to 6 minutes. However, if cardiac arrest occurs first, no oxygen is supplied to the vital organs. A patient whose heart and respirations have ceased for less than 4 minutes has an excellent chance of recovery with CPR and advanced cardiac life support (ACLS). Brain damage may occur after 4 minutes, and becomes certain after 6 minutes. The initial goals of CPR, therefore, are to deliver oxygen to the lungs and perfuse the vital organs. These goals are achieved by performing the "C-A-B-Ds" of the primary and secondary surveys.[9]

The primary survey consists of airway management using noninvasive techniques, positive pressure ventilation, and performing CPR until an automated external defibrillator (AED) arrives. The secondary survey requires the use of advanced, invasive techniques to further resuscitate and stabilize the patient (Table 1). For full details regarding basic life support (BLS) and ACLS, the reader is referred to the guidelines published by the American Heart Association (AHA).[9] However, a brief review is provided here.

In 1960, Kouwenhoven and colleagues[10] first described external chest compressions as a means to provide circulation in a pulseless patient. Current understanding of the primary mechanism of blood movement involves fluctuations in the intrathoracic pressure caused by compressions that then leads to a peripheral arteriovenous pressure gradient.[11] External chest compressions increase the intrathoracic pressure, which is distributed to all intrathoracic structures. However, competent venous valves prevent transmission of this pressure to extrathoracic veins, whereas arteries transmit the increased pressure, creating an artificial gradient and forward blood flow. The mitral and tricuspid valves remain open during CPR, supporting the notion that the heart acts as a passive conduit at this time.[12]

When chest compressions are required in a pulseless patient, they should be given at a rate of 100 times per minute and interrupted only for brief assessments and application of electrical therapy when necessary. Defibrillators can be used without significant complications to the fetus in pregnant women, and no modifications to the current recommendations are necessary.[13,14]

Opening the airway and beginning rescue breathing achieves delivery of oxygen to the patient. However, in the unconscious patient the tongue and epiglottis often obstruct the airway, and must be relieved with either the head-tilt with chin-lift maneuver or the jaw-thrust maneuver.[9] Foreign material may also cause obstruction, and should be removed manually or with active suction if available. If air does not appear to enter the lungs with rescue breathing, it is important to reposition the head and attempt rescue breathing again. Persistent obstruction may require the Heimlich maneuver (subdiaphragmatic abdominal thrusts), chest thrusts, removal of a foreign body if visible, and rescue breathing. The Heimlich maneuver is contraindicated in the later stages of pregnancy or in an obese patient. A patient who is conscious but struggling with a partial airway obstruction should attempt removal of the obstruction herself. If appropriate equipment is available and nonsurgical procedures fail to relieve the airway obstruction, emergency cricothyroidotomy or jet-needle insufflation are indicated.

Abdominal thrusts are performed by wrapping the rescuer's hands around the victim's waist,

Table 1
Primary and secondary surveys of emergency cardiac care

	Primary	Secondary
C (Circulation)	Chest compressions/Doppler fetal heart tones	Intravenous access, pharmacologic interventions, assess rhythm
A (Airway)	Open	Intubate/advanced airway devices
B (Breathing)	Positive pressure ventilation (PPV)	Assess bilateral chest rise and ventilation/PPV
D (Defibrillate)	Shock ventricular fibrillation, pulseless ventricular tachycardia	Differential diagnosis: treat reversible causes; consider delivery

Adapted from Hueppchen NA, Satin AJ. Cardiopulmonary resuscitation. In: Dildy GA, Belfort MA, Saade G, et al, editors. Critical care obstetrics. 4th edition. Wiley-Blackwell Publishing Ltd; 2008. p. 88; with permission.

making a fist with one hand and placing the thumb side of the fist against the victim's abdomen in the midline, slightly above the umbilicus and well below the top of the xiphoid process. The rescuer grasps the fist with the other hand and presses the fist into the victim's abdomen with quick, upward thrusts. The thrusts are continued until the obstructing object is expelled or the victim becomes unconscious, at which time the victim is placed in a supine position and upward thrusts are administered using the heel of one hand against the victim's abdomen with the second hand on top of the first.

Chest thrusts are necessary in later pregnancy or in obese patients. In a victim who is conscious, sitting, or standing, the rescuer's fist is placed on the middle of the sternum, thumb side down, avoiding the xiphoid and ribs. The rescuer grabs the fist with the other hand and performs chest thrusts until the object dislodges or the victim becomes unconscious. Once unconscious, the victim is placed in the supine position and the rescuer's hand is placed 2 fingerbreadths above the xiphoid. The long axis of the heel of the hand should rest along the long axis of the sternum. The second hand is placed over the first and the chest is compressed 1.5 to 2 inches. After 5 abdominal or chest thrusts, the jaw-lift should be repeated, and visualization of the foreign body and ventilation attempted again.

If the patient is unresponsive but breathing spontaneously, she should be placed in the recovery position to keep the airway open. The pregnant patient is placed on her left side with the left arm placed at a right angle to the victim's torso and the right arm placed across her chest with the back of her hand under the lower cheek. The right thigh should be flexed at a right angle to the torso, across the left leg, with the right knee resting on the surface. The victim's head should be tilted back to maintain the airway. Fetal monitoring should be initiated as soon as possible and breathing should be monitored regularly.

If a respiratory arrest is witnessed when the airway is known to be clear, the airway must be protected from aspiration and kept patent. Endotracheal intubation by direct laryngoscopy is preferred for maintaining the airway of a gravid victim. Alternative techniques include endotracheal intubation by light stylet, esophageal tracheal combitube, laryngeal mask airway, and transtracheal ventilation. Tracheal intubation protects the airway, facilitates oxygenation and ventilation, and provides a route for administration of medications during a cardiac arrest. Tracheal-tube placement is typically confirmed with end-tidal carbon dioxide indicators, but may also be performed with esophageal detector devices. These devices, however, may produce false-negative results in late pregnancy because of the decreased functional residual capacity (FRC) and tracheal compression. Direct visualization remains the gold standard for confirmation in pregnant women.

Rescue breathing may be performed via mouth-to-mouth, mouth-to-nose, mouth-to-mask, bag-valve-to-mask, or endotracheal intubation. The current guidelines recommend a ratio of 2 ventilations to 30 compressions in 1- or 2-person CPR, pausing for ventilations in the absence of an advanced airway. With a protected airway, the guidelines call for continuous chest compressions at a rate of 100 per minute with rescue breaths delivered at a rate of 8 to 10 per minute (1 breath every 6–8 seconds).[9]

Adequate blood volume is necessary for maintaining circulatory function. Although volume administration is generally not recommended in cardiac arrest, it should be considered when cardiopulmonary arrest occurs secondary to postpartum hemorrhage or circulatory collapse, as seen in anaphylaxis of pregnancy. At present, whole blood or reconstitutions thereof are recommended for massive hemorrhage; overzealous use of crystalloid fluids before control of hemorrhage and in the early stages of resuscitation has actually led to decreased survival.[15]

Assessment of the fetal status and whether delivery of the fetus would benefit the mother and/or fetus should be evaluated at this time as well. If fetal heart tones are not present, treatment should be directed toward maternal survival, which may include uterine evacuation to improve CPR efforts. If fetal heart tones are present, delivery may again be indicated to improve survival of both patients, but gestational age also plays a significant role in this decision (see the section Perimortem Cesarean Delivery).

EFFECTS OF PREGNANCY ON CARDIOPULMONARY RESUSCITATION

The normal physiologic changes of pregnancy may have a profound effect on CPR (**Table 2**). Airway access and maintenance can be difficult in the gravid patient secondary to enlarged breasts and increased pharyngeal edema. A smaller endotracheal tube may be necessary. Also, progesterone relaxes the lower esophageal sphincter, increasing the risk of reflux and aspiration. The expanding breast tissue decreases chest wall compliance, hindering ventilation. The enlarging uterus also displaces the diaphragm upwards, leading to the decrease in FRC. The increased oxygen demand of the fetal-maternal unit, as well

Table 2
Maternal physiologic changes of pregnancy

Parameter	Direction of Change	Values in Normal Pregnancy	Effect on CPR
Respiratory			
Pharyngeal edema	↑		May need smaller endotracheal tube
Minute ventilation	↑ 50%		Increased development of hypercarbia
Oxygen consumption	↑ 20%		More rapid development of hypoxia
FRC	↓ 20%		More rapid development of hypoxia
Arterial P_{CO_2}	↓	28–32 torr	
Serum bicarbonate	↓	18–21 mEq/L	Decreased acid buffering capability
Chest wall compliance	↓		More difficult intubation, increased ventilation pressures
Cardiovascular			
Cardiac output	↑ 50%	6.2 ± 1.0 L/min	Increased circulatory demand
Blood volume	↑ 30%–50%		Dilutional anemia with decreased O_2-carrying capacity
Heart rate	↑ 15%–30%	83 ± 10 beats/min	
SVR	↓ 20%	1210 ± 256 dyne/s/cm^5	
COP	↓ 15%	18 ± 1.5 mm Hg	Propensity to pulmonary edema
PCWP	↓	7.5 ± 1.8 mm Hg	
Aortocaval compression	↑		Lateral uterine displacement required
Hematologic			
Most clotting factors	↑		Propensity to thrombosis
Gastrointestinal			
Motility	↓		Increased risk of aspiration
Lower esophageal sphincter tone	↓		Increased risk of aspiration
Renal			
Compensated respiratory alkalosis	↑		Modification of target values and increased ventilation required, avoid bicarbonate in CPR
Glomerular filtration rate	↑		Drug clearance may be modified

Abbreviations: COP, colloid osmotic pressure; CPR, cardiopulmonary resuscitation; FRC, functional residual capacity; P_{CO_2}, partial pressure of carbon dioxide; PCWP, pulmonary capillary wedge pressure; SVR, systemic vascular resistance.

Adapted from Shields A, Fausett MB. Cardiopulmonary resuscitation in pregnancy. In: Belfort M, Saade G, Foley M, et al, editors. Critical care obstetrics. 5th edition. West Sussex: Blackwell Publishing Ltd; 2010. p. 93–107; with permission.

as the decrease in FRC, predisposes the pregnant woman to rapid decreases in arterial and venous oxygen tension during periods of decreased ventilation.

Centrally, progesterone increases minute ventilation, leading to a decline in arterial carbon dioxide, thus causing renal compensation via reduction in serum bicarbonate concentration.

This normal state of maternal respiratory alkalosis enhances fetal excretion of carbon dioxide. Therefore, when maternal carbon dioxide levels increase, fetal acidosis increases as well. Fetal acidosis is also promoted by decreased utero-placental blood flow during hypoxic events. Fetal demands and the normal maternal adaptations to these demands lead to rapid maternal hypoxia and acidosis in the presence of hypoventilation, further impeding the resuscitative efforts.

Pregnancy represents a high-flow, low-resistance state characterized by a high cardiac output (CO) and low systemic vascular resistance (SVR). CO increases by 50% compared with nonpregnant values and the uterus, normally receiving 2% to 3% in the nonpregnant state, now receives 30% of that CO. This increase in CO satisfies the oxygen demands of the growing fetus, placenta, and mother.

In the later half of pregnancy, the gravid uterus compresses the inferior vena cava, iliac vessels, and abdominal aorta, leading to sequestration of up to 30% of the circulating blood volume.[16] Decreased venous return leads to supine hypotension, which then decreases the effectiveness of thoracic compressions. The enlarged uterus also obstructs forward blood flow, especially in cardiac arrest whereby arterial pressure and volume are already decreased.

MODIFICATIONS OF LIFE SUPPORT IN PREGNANCY

In general, resuscitative algorithms[15] during cardiac arrest are the same for pregnant as for nonpregnant victims, with a few exceptions:

- Heimlich maneuver is contraindicated in later pregnancy; chest thrusts may be necessary.
- Left uterine displacement to increase venous return is achieved via: (1) manual displacement of the uterus by a team member, (2) positioning the patient with a left lateral tilt on the operating room table, (3) placing a rolled towel or blanket under the patient's right hip, (4) using a human wedge or the back of an upside-down chair, or (5) use of a Cardiff wedge. This wedge is one made specifically for CPR on a pregnant patient with a 27° angle, calculated when Rees and Willis measured the resuscitative force on manikins in the supine position to be 67% of the rescuer's body weight compared with 36% in the full lateral position. At a 27° angle, the maximal

resuscitative force was 80% of that which could be achieved in the supine position.[17]
- Aggressive airway management with early intubation if possible.
- Continuous cricoid pressure to avoid aspiration.
- Increased chest wall compression force.
- Delivery within 5 minutes if the fetus is viable.
- Aggressive restoration of circulatory volume if appropriate.
- Do not administer sodium bicarbonate (NaHCO$_3$): according to animal studies, NaHCO$_3$ crosses the placenta slowly. With rapid correction of maternal metabolic acidosis, the patient's respiratory compensation will cease when her partial pressure of carbon dioxide (P$_{CO_2}$) normalizes. Therefore, the fetal P$_{CO_2}$ will also increase, leading to a reduction in the fetal pH. Instead, adequate ventilation and restoration of perfusion will effectively restore the acid-base balance.[17]
- Thrombolytic therapy: Several case reports have indicated that recombinant tissue plasminogen activators (TPA) may be indicated in certain situations. However, the use of such agents increases the risk of hemorrhage, an important caveat when an operative delivery has or is likely to occur.
- Do not use the femoral vein or other lower extremity sites for venous access, because medications administered there may not reach the maternal heart unless or until the fetus is delivered.

PERIMORTEM CESAREAN DELIVERY

Blood is sequestered by the low-resistance, high-volume uteroplacental unit, hindering effective CPR. Reports of perimortem cesareans found that optimal fetal outcomes were achieved if delivery was implemented within 5 minutes of maternal death (**Table 3**).[18,19] Delivery leads to decreased aortocaval obstruction, increased effectiveness of compressions, and an increase in maternal CO of up to 25%. In a recent review, Katz and colleagues[18] reported 12 of 22 cases with sudden and dramatic improvements in pulseless pregnant patients following uterine evacuation. Although optimal outcomes were achieved within 4 to 5 minutes of maternal asystole, multiple reports of neonatal survival without adverse neurologic sequelae suggest that this rule should not be considered absolute.

When determining whether to perform a perimortem cesarean, several factors must be rapidly

Table 3
Perimortem cesarean delivery fetal outcomes from time of death until delivery

Time Interval (min)	No. of Surviving Infants	Intact Neurologic Status of Survivors (%)
0–5	45	98
6–15	18	83
16–25	9	33
26–35	4	25
36+	1	0

Data from Clark SL, Hankins GD, Dudley DA, et al. Amniotic fluid embolism: analysis of the national registry. Am J Obstet Gynecol 1995;172(4 Pt 1):1158–67; and Katz V, Dotters DJ, Droegemueller W. Perimortem cesarean delivery. Obstet Gynecol 1986;68:571–6.

accounted for, including the gestational age, features of the cardiac arrest, and the setting of the arrest. Whereas the gravid uterus at 20 weeks' gestation already has begun to compromise venous return, fetal viability begins at approximately 24 weeks.

- Gestational age less than 20 weeks: an emergency hysterotomy likely will not improve the situation.
- Gestational age 20 to 23 weeks: an emergency hysterotomy may improve survival of the mother, although survival of the fetus is extremely unlikely.
- Gestational age greater than 24 weeks: emergent cesarean will likely rescue both mother and infant.

Features of the cardiac arrest that may increase the infant's chance of survival after a perimortem cesarean include:

- Short interval between mother's arrest and infant's delivery
- No sustained prearrest hypoxia in the mother
- Minimal or no signs of fetal distress prearrest
- Aggressive and effective resuscitative efforts for the mother
- The presence of a neonatal intensive care unit.

The setting for the perimortem cesarean is essential for survival of mother and infant. Appropriate equipment as well as skilled medical personnel for both the mother and the infant (especially if preterm) are critical. If the health care team deems that perimortem cesarean is feasible at its medical center, the protocol for

such an emergency should be activated immediately on arrest of a pregnant patient so that all team members can be assembled rapidly and delivery expedited, ideally within 4 to 5 minutes of the initial arrest. CPR should continue during delivery.

PHARMACOLOGY OF CARDIOPULMONARY RESUSCITATION

Clinical experience with the usual medications used for ACLS is limited in pregnancy, particularly in acute life-threatening situations. Vasopressors, in particular α-adrenergic or combined α and β agents, may lead to uteroplacental vasoconstriction. However, in the acute situation the benefits of restoring maternal circulation outweigh their risks.

At present, the consensus regarding the first-line pressor agent to be used in asystole or pulseless arrest favors regular-dose epinephrine (an α-adrenergic stimulator), but higher doses (>1 mg) for prolonged, resistant cardiac arrest. The second-line medication is vasopressin. Atropine reverses cholinergic-mediated decreases in heart rate, SVR, and blood pressure. However, studies to support or refute its use in cardiac arrest are sparse. Therefore, although it may be considered for asystole or pulseless activity, it is not a first-line agent.

In 2000, the AHA recommended amiodarone (a category D drug) as the medication of choice for treatment of wide-complex tachycardia, stable narrow-complex tachycardia, monomorphic and polymorphic ventricular tachycardia, and potentially shock-refractory ventricular fibrillation/tachycardia. With chronic use, fetal effects of amiodarone include growth restriction, hypothyroid goiter, enlarged fontanels, and transient bradycardia in the newborn. This medication has been used to successfully treat resistant fetal tachycardia both transplacentally and via direct insertion into the umbilical cord. As with vasopressors, the benefits of amiodarone in acute maternal resuscitation outweigh the risks seen with chronic use. Lidocaine, another antiarrhythmic, appears to be safe in pregnancy, but has a higher incidence of asystole than amiodarone and is considered a second-line agent. Magnesium may be administered for torsades de pointes (irregular/polymorphic ventricular tachycardia with prolonged QT interval). Although procainamide appears to be safe in pregnancy, its use is limited by the need for slow infusion and uncertain efficacy.

Other medications indicated in the treatment of tachyarrhythmias, including adenosine, calcium-channel blockers, and β-blockers, appear to be safe in pregnancy as well. Adenosine is recommended for stable narrow-complex atrial ventricular nodal or sinus nodal reentry tachycardia, unstable reentry supraventricular tachycardia before cardioversion, stable narrow-complex supraventricular tachycardia, and stable wide-complex tachycardia in patients with recurrence of a known reentry pathway. Calcium-channel blockers such as verapamil and diltiazem slow conduction and increase refractoriness in the atrial ventricular node, making these medications useful for stable narrow-complex tachycardia not controlled by adenosine or vagal maneuvers as well as for controlling the ventricular response in atrial fibrillation or flutter. β-Blockers are indicated for narrow-complex tachycardia originating from a reentry mechanism or an automatic focus, or for controlling the rate in atrial flutter or fibrillation in patients with preserved ventricular function.

The volume of distribution and drug metabolism varies in pregnancy from the nonpregnant state. Increased intravascular volume, reduced drug-protein binding, increased clearance of renally excreted drugs, progesterone-activated increased hepatic metabolism, and altered gastrointestinal absorption all affect the blood levels of medications. Higher doses should be considered in the gravid patient if standard doses do not produce a response.

COMPLICATIONS AND PROGNOSIS OF CARDIOPULMONARY RESUSCITATION IN PREGNANCY

Successful resuscitation is reported in 6% to 15% of patients who suffer an in-hospital cardiac arrest, and the survival is likely lower in pregnant patients secondary to the normal maternal physiologic changes and complicated resuscitative efforts. The demographics of the reproductive-age woman, however, with her overall general good health, may improve the likelihood of success.

Secondary complications of CPR may occur, including maternal injuries (fractures of ribs and sternum, hemothorax, and hemopericardium, rupture of internal organs, especially the spleen and uterus, lacerations of organs, most often the liver) and fetal injuries (central nervous toxicity from medications, hypoxemia, and acidemia from reduced uteroplacental perfusion).

Rarely, a patient is successfully resuscitated but continues in a brain-dead state and a cesarean has not been performed. Multiple medical, social, ethical, and legal principles now come into play. If an advance directive is available and deemed lawful, it should be interpreted with the patient's

values in mind in the setting of the particular situation. Legal counsel is recommended if there is conflict.

Eleven published case reports have demonstrated that pregnancy may be prolonged as long as 204 days following severe neurologic injury and as early as 15 weeks' gestation in brain-dead patients.[20,21] However, no reports describe an unfavorable outcome, likely attributable to publication bias rather than lack of actual poor outcomes. If the decision is made to prolong a pregnancy, a unique set of medical complications (termed somatic support[17]) must also be addressed, including support of maternal cardiovascular, endocrine, and respiratory systems, temperature regulation, nutrition, and prevention of infection.

Severe hypertension often occurs immediately after brain death, followed by normotension or, more commonly, hypotension requiring treatment. Brainstem herniation causes massive sympathetic discharge leading to severe vasoconstriction, which is then followed by a dramatic drop in sympathetic tone. Impaired cardiac contractility and decreased CO are reflected in the hypotensive period. The uterus, as a result, lacks autoregulation of its blood supply, and the fetus can be adversely affected. Therefore, optimizing intravascular volume with intravenous fluids and CO via inotropic medications is necessary to maintain adequate uteroplacental perfusion.

Disruption of the hypothalamic-pituitary axis leads to panhypopituitarism, commonly evidenced by diabetes insipidus and requiring administration of vasopressin. Measurements of adrenal and thyroid function can aid in replacement of these hormones, as well as cortisol levels to determine the need for treatment. Prednisone or methylprednisolone were recommended in one study because these medications do not cross the placenta easily.[20] Maternal hyperglycemia should be managed closely with serum glucose levels and titrated insulin therapy.

The diagnosis of brain death includes absence of spontaneous respirations resulting from cessation of brainstem function. Therefore, somatic support requires continued mechanical ventilation, with adjustments made for normal physiology of pregnancy. Heated humidified gas also assists with poikilothermia (body temperature dependent on the environmental temperature) resulting from loss of hypothalamic function. Poikilothermia most often leads to hypothermia, the fetal effects of which remain uncertain.

Adequate maternal nutrition is critical to fetal growth and well-being. Most reports recommend aggressive nutritional support, via enteral feeds, parenteral feeds, or both. However, exact estimations for caloric intake or protein requirements are difficult secondary to the physiologic changes in brain-dead patients.

It is vital for the physician to extensively counsel the family in their understanding of what prolongation of the pregnancy means, with regard to the potential economic, physical, and emotional costs of weeks in the intensive care unit on somatic support; and that the fetal outcome cannot be guaranteed despite expert medical care. The family must have a comprehensive understanding of these issues before proceeding with any decisions affecting the continuation or termination of the pregnancy.

SUMMARY

Cardiac arrest in pregnancy is uncommon as well as catastrophic. Early aggressive resuscitation by well-trained health care providers improves the chances of successful outcomes for both the patient and her fetus. Several modifications to standard CPR are necessary in the pregnant patient, and urgent cesarean delivery may be indicated to benefit both the mother and the infant.

REFERENCES

1. Mathews TJ, Hamilton BE. Delayed childbearing: more women are having their first child later in life. NCHS Data Brief 2009;21:1–8.

2. Einav S, Matot I, Berkenstadt H, et al. A survey of labour ward clinicians' knowledge of maternal cardiac arrest and resuscitation. Int J Obstet Anesth 2008;17:238–42.

3. Cohen SE, Andes LC, Carvalho B. Assessment of knowledge regarding cardiopulmonary resuscitation of pregnant women. Int J Obstet Anesth 2008;17:20–5.

4. Heit JA, Kobbervig CE, James AH, et al. Trends in the incidence of venous thromboembolism during pregnancy or postpartum: a 30-year population-based study. Ann Intern Med 2005;143:697–706.

5. James AH, Jamison MG, Biswas MS, et al. Acute myocardial infarction in pregnancy. Circulation 2006;113:1564–71.

6. Phillips LM, Makaryus AN, Beldner S, et al. Coronary artery dissection during pregnancy treated with medical therapy. Cardiol Rev 2006;14:155–7.

7. Martin SR, Foley MR. Intensive care in obstetrics: an evidence-based review. Am J Obstet Gynecol 2006; 195:673–89.

8. Clark SL, Hankins GD, Dudley DA, et al. Amniotic fluid embolism: analysis of the national registry. Am J Obstet Gynecol 1995;172(4 Pt 1):1158–67.

9. ECC Committee, Subcommittees and Task Forces of the American Heart Association. 2010 American Heart Association Guidelines for Cardiopulmonary Resuscitation and Emergency Cardiovascular Care. Circulation 2010;122:S640–861.

10. Kouwenhoven WB, Jude JR, Knickerbocker GG. Closed-chest cardiac massage. JAMA 1960;173(10): 1064–7.

11. Rudikoff MT, Maughan WL, Effron M, et al. Mechanisms of blood flow during cardiopulmonary resuscitation. Circulation 1980;61(2):345–52.

12. Werner JA, Greene HL, Janko CL, et al. Visualization of cardiac valve motion in man during external chest compression using two-dimensional echocardiography. Implications regarding the mechanism of blood flow. Circulation 1981;63:1417–21.

13. Ogburn PL, Schmidt G, Linman J, et al. Paroxysmal tachycardia and cardioversion during pregnancy. J Reprod Med 1982;27:359–62.

14. Nanson J, Elcock D, Williams M, et al. Do physiological changes in pregnancy change defibrillation energy requirements? Br J Anaesth 2001;87(2): 237–9.

15. Shields A, Fausett MB. Cardiopulmonary resuscitation in pregnancy. In: Belfort M, Saade G, Foley M, et al, editors. Critical care obstetrics. 5th edition. West Sussex: Wiley-Blackwell; 2010. p. 93–107.

16. Lee RV. Cardiopulmonary resuscitation of pregnant women. In: Elkayam U, Gleicher N, editors. Cardiac problems in pregnancy. 3rd edition. West Sussex: Wiley-Liss, Inc; 1998. p. 315–26.

17. Mallampalli A, Powner DJ, Gardner MO. Cardiopulmonary resuscitation and somatic support of the pregnant patient. Crit Care Clin 2004;20:747–61.

18. Katz V, Balderston K, DeFreest M. Perimortem cesarean delivery: were our assumptions correct? Am J Obstet Gynecol 2005;192:1916–20.

19. Katz V, Dotters DJ, Droegemueller W. Perimortem cesarean delivery. Obstet Gynecol 1986;68:571–6.

20. Bernstein IM, Watson M, Simmons GM, et al. Maternal brain death and prolonged fetal survival. Obstet Gynecol 1989;74:734–7.

21. Sim KB. Maternal persistent vegetative state with successful fetal outcome. J Korean Med Sci 2001; 16:669–72.

Cardiovascular Drugs in Pregnancy

William H. Frishman, MD[a,]*, Uri Elkayam, MD[b],
Wilbert S. Aronow, MD[c]

KEYWORDS

- Pregnancy • Gestation • Teratogenic fetal risk • Pharmacotoxicity • Adverse reactions

KEY POINTS

- The physiologic changes that occur in pregnancy can affect the pharmacokinetic properties of cardiovascular drugs in the mother. These affects can influence the dosing of drugs and the potential loss of pharmacologic efficacy over a dosing interval.
- During pregnancy, drug transfer across the placenta and the pharmacokinetic properties of certain drugs may influence the rate of passage to the fetus and fetal drug concentrations.
- Most cardiovascular drugs are relatively safe to use in pregnancy when used for appropriate indications. However, drugs that block the renin-angiotensin system (angiotensin-converting enzyme inhibitors, angiotensin receptor blockers, and direct renin inhibitors) and warfarin are fetotoxic and are contraindicated in pregnancy.
- Some antiarrhythmic drugs can be administered to the mother (eg, digoxin, quinidine), and through placental transfer, can treat fetal tachyarrhythmias.

CLINICAL PHARMACOLOGY

During pregnancy, certain physiologic changes occur in the cardiovascular, renal, gastrointestinal (GI), and endocrine systems that may influence the pharmacokinetics of drugs (**Table 1**),[1] thereby affecting drug transfer across the maternofetal unit.

Decreased motility in the GI tract may influence drug absorption. Drug stagnation may occur as a result of reduced gastric motility.[2] Increased gastric pH due to decreased acid secretion and increased production of alkaline mucus may affect the degree of ionization and solubility of drugs.[3] Longer transit time through the GI tract may also allow for increased metabolism of drugs in the gut wall, or conversely, more complete drug absorption leading to increased bioavailability.[4,5]

During pregnancy, increases in maternal intravascular and extravascular fluid volumes by 5–8 L also may affect drug distribution.[6,7] Because of the greater physiologic volume, higher loading doses may be required to produce expected serum drug concentrations. However, steady-state concentrations resulting from chronic drug administration do not differ from the nonpregnant state.[4] The plasma volume in a pregnant woman is increased progressively by 50% and is associated with a progressive decrease in the plasma protein concentration.[6–8] Serum albumin, the principal drug-binding protein, decreases progressively throughout pregnancy.[4] Together with the altered binding of α_1-acid glycoprotein,[9,10] the increase in fatty acids, lipids, and hormones leads to an increase in the unbound drug fraction.[4] This may partially explain the increased clearance seen

Disclosures: None.
[a] Department of Medicine, New York Medical College/Westchester Medical Center, Munger Pavilion, Room 263, Valhalla, NY 10595, USA; [b] Department of Medicine, USC School of Medicine, 2025 Zonal Avenue, Los Angeles, CA 90033, USA; [c] Department of Medicine, Cardiology Division, New York Medical College/Westchester Medical Center, Macy Pavilion, Room 138, Valhalla, NY 10595, USA
* Corresponding author.
E-mail address: William_Frishman@nymc.edu

cardiology.theclinics.com

Table 1
Factors affecting drug kinetics during pregnancy

Process	Mother	Placental-Fetal Unit
Absorption	Increased plasma progesterone level reduces intestinal motility resulting in a 30%–50% increase in gastric and intestinal emptying time Gastric acid and mucus secretions are reduced resulting in increased gastric pH Increased cardiac output and tidal flow increase pulmonary absorption of drugs	Only free (unbound) drug can cross the placental barrier Nonionized, highly lipid-soluble molecules penetrate biological membranes more quickly than less lipid-soluble ionized molecules Maternal and fetal pH are important determinants of placental transfer, especially for weakly acidic or basic drugs (weakly basic drugs cross the placenta easily in the nonionized form but ionize in the relatively acidic fetal blood, resulting in more drug transfer to the fetus (this is referred to as ion trapping)
Distribution	A 50% plasma volume expansion may result in altered volume of distribution of some drugs Mean total body water increases by 8 L, of which 40% is to maternal tissue (remainder to placenta, fetus and amniotic fluid)	Half the fetal circulation (umbilical vein) directly reaches the heart and brain, bypassing the liver
Protein binding	Reduced number of available binding sites because of occupancy by steroid and placental hormones Dilutional hypoalbuminemia occurs, decreasing protein binding	Drug affinity for fetal plasma proteins can be less (eg, ampicillin) or greater (eg, salicylates) than affinity for maternal proteins
Elimination	Changes in levels of endogenous substance may result in increases or decreases in hepatic elimination of drugs (eg, phenytoin metabolism is increased, possibly caused by stimulation of microsomal enzymes by progesterone; theophylline metabolism is decreased, possibly because of competitive inhibition by progesterone and estradiol) A 25%–50% increase in renal plasma flow and a 50% increase in glomerular filtration rate may increase renal elimination of drugs[a]	Elimination of drugs from the fetus is primarily by diffusion of the drug back to the maternal compartment (although there is some evidence that both the placenta and fetus are capable of metabolizing drugs) As the fetal kidney matures, more drugs are excreted into the amniotic fluid

[a] The changes in renal drug elimination are usually clinically insufficient to require dosage alteration.

Data from Loebstein R, Lalkin A, Koren G. Pharmacokinetic changes during pregnancy and their clinical relevance. Clin Pharmacokinet 1997;33:328–43.

with some drugs and the resultant decrease in total drug concentration. Tissue-to-plasma distribution of drugs also is increased.[11] Because the bound drug concentration is decreased, the average total drug concentration at steady state is less, although the mean steady-state serum concentration of the unbound drug that is therapeutically active remains unchanged. Therefore, the serum concentration of total drug in pregnant women underestimates the concentration of free drug, and may lead to unnecessary increases in drug dosage.[12] Although the mean steady-state concentration does not change, a greater fluctuation in the unbound drug concentration occurs within a dosing interval, potentiating toxic effects at the beginning of a dosing interval, or loss of therapeutic effect at the end of an interval. Consequently, more frequent dosing without change in daily dosage may be required.[12]

The metabolism of many drugs is altered during pregnancy. The principal change in cardiovascular hemodynamics is an increase of 30% to 50% in cardiac output.[6,8,13] Consequently, renal blood flow and glomerular filtration rate increase rapidly, increasing by 50% by the fourth month of gestation.[14] Therefore, certain drugs and their metabolites that principally are excreted by the kidneys are cleared more rapidly during pregnancy, resulting in subtherapeutic concentrations with the usual nonpregnant dosage regimen. The liver is another major organ of drug metabolism. Hepatic clearance depends on hepatic blood flow, the binding affinity of drugs, and the metabolizing enzyme system.[4] Progesterone increases maternal hepatic enzymatic activity, resulting in increased drug clearance. The cytochrome P450 system may also be activated in pregnancy, leading to increased drug clearance.[15] Also, some drug biotransformation may occur in the placenta and the fetal liver.[16] The placenta contains several enzymatic systems that transform certain drugs into toxic and nontoxic metabolites.[4] The fetus also may participate in drug metabolism after the eighth week of gestation.[17]

Drug transfer across the placenta can occur by simple diffusion for almost all drugs when taken in significant amounts by the mother.[4] The rate of diffusion obeys Fick's Law which states that the diffusion rate is directly proportional to the maternal-fetal concentration gradient and the surface area of the placenta, and is inversely proportional to the thickness of the placental membrane. Drug properties such as degree of lipid solubility, molecular weight, degree of ionization, and the pH difference between maternal and fetal fluids also may influence the rate of passage. Therefore, diffusion is facilitated by a drug's high degree of lipid solubility, low degree of ionization, and low molecular weight. The transfer of weak acids and bases also depends on their pKa and the pH of the maternal and fetal fluids. Fetal plasma tends to be slightly more acidic than maternal plasma. Weak bases become ionized after crossing the placental membrane and therefore become trapped in the more acidic fetal circulation. In fetal acidosis, such drug trapping may lead to higher drug concentrations in the fetus than in the mother.

In this article, various classes of cardiac drugs are discussed with regard to pregnancy.

CARDIAC GLYCOSIDES

Numerous animal and human studies have shown that both digoxin and digitoxin are transferred readily across the placenta. Okita and colleagues[18] observed low levels of transplacental digitoxin present in the fetus after 3 to 5 hours of an intravenous injection of digitoxin to the mother. Increasing transplacental passage of digoxin is observed as pregnancy progresses, presumably as the maternofetal placental unit becomes more developed. Saarikoski[19] injected a single dose of radioactive digoxin into pregnant women before legal abortion and observed low levels in fetal tissues. He concluded that in the first half of gestation, digoxin uptake by the fetus is limited. No teratogenicity has been associated with the use of the cardiac glycosides. However, adverse effects on the fetus have been found in mothers who developed digitalis toxicity. Digoxin is a mainstay in the treatment of fetal arrhythmias, providing an 80% success rate in cardioverting supraventricular tachycardias (SVT).[20,21]

ANTIARRHYTHMICS
Class IA Antiarrhythmics

Quinidine has been used to treat pregnant women with ectopic rhythms since the 1930s. The drug has also been used successfully, alone or in combination with other antiarrhythmics, for transplacental treatment of fetal SVT[22] and fetal atrial flutter.[23] Its relative safety has been demonstrated repeatedly.[24]

Procainamide has no known teratogenic effects.[25] It can be used with relative safety to treat a variety of maternal and fetal arrhythmias. However, because of the high incidence of antinuclear antibodies and the lupuslike syndrome observed with chronic therapy, its use in long-term therapy should be reserved for patients who are refractory to or who do not tolerate quinidine.

Disopyramide readily crosses the placenta.[25,26] Neonatal concentrations have been found to be approximately 40% of maternal concentrations. Disopyramide has not been shown to be teratogenic in animal studies when given orally in doses less than 150 mg/kg body weight. However, low fetal weight was reported after higher dosing of the drug.[25,26] Because of limited experience regarding its use and compelling evidence of its oxytocic properties, disopyramide should be used with caution during pregnancy as it may induce premature uterine contractions. It should be reserved for use in selected patients who do not respond to other antiarrhythmic agents.

Class IB Antiarrhythmics

Lidocaine has been used primarily for epidural or local anesthesia during pregnancy. Investigators have shown that lidocaine rapidly crosses the placenta after intravenous or epidural administration.[27–29] Despite the small amount of information on the actual use of lidocaine as an antiarrhythmic agent during pregnancy, data gathered from its clinical application as a local and epidural anesthetic agent indicate that it is relatively safe to use in pregnancy with careful blood monitoring. To avoid any possible side effects, fetal acid-base status should be within the normal range and maternal lidocaine blood levels should be kept within the mid to low therapeutic range. Because it is metabolized mainly by the liver, pregnant women with decreased hepatic flow should have their dosing regimen reduced accordingly.

Mexiletine is well absorbed from the GI tract. Because it is absorbed almost completely from the proximal bowel, the delayed gastric emptying that occurs in pregnancy may retard its absorption. Mexiletine administration during pregnancy is associated with no consequent adverse effects.[30] However, isolated reports of fetal bradycardia, small size for gestational age, low Apgar scores, and neonatal hypoglycemia have been associated with its use.[30,31] Nevertheless, no teratogenic or long-term adverse effects have been observed in these or other reported cases.

Tocainide is not recommended for use in pregnancy until there is more evidence documenting its safety.

Class IC Antiarrhythmics

Flecainide has been used with clinical effectiveness and safety to treat several cases of maternal tachyarrhythmias[32,33] and fetal tachycardias.[34–36] Flecainide readily crosses the placenta[33] with approximately 70% to 80% of the drug being transferred to the fetus.[33,35,36]

Flecainide has become the treatment of choice for fetal SVT.[37] It is especially useful in treating cases refractory to digoxin and in those complicated by hydrops fetalis.[38] Although most reported cases have good outcomes, caution is still advised with flecainide use.[37] Class 1C antiarrhythmic agents have been described favorably in pregnancy, however, the absence of information gathered from controlled studies involving the use of these drugs during pregnancy and breast feeding does not permit clear recommendations at this time.

Class II Antiarrhythmics: β-Adrenergic Blocking Agents

β-Adrenergic blocking agents act by blocking β1 and β2 receptors. Cardiac effects are mediated primarily by β1 receptors, whereas β2 receptors are found in the bronchi and the blood vessels. β2 receptor–mediated myometrial relaxation also occurs in pregnancy. Nonselective β-blockers include propranolol, nadolol, pindolol, timolol,

sotalol, carvedilol, and labetalol (carvedilol and labetalol also have α-blocking activity); β1-selective antagonists include atenolol, metoprolol, nebivolol, and esmolol (available in intravenous form). β-Blockers are useful in the management of supraventricular and ventricular tachycardia. They are also used to control the rate of ventricular response in atrial flutter and atrial fibrillation. The antiarrhythmic effects of these agents have been attributed to the β-adrenergic blocking activity rather than the membrane-stabilizing properties possessed by some of these agents.[39]

Although no systematic study has been conducted to assess the treatment of β-blockers for arrhythmias during pregnancy, growing documentation of their use in the past few years has accumulated with regard to treatment of pregnant patients with hypertension,[40,41] hereditary long QT syndrome,[42] thyrotoxicosis,[43] idiopathic hypertrophic subaortic stenosis,[44] and fetal tachycardia.[45] To date, none of the β-blockers has been implicated as a causative agent of fetal malformation. At least 2 studies included women on β-blocker therapy before conception and no fetal abnormalities were observed in either study.[40,46] Both nonselective and selective β-blockers readily cross the placenta.[47] At delivery, similar serum drug concentrations are found in the mother and the umbilical cord, although lower fetal concentrations than maternal concentrations have been reported. The effects of α-adrenergic and β-adrenergic receptor stimulation and blockade on maternal-fetal physiology are shown in **Table 2**.

Hurst and colleagues[48] have made the following recommendations when using β-blockers in pregnancy:

1. Try, when possible, to avoid initiating long-term therapy during the first trimester.
2. Use the lowest dose possible. The use of adjunctive antihypertensive drugs might help achieve this goal.
3. Discontinue, if possible, therapy at least 2–3 days before delivery to limit the effect of the drug on uterine contractility and to prevent possible neonatal complications.
4. Neonates born to mothers on β-blockers should be closely observed for 72 to 96 hours after parturition unless the drug was stopped well before delivery.
5. To avoid interference with β_2-mediated uterine relaxation and peripheral vasodilation, blockers with β_1 selectivity, intrinsic sympathetic activity, or α-adrenergic blocking activity are preferred.
6. Mothers should avoid nursing their infants at the time of expected peak maternal β-blocker

Table 2
Adrenergic influences on maternal-fetal physiology

	Stimulation		Blockade	
	α Receptor	β Receptor	α Receptor	β Receptor
Fetal heart rate	↔	↑	↔	↔ ↓
Maternal heart rate	↔	↑	↔	↓
Umbilical blood flow	↔	↑	↔	↓
Myometrial activity	↑	↓	↓	↑

↔ no effect; ↑ increases; ↓ decreases.
Data from Widerhorn J, Rubin JN, Frishman WH, et al. Cardiovascular drugs in pregnancy. Cardiol Clin 1987;5:651–74.

plasma concentrations, usually occurring 3 to 4 hours after a dose.

Propranolol use in pregnancy has been favorably documented in the past 4 decades since it was introduced.[40,44,46,49,50] However, adverse fetal effects have been described, including bradycardia,[51] birth apnea,[52] hypoglycemia,[51] intrauterine growth retardation (IUGR),[51,53,54] hyperbilirubinemia,[51] polycythemia,[51] prolonged labor,[51] and a single case of fetal death.[55] None of these complications, however, were reported consistently in chronic therapy studies.

Esmolol is a β₁-adrenergic receptor blocker that has been used in pregnancy to control heart rate in thyrotoxicosis, to treat increased blood pressure, and to treat supraventricular arrhythmias.[48] It has a rapid onset of action and maximum effect (within 5–10 minutes), a plasma half-life of only 9 minutes, and a duration of action lasting 20 minutes. Esmolol has a rapid transplacental passage and its administration lowers both maternal and fetal heart rate.[48] However, the heart rate returns to normal once the drug is discontinued.

Sotalol is a nonselective β-adrenergic antagonist with class III electrophysiologic properties. It has been used in pregnancy to manage chronic hypertension and maternal and fetal arrhythmias. Third trimester pharmacokinetics demonstrated a plasma half-life of 11 and 7 hours after a single oral and intravenous dose of sotalol, respectively, similar to the half-life obtained 6 weeks postpartum.[56] Drug clearance was significantly greater in the third trimester but the volume of distribution did not change compared with postpartum. Sotalol readily crosses the human placenta.[56]

Transplacental therapy with sotalol has been used to treat fetal SVT. In 1 study, 14 fetuses diagnosed with SVT at gestational ages ranging from 24 to 35 weeks were first treated with digoxin before oral sotalol (80–160 mg × 2) was given to the mother.[57] Cardioversion was obtained in 10 fetuses. Two of the nonresponding fetuses did

not cardiovert even after using different combinations of digoxin, sotalol, flecainide, and/or propafenone after birth. These fetuses were found to have a long RP tachycardia. In another study looking at 43 fetuses with perinatal atrial flutter, digoxin failed to prevent recurrence of atrial flutter at the time of delivery in a quarter of the patients, whereas no recurrence of atrial flutter was reported in the sotalol group.[58]

Class III Antiarrhythmics

No consequent adverse effects have been documented with the use of amiodarone early in gestation.[59–61] However, the high content of iodine in amiodarone, approximately 40% of its molecular weight, has been implicated in causing fetal hypothyroidism in several pregnant women receiving amiodarone therapy.[62–67] A similar incidence was found for hyperthyroidism.

In view of the conflicting literature regarding the adverse effects of amiodarone use in pregnancy, and until experience with its use is documented more widely, amiodrarone should be used with great caution in pregnancy. Because of the potent side effects, which include neonatal hypothyroidism, hyperthyroidism, bradycardia, small size for gestational age, prematurity, and possibly neurodevelopmental problems, it should be used as a second-line drug in cases resistant to those antiarrhythmic agents with a more established safety profile. Physicians using amiodarone in pregnant women should be wary of possible thyroid dysfunction and fetal thyroid hormone levels should be monitored regularly.

Class IV Antiarrhythmics: Calcium Channel Antagonists

Verapamil has been reported to be successful in the management of maternal supraventricular arrhythmias,[68–70] in the treatment of severe maternal hypertension,[71,72] preeclampsia,[73] premature labor,[74] and fetal SVT.[74–76] No adverse pregnancy or fetal outcomes were reported.

Diltiazem's electrophysiologic action is similar to verapamil. To date, there are no reported adverse effects of diltiazem use in human pregnancy. Several animal studies have documented the tocolytic properties of diltiazem.[77,78] Significant reduction in mean blood pressure with little change in heart rate has also been observed.[77,78]

Nifedipine and its indications in pregnancy have been reviewed in detail by Childress and Katz.[79] The investigators found that nifedipine demonstrated safety and efficacy in multiple studies involving pregnant women when used as an antihypertensive and tocolytic agent. Its role in the treatment of primary dysmenorrhea, bladder instability, and Raynaud syndrome was also discussed. Its successful use in the management of primary pulmonary hypertension has also been reported.[80] Studies of pregnant women on oral nifedipine have not described significant increases in maternal heart rate.[81] This may be related to the increase in plasma volume that occurs during the pregnancy and the gradual onset of oral administration.

Nicardipine is used for the treatment of angina and hypertension. Similar to nifedipine, it is also used as a tocolytic agent. However, compared with nifedipine, nicardipine is a more potent tocolytic agent but the onset of action is slower.[82]

Other Antiarrhythmic Drugs

Adenosine is a purine nucleoside that is effective in treating paroxysmal SVT (**Fig. 1**).[25] Although the data regarding the use of adenosine in pregnancy is limited, this drug seems to be safe because it is naturally occurring and short acting. The case reports describing its use in pregnancy thus far have been positive, showing both efficacy and a lack of any direct adverse or teratogenic side effects on the fetus.[83]

DRUGS USED TO TREAT ACUTE HYPERTENSION

Hydralazine, used extensively in pregnancy since the early 1950s, is one of the agents of choice for the management of hypertensive emergencies in pregnancy, as well as for maintenance therapy, to be used alone or in combination with other antihypertensive drugs (**Table 3**).[84–89] It has a direct relaxing effect on arteriolar vascular smooth muscle, producing a decrease in systemic vascular resistance and vasodilation.[90]

The use of intravenous hydralazine in hypertensive emergencies such as preeclampsia and eclampsia has been shown to be effective in lowering blood pressure and in preventing hypertensive encephalopathy or intracranial hemorrhages. Hydralazine therapy is associated with a risk of fetal distress, particularly in patients with a reduced uteroplacental reserve. In these patients, a precipitous decrease in blood pressure clearly is associated with fetal distress and should be avoided. Some investigators[91] believe that the observed reduction in uterine blood flow is caused by catecholamine-induced vasoconstriction rather than a reduction in perfusion pressure alone. They suggest that the concomitant administration of an antiadrenergic agent, such as methyldopa, as well as avoidance of an unnecessary reduction in blood pressure, may explain the low incidence of fetal distress noted in their patients.

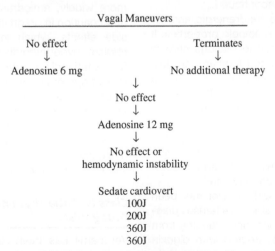

Fig. 1. Management of reentrant supraventricular tachycardia with adenosine in pregnant patients. (*From* Burkart TA, Conti JB. Arrhythmias in the pregnant patient: evaluation and management. ACC Curr J Rev 1999; 8:41; with permission.)

Table 3
Drug therapy for acute and severe hypertension in pregnancy[a]

Drug	Dose and Route	Onset of Action	Adverse Effects[b]	Comments
Hydralazine (C)	5 mg IV or IM, then 5–10 mg every 20–40 min; constant infusion of 0.5–10 mg/h	IV: 10 min IM: 10–30 min	Headache, flushing, tachycardia, and possibly arrhythmias, nausea, vomiting	Drug of choice according to NHBPEP Working Group, broad experience of safety and efficacy
Labetalol (C)	20 mg IV, then 20–80 mg every 20–30 min, up to 300 mg; constant infusion of 1–2 mg/min to desired effect, then stop or reduce to 0.5 mg/min	5–10 min	Flushing, nausea, vomiting, tingling of scalp, older literature noted retroplacental bleeding	Experience in pregnancy considerably less than that of hydralazine
Nifedipine (C)	5–10 mg by mouth; repeat in 30 min if necessary, then 10–20 mg by mouth every 3–6 h	10–15 min	Flushing, headache, tachycardia, nausea, inhibition of labor	May have synergistic interaction with magnesium sulfate; experience in pregnancy limited
Sodium nitroprusside[c] (C)	0.5–10 µg/kg/min by constant IV infusion	Instant	Cyanide toxicity, nausea, vomiting	Use only in critical care unit at low doses for briefest time feasible; may cause fetal cyanide toxicity

(C) Pregnancy risk per FDA, adverse effects in animals, no controlled trials in humans, use if risk seems justified.
Abbreviations: IM, intramuscular; IV, intravenous; NHBPEP, National High Blood Pressure Education Program.
[a] Indicated for acute increase of Korotkoff phase V blood pressure >105 mm Hg; goal is gradual reduction to 90–100 mm Hg.
[b] All agents may cause marked hypotension, especially in severe preeclampsia.
[c] Relatively contraindicated.
Adapted from Barron WM. Hypertension. In: Barron WM, Lindheimer MD, editors. Medical disorders during pregnancy. 3rd edition. St Louis (MO): Mosby Year Book; 2000. p. 16; with permission.

Labetalol is a potent antihypertensive agent, unique in that in addition to blocking both β1 and β2 adrenoceptors, it also has α1-adrenergic blocking properties and direct vasodilating activity. Its safe use in pregnancy has been documented favorably in several reports.[92,93] Clinically significant β-blocker effects, such as fetal hypoglycemia and bradycardia, have not been observed. When given in the early stages of pregnancy-induced hypertension, labetalol may slow the progression to preeclampsia.[94] However, the use of intravenous labetalol for the treatment of preeclampsia shortly before delivery has been associated with a few cases of bradycardia, inadequate breathing, hypotonia, and circulatory collapse in the newborn.[95,96]

Labetalol has also been used successfully in the treatment of maternal and fetal thyrotoxicosis.[97]

Compared with methyldopa, labetalol was quicker and more efficient in controlling blood pressure in 100 women with pregnancy-induced hypertension.[98] Eighteen percent of the patients receiving methyldopa developed proteinuria, whereas none developed proteinuria in the labetalol group. In addition, the labetalol group had a lower rate of induction of labor and cesarean delivery, a higher Bishop score at induction, and less side effects than the methyldopa group. Parenteral labetalol seems to reduce blood pressure as effectively as hydralazine.[99]

Sodium nitroprusside is one of the most potent drugs for the treatment of hypertensive emergencies, especially in patients unresponsive to intravenous hydralazine or calcium channel blockers.[1] During pregnancy, sodium nitroprusside has been used to control blood pressure during intracranial aneurysm surgery[100] or severe gestational hypertension.[101] Sodium nitroprusside was demonstrated to cross the placenta in both human[102] and animal studies.[103–105] Nitroprusside is a very effective but toxic drug. Although there is no evidence of it having any teratogenic effects, until further studies clarify its pharmacodynamics, kinetics, and safety during pregnancy, caution is recommended with its use.

Intravenous nitroglycerin was used during pregnancy to control severe pregnancy-induced hypertension and for relaxation of the uterus in the postpartum patient with retained placenta.[106,107] It may also be used when pregnancy is complicated by myocardial infarction[108] or when pulmonary edema is associated with severe preeclampsia.[109] Nitroglycerin has also been used intravenously as an effective tocolytic agent with minimal complications.[110] However, it seems that the use of nitrates in pregnancy is not without side effects, especially hypotension. Further studies are needed to fully clarify its effects and safety during pregnancy.

Minoxidil is a direct-acting vasodilator that reduces systolic and diastolic blood pressure. The reduction of arteriolar resistance and decrease in blood pressure with the drug elicits a sympathetic response followed by an activation of renin secretion. Limited information is available in the literature concerning the use of minoxidil use in pregnancy. There is no clear evidence of minoxidil being a teratogen although hypertrichosis, a generalized increase in the growth and pigmentation of body hair, was noted in newborns.[109] Thus, minoxidil use is not recommended in pregnancy.

Nifedipine has also been used for the acute treatment of hypertension. Nifedipine seems to have no significant adverse effects on fetal well-being, as long as the maternal blood pressure is not lowered excessively.[87] The usual dose for nifedipine is 5 to 10 mg by mouth, repeated in 30 minutes.

ANTIHYPERTENSIVES FOR CHRONIC TREATMENT

The treatment of mild to moderate hypertension in pregnancy may provide some maternal advantage, but is unlikely to benefit the fetus.[87,111–115] Treatment-induced decreases in mean arterial pressure in pregnant women may be associated with an increased percentage of small-for-gestational-age infants, and a minor decrease in birthweight.[111,116]

Methyldopa, an α_2 agonist, has been used long term to treat hypertension in pregnancy.[117]

There seems to be no fetal or neonatal risk with treatment.

Clonidine, another central α_2 agonist agent, has been compared with methyldopa for the treatment of hypertension in pregnancy, and seems to have comparable efficacy and safety profiles.[118] However, there is much less long-term experience with clonidine compared with methyldopa.

Angiotensin-converting enzyme (ACE) inhibitors have shown fetotoxic effects during the latter half of pregnancy in numerous animal studies. The earliest animal data came from Broughton-Pipkin and colleagues[119] in 1980 who reported on an increased fetal mortality associated with the use of captopril in pregnant ewes during the third trimester. Subsequent similar studies in which captopril was administered in middle to late gestation have substantiated the initial finding of an increased number of stillborn fetuses.[120–122] Various investigators postulated that the decreased uterine perfusion secondary to the effects of ACE inhibitors on maternal blood pressure, rather than direct inhibition of fetal renal blood flow, is the mechanism responsible for the poor fetal outcome observed.[120,123,124]

In humans, it is well established that the drugs cross the placenta in significant amounts.[125] In the fetus, ACE inhibitors are most likely excreted by the fetal kidneys in urine, which then may be re-swallowed and recirculated. Consequently, it is reasonable to conclude that there would be pharmacologic toxic effects on the fetal renal system. The first reports documenting the harmful effects of ACE inhibitors on the human fetus appeared in the early 1980s. Duminy and Burger[126] published the first report of the teratogenic effects of ACE inhibitor exposure in the human fetus. They described a 30-year-old woman with renovascular hypertension treated with captopril, propranolol, and amiloride throughout her pregnancy. She delivered a malformed fetus with a shortened left leg ending in midthigh and a defective skull vault. Many other case reports implicating ACE inhibitors as fetotoxins have appeared in the literature.[127,128] Official warnings about the use of these drugs began to appear in the mid-1980s.[129]

In 1992, the US Food and Drug Administration (FDA) issued a warning against the use of ACE inhibitors in the second and third trimesters of pregnancy.[130] The first trimester was intentionally left out of this warning because several studies showed that exposure to ACE inhibitors need not be harmful if given early in pregnancy. However, because the number of exposures assessed in these and other early pregnancy studies are small, it cannot be determined conclusively that first trimester administration of ACE inhibitors is not associated with typical ACE inhibitor fetopathy. Thus, these agents should still be avoided whenever possible throughout pregnancy. Reported cases in the literature show that ACE inhibitors produce fetotoxic effects principally affecting the developing fetal kidneys. Adverse consequences of ACE inhibitors also include oligohydramnios, IUGR, premature labor, fetal and neonatal failure, bony malformations, limb contractures, patent ductus arteriosus, pulmonary hypoplasia, respiratory distress syndrome, hypotension, anuria, and neonatal death.[131] The potential of ACE inhibitors to produce teratogenic effects is high, but additional evidence needs to be provided. Nevertheless, when the patient has failed other safer antihypertensive medications, ACE inhibitors should be administered during pregnancy only as a last resort.

Angiotensin receptor blocker (ARB) drugs can potentially cause fetal morbidity and mortality, similar to ACE inhibitors. Fetal hypotension, neonatal skull hypoplasia, oligohydramnios, anuria, and death have been associated with fetal exposure to ACE inhibitors in the second and third trimesters. Because of the documented evidence of toxicity associated with use in the second and third trimesters, ARBs are not recommended for use during pregnancy, even during the first trimester. Pregnant women exposed to the drug should be monitored closely for signs of fetal renal toxicity (eg, oligohydramnios or fetal hypotension).

Direct renin inhibitors, similar to ACE inhibitors and ARBs, are contraindicated in pregnancy and lactation.

Thiazide diuretics are used in the treatment of hypertension either alone or as adjunctive therapy. They cross the placenta and appear in cord serum. Although human studies have not been conducted, they can cause injury to the fetus. Possible adverse effects include fetal or neonatal jaundice, thrombocytopenia, hypoglycemia, hemolytic anemia, hyponatremia, and fetal bradycardia (due to chlorothiazide-induced maternal hypokalemia).[132] Uterine blood flow and placental perfusion may also be impaired. In other animal studies conducted with chlorothiazide and chlorthalidone using doses 25 times and 420 times the recommended human dose, no adverse fetal effects were seen.[133]

Loop diuretics, such as furosemide, bumetanide, ethacrynic acid, and torsemide, are indicated in the management of edema associated with congestive heart failure, renal disease, hepatic cirrhosis, or toxemia of pregnancy. They should be used with caution in pregnancy, as adequate and well-controlled studies using these drugs have not been conducted on pregnant women.

Potassium-sparing diuretics are used in the management of edematous states, especially when a potassium-sparing diuretic effect is desired. They include amiloride, spironolactone, and triamterene. All 3 drugs cross the placenta, however, there is a lack of adequate and well-controlled studies in pregnant women. Animal teratogenicity studies using the 3 drugs separately at doses 20 to 30 times the recommended maximum human dose have demonstrated no fetal injury.[133] There are few data regarding the effects on pregnancy of the new selective aldosterone antagonist, eplerenone.

Carbonic anhydrase inhibitors, such as acetazolamide, are mainly used for glaucoma and are rarely used as a diuretic.[134] During pregnancy, however, they have been used in the treatment of pseudotumor cerebri.[135] The administration of acetazolamide during pregnancy has been possibly associated with metabolic acidosis, hypocalcemia, and hypomagnesemia in the newborn.[135] The US National High Blood Pressure Education Working Group has indicated that diuretics may be used in the chronically hypertensive pregnant patient who seems to be salt sensitive.[84] Diuretics do not prevent preeclampsia or perinatal death and are hazardous in preeclampsia.[132] They are contraindicated when uteroplacental perfusion is already reduced, as seen in preeclampsia. They can be used in the treatment of chronic hypertension, but not as first-line agents and only in combination with antiadrenergic agents and vasodilators. With respect to congestive heart failure during pregnancy, furosemide and thiazides, with or without digoxin, are considered the best therapy.

α-Adrenergic blockers have not been reported on much, except for the treatment of pheochromocytoma[136] in pregnancy or drug-resistant hypertension.[137]

CHOLESTEROL-LOWERING AGENTS

Hydroxymethylglutaryl-coenzyme A (HMG-CoA) reductase inhibitors (statins) are used in the treatment of patients with primary hypercholesterolemia (types IIa and IIb) with increased low-density lipoprotein (LDL) cholesterol concentrations. They inhibit the synthesis of mevalonic acid, a principal cholesterol precursor. Because mevalonic acid may play an important role in DNA replication, and is essential to the synthesis of steroids and cell membranes in fetal development, HMG-CoA reductase inhibitors are potential fetotoxins and are not recommended for use during pregnancy.[138]

Bile acid sequestrants such as cholestyramine, colesevalam, and colestipol are also used in the treatment of hyperlipidemia (type IIa) associated with increased LDL cholesterol. They are almost completely unabsorbed after oral ingestion. Problems in pregnant humans have not been documented. Theoretic adverse effects on the fetus can occur secondary to reduced maternal absorption of vitamins and nutrients with these drugs. Cholestyramine has been used to treat cholestasis in pregnancy.[139]

The National Cholesterol Education Program guidelines for adults note that such agents may be suitable for treating women during pregnancy because bile acid sequestrants are not absorbed and lack systemic toxicity.[140] The same report mentions that lipid-lowering agents, in general, should be discontinued in pregnancy because their effects on the fetus have not been well studied.

Niacin (nicotinic acid) is indicated in the treatment of primary hyperlipidemia (types IIa, IIb, III, IV, and V). It increases high-density lipoprotein (HDL) and lowers very-low-density lipoprotein (VLDL), LDL, and triglycerides plasma concentrations. No studies have been conducted in either pregnant animals or humans. However, no adverse effects have been reported with the normal daily recommended amounts. Given this lack of data, this drug is best avoided during pregnancy.

Gemfibrozil is used as a second-line drug in the management of patients with type IIb hyperlipidemia who have the triad of low HDL, high LDL, and high triglyceride levels. It is also recommended for use in severe primary hyperlipidemias, types III, IV, and V. Studies in pregnant humans have not been performed. Animal studies have demonstrated fetal adverse effects resulting in the recommendation that gemfibrozil not be used during pregnancy.[133]

Fenofibrate is also recommended as an adjunctive therapy in the management of severe primary hyperlipidemia. Potential adverse effects include cholelithiasis and carcinogenicity, as was seen with clofibrate. Although there are no adequate studies in humans, fenofibrate has been shown to be embryocidal and teratogenic in rats when given at doses 7 to 10 times the maximum recommended human dose (based on mg/m^2 surface area).[141]

Ezetimibe is a antihyperlipidemic that inhibits the absorption of cholesterol. Its use is contraindicated in pregnancy.

ANTICOAGULANT AGENTS

Heparin is a naturally occurring glycosaminoglycan synthesized by mast cells and produced by extraction from bovine and porcine intestinal mucosa. Unfractionated heparin does not cross the placenta. Although an earlier study conducted by Hall and colleagues[142] suggested a high incidence of fetal waste and prematurity associated with heparin therapy, this was later shown to be secondary to other factors separate from the condition indicated for heparin therapy.[143] Several groups have reported the successful use of prophylactic heparin during pregnancy without fetal adverse effects.[144,145] Although there has been no controlled human study, clinical observation suggests that the use of heparin for prophylaxis and for thrombosis during pregnancy has a low potential for fetal risk. However, other serious potential side effects of heparin use that warrant caution include severe thrombocytopenia and osteopenia.

Low-molecular-weight heparin (LMWH) can be manufactured from unfractionated heparin by depolymerization processes, and has the advantage of a longer half-life (2 hours vs 45–60 minutes) and greater bioavailability from subcutaneous tissue than heparin (100% vs 50%). Both animal and human studies also indicate that LMWH does not undergo placental transfer.[146,147] LMWH has become the anticoagulant of choice during pregnancy because of its lower incidence of thrombocytopenia and osteoporosis.[145]

Warfarin is an orally active 4-hydroxycoumarin. Its anticoagulating effect is caused by inhibition of the γ-carboxylation step of glutamic residues of vitamin K-dependent precursor proteins of coagulation factors II, VII, IX, and X, synthesized in the liver, which causes a net antithrombotic state. It is well known that exposure to warfarin during organogenesis results in a characteristic warfarin embryopathy.[148] Characteristic features include nasal hypoplasia with a depressed nasal bridge, which may result in respiratory distress, and stippling in uncalcified epiphyseal regions seen on radiographs. These complications are dose dependent.[149] Inhibition of γ-carboxylation of vitamin-K-dependent proteins and disturbance of calcification during embryonic development has been postulated as the cause.[150,151] Central nervous system abnormalities, such as microcephaly, mental retardation, optic atrophy, and blindness, have been attributed to fetal exposure to warfarin after the first trimester of pregnancy.[152,153] Some controversial long-term effects on children exposed to warfarin in utero may include low scores on neurologic assessment and IQ tests.[154] For these reasons, oral anticoagulants should be avoided throughout pregnancy provided there is adequate alternative therapies to protect the mother from thrombosis.

Antithrombotic therapy during pregnancy is used for the treatment and prophylaxis of venous thromboembolic disease, for the prevention and treatment of systemic embolism associated with valvular heart disease and/or prosthetic heart valves, and for the prevention of IUGR and pregnancy loss in patients with antiphospholipid lipid antibodies.[145,155]

The studies on antithrombotic use in pregnancy are, for the most part, of poor quality. Heparin is safe for the fetus and its efficacy has been established in the prophylaxis and treatment of venothromboembolic disease.[145] Although heparin in full doses has been suggested for the prevention of systemic embolism in patients with prosthetic heart valves, its actual benefit has not been well established.[145,155–157] Clearly, low doses of heparin are not as effective in preventing systemic embolization in patients with mechanical heart valves.

For venothromboembolic prophylaxis during pregnancy, either 5000 U or an adjusted heparin dose administered every 12 hours to produce a heparin level of 0.1 to 0.2 U/mL followed by 4 to 6 weeks of warfarin after delivery for low-risk patients is recommended. However, such prophylaxis has been shown to be ineffective in patients with recurrent venous thrombosis.[158] Higher subcutaneous adjusted doses of heparin provide protection equivalent to warfarin and are advised for patients at high risk. As an alternative, the use of the LMWH, enoxaparin, at 40 mg once daily throughout pregnancy, provides antifactor Xa levels effective enough to prevent venous thromboembolisms.

For venous thrombosis or pulmonary embolism, an intravenous bolus dose of 5000 U of heparin should be given followed by continuous intravenous infusion for 5 to 10 days and then by an adjusted dose by subcutaneous injection every 12 hours until term.[145,158] Heparin should be discontinued just before delivery and then both heparin and warfarin can be started in the postpartum period. Once warfarin reaches therapeutic levels (internationalized normalized ratio of 2–3), heparin can be discontinued while oral anticoagulation is maintained for 3 to 6 months.

In patients who become pregnant while receiving oral anticoagulant treatment, warfarin should be discontinued as soon as possible and heparin substituted.[145] In patients with mechanical heart valves, either full-dose heparin is used throughout pregnancy or heparin is used until the 13th week of pregnancy when warfarin can be substituted. Chan[159] has shown that the use of oral anticoagulants throughout pregnancy in women with a mechanical valve is associated

with warfarin embryopathy in 6.4% of live births (95% confidence interval, 4.6%–8.9%). The study found that replacing oral anticoagulants with heparin in the first trimester (between weeks 6 and 12) eliminates this risk but with an increased risk of thromboembolic complications. In addition, the overall risk for spontaneous abortion, stillbirth, and neonatal death remains similar to those treated with warfarin throughout pregnancy. The best management of women with mechanical heart valves may involve the use of warfarin throughout pregnancy except for the periods between 6 and 12 weeks' gestation and after 36 weeks' gestation. During these times, adjusted-dose unfractionated heparin should be used to maintain an activated partial thromboplastin time of 2.0 to 2.5 times the control. Low-dose aspirin (80–100 mg) should be considered in combination with anticoagulants in patients with prosthetic heart valves.[160]

For the pregnant patient with antiphospholipid antibodies, aspirin plus heparin or aspirin with or without prednisone has been suggested. Heparin should be used in patients who have developed a venothromboembolism.[145]

The direct thrombin inhibitor (dabigatran) and the factor 10A inhibitors (rivaroxaban, apixiban) are new oral anticoagulants that have become available.[161] Their use in pregnancy has not been established.

ANTIPLATELET DRUGS

Aspirin acetylates the cyclooxygenase enzyme responsible for the synthesis of prostaglandin endoperoxides, which results in marked inhibition of the synthesis of thromboxane A2 in platelets, thus exerting an inhibitory effect on primary hemostasis. Although an initial recommendation[144] suggests that aspirin should be avoided during pregnancy because of a potential risk of premature closure of the ductus arteriosus, a recent meta-analysis[162] and a large randomized trial[163] found no observed risk of fetal or maternal side effects in 394 pregnant women given aspirin 60 to 150 mg daily.

Clopidogrel, prasugrel, ticagrelor, and ticlopidine are inhibitors of platelet aggregation induced by adenosine diphosphate. There is no evidence of impaired fertility or fetotoxicity in animal studies. There are, however, no adequate or well-controlled studies in pregnant women.

THROMBOLYTIC AGENTS

The thrombolytics, streptokinase, urokinase, recombinant tissue plasminogen activator (rtPA),

Table 4
Guide to cardiovascular drug use in pregnancy and with nursing

Drugs	Pregnancy	Lactation	Pregnancy Category
α-Adrenergic Antagonists			
Doxazosin	Weigh benefits vs risk	Breastfeeding not recommended; excretion in milk unknown	C
Phenoxybenzamine	Weigh benefits vs risk	Breastfeeding not recommended; excretion in milk unknown	C
Phentolamine	Weigh benefits vs risk	Breastfeeding not recommended; excretion in milk unknown	C
Prazosin	Weigh benefits vs risk	Breastfeed with caution; drug excreted in breast milk	C
Terazosin	Weigh benefits vs risk	Breastfeeding not recommended; excretion in milk unknown	C
α₂-Adrenergic Agonists			
Clonidine	Weigh benefits vs risk	Breastfeed with caution; drug excreted in breast milk	C
Guanabenz	Weigh benefits vs risk	Breastfeeding not recommended; excretion in milk unknown	C
Guanfacine	Use only if clearly indicated	Breastfeeding not recommended; excretion in milk unknown	C
Methyldopa	Weigh benefits vs risk	Breastfeed with caution; drug excreted in breast milk	B(PO), C(IV)
ACE Inhibitors			
Benazepril	The use of ACE inhibitors during the second and third trimesters of pregnancy has been associated with fetal and neonatal injury, including hypotension, neonatal skull hypoplasia, anuria, reversible or irreversible renal failure and death	Breastfeeding not recommended; excretion in milk unknown	C (first trimester)
Captopril		Breastfeeding not recommended; drug excreted in breast milk	D (second, third trimesters)
Enalapril		Breastfeeding not recommended; drug excreted in breast milk	
Fosinopril		Breastfeeding not recommended; drug excreted in breast milk	
Lisinopril		Breastfeeding not recommended; excretion in milk unknown	
Moexipril		Breastfeeding not recommended; excretion in milk unknown	

Drug	Comments	Category	Breastfeeding
Perindopril			Breastfeeding not recommended; excretion in milk unknown
Quinapril			Breastfeeding not recommended; drug excreted in breast milk
Ramipril			Breastfeeding not recommended; excretion in milk unknown
Trandolapril			Breastfeeding not recommended; excretion in milk unknown
Angiotensin-II-Receptor Blockers			
Azilsartan	The use of medications that act directly on the renin-angiotensin system during the second and third trimesters of pregnancy has been associated with fetal and neonatal injury including hypotension, neonatal skull hypoplasia, anuria, reversible or irreversible renal failure, and death	C	Breastfeeding not recommended; excretion in milk unknown
Candesartan		C (first trimester)	Breastfeeding not recommended; excretion in milk unknown
Eprosartan		D (second, third trimesters)	Breastfeeding not recommended; excretion in milk unknown
Irbesartan			Breastfeeding not recommended; excretion in milk unknown
Losartan			Breastfeeding not recommended; excretion in milk unknown
Olmesartan			Breastfeeding not recommended; excretion in milk unknown
Telmisartan			Breastfeeding not recommended; excretion in milk unknown
Valsartan			Breastfeeding not recommended; excretion in milk unknown
Antianginal Agent			
Ranolazine	Weigh benefits vs risk	C	Breastfeeding not recommended; excretion in milk unknown
Antiarrhythmic Agents			
Class IA			
Disopyramide	Weigh benefits vs risk	C	Breastfeeding not recommended; drug excreted in breast milk
Procainamide	Weigh benefits vs risk	C	Breastfeeding not recommended; drug excreted in breast milk
Quinidine	Weigh benefits vs risk	C	Breastfeeding not recommended; drug excreted in breast milk

(continued on next page)

Table 4
(continued)

Drugs	Pregnancy	Lactation	Pregnancy Category
Class IB			
Lidocaine	Use only if clearly indicated	Breastfeed with caution; drug excreted in breast milk	B
Mexiletine	Weigh benefits vs risk	Breastfeeding not recommended; drug excreted in breast milk	C
Tocainide	Weigh benefits vs risk	Breastfeeding not recommended; drug excreted in breast milk	C
Class IC			
Flecainide	Weigh benefits vs risk	Breastfeeding not recommended; drug excreted in breast milk	C
Moricizine	Use only if clearly indicated	Breastfeeding not recommended; drug excreted in breast milk	B
Propafenone	Weigh benefits vs risk	Breastfeeding not recommended; excretion in breast milk unknown	C
Class II (β-Blockers)			
Acebutolol	Use only if clearly indicated	Breastfeeding not recommended; drug excreted in breast milk	B
Atenolol	Weigh benefits vs risk	Breastfeeding not recommended; drug excreted in breast milk	D
Betaxolol	Weigh benefits vs risk	Breastfeed with caution; drug excreted in breast milk	C
Bisoprolol	Weigh benefits vs risk	Breastfeeding not recommended; excretion in milk unknown	C
Carteolol	Weigh benefits vs risk	Breastfeeding not recommended; excretion in milk unknown	C
Carvedilol	Weigh benefits vs risk	Breastfeeding not recommended; excretion in milk unknown	C
Esmolol	Weigh benefits vs risk	Breastfeeding not recommended; excretion in milk unknown	C
Labetalol	Weigh benefits vs risk	Breastfeed with caution; drug excreted in breast milk	C
Metoprolol	Weigh benefits vs risk	Breastfeeding not recommended; drug excreted in breast milk	C

Drug			
Nadolol	Weigh benefits vs risk	Breastfeed with caution; drug excreted in breast milk	C
Nebivolol	Weigh benefits vs risk	Breastfeeding not recommended; excretion in milk unknown	C
Penbutolol	Weigh benefits vs risk	Breastfeeding not recommended; excretion in milk unknown	C
Pindolol	Use only if clearly indicated	Breastfeed with caution; drug excreted in breast milk	B
Propranolol	Weigh benefits vs risk	Breastfeed with caution; drug excreted in breast milk	C
Timolol	Weigh benefits vs risk	Breastfeed with caution; drug excreted in breast milk	C
Class III			
Amiodarone	Not recommended	Breastfeeding not recommended; drug excreted in breast milk	D
Bretylium	Weigh benefits vs risk	Breastfeeding not recommended; excretion in milk unknown	C
Dofetilide	Weigh benefits vs risk	Breastfeeding not recommended; excretion in milk unknown	C
Dronedarone	Contraindicated	Breastfeeding not recommended; excretion in milk unknown	X
Ibutilide	Weigh benefits vs risk	Breastfeeding not recommended; excretion in milk unknown	C
Sotalol	Use only if clearly indicated	Breastfeeding not recommended; drug excreted in breast milk	B
Class IV (Calcium Antagonists)[a]			
Amlodipine	Weigh benefits vs risk	Breastfeeding not recommended; excretion in milk unknown	C
Clevidipine	Weigh benefits vs risk	Breastfeeding not recommended; excretion in milk unknown	C
Diltiazem	Weigh benefits vs risk	Breastfeeding not recommended; drug excreted in breast milk	C
Felodipine	Weigh benefits vs risk	Breastfeeding not recommended; excretion in milk unknown	C

(continued on next page)

Table 4
(continued)

Drugs	Pregnancy	Lactation	Pregnancy Category
Isradipine	Weigh benefits vs risk	Breastfeeding not recommended; excretion in milk unknown	C
Nicardipine	Weigh benefits vs risk	Breastfeeding not recommended; excretion in milk unknown	C
Nifedipine	Weigh benefits vs risk	Breastfeeding not recommended; drug excreted in breast milk	C
Nimodipine	Weigh benefits vs risk	Breastfeeding not recommended; excretion in milk unknown	C
Nisoldipine	Weigh benefits vs risk	Breastfeeding not recommended; excretion in milk unknown	C
Verapamil	Weigh benefits vs risk	Breastfeeding not recommended; drug excreted in breast milk	C
Antithrombotic Agents			
Anticoagulants			
Argatroban	Use only if clearly needed	Breastfeeding not recommended; excretion in milk unknown	B
Bivalirudin	Use only if clearly needed	Breastfeeding not recommended; excretion in milk unknown	B
Dabigatran	Weigh benefits vs risk	Breastfeeding not recommended; excretion in milk unknown	C
Dalteparin	Use only if clearly needed	Breastfeeding not recommended; excretion in milk unknown	B
Enoxaparin	Use only if clearly needed	Breastfeeding not recommended; excretion in milk unknown	B
Fondaparinux	Use only if clearly needed	Breastfeeding not recommended; excretion in milk unknown	B
Heparin	Weigh benefits vs risk	Not excreted in breast milk	C
Lepirudin	Use only if clearly needed	Breastfeeding not recommended; excretion in milk unknown	B
Rivaroxaban	Weigh benefits vs risk	Breastfeeding not recommended; excretion in milk unknown	C

Drug	Pregnancy	Breastfeeding	Category
Tinzaparin	Use only if clearly needed	Breastfeeding not recommended; excretion in milk unknown	B
Warfarin	Contraindicated	Breastfeeding not recommended; drug excreted in breast milk	X
Antiplatelets			
Anagrelide	Weigh benefits vs risk	Breastfeeding not recommended; excretion in milk unknown	C
Aspirin	Contraindicated in third trimester	Breastfeed with caution; drug excreted in breast milk	D
Abciximab	Weigh benefits vs risk	Breastfeeding not recommended; excretion in milk unknown	C
Clopidogrel	Use only if clearly needed	Breastfeeding not recommended; excretion in milk unknown	B
Dipyridamole	Use only if clearly needed	Breastfeed with caution; drug excreted in breast milk	B
Eptifibatide	Use only if clearly needed	Breastfeeding not recommended; excretion in milk unknown	B
Prasugrel	Use only if clearly needed	Breastfeeding not recommended; excretion in milk unknown	B
Ticagrelor	Use only if clearly needed	Breastfeeding not recommended; excretion in milk unknown	C
Ticlopidine	Use only if clearly needed	Breastfeeding not recommended; excretion in milk unknown	B
Tirofiban	Use only if clearly needed	Breastfeeding not recommended; excretion in milk unknown	B
Thrombolytics			
Alteplase (t-PA)	Weigh benefits vs risk	Breastfeeding not recommended; excretion in milk unknown	C
Anistreplase	Weigh benefits vs risk	Breastfeeding not recommended; excretion in milk unknown	C
Reteplase	Weigh benefits vs risk	Breastfeeding not recommended; excretion in milk unknown	C
Streptokinase	Weigh benefits vs risk	Breastfeeding not recommended; excretion in milk unknown	C
Tenecteplase	Weigh benefits vs risk	Breastfeeding not recommended; excretion in milk unknown	C

(continued on next page)

Table 4
(continued)

Drugs	Pregnancy	Lactation	Pregnancy Category
Diuretics			
Loop			
Bumetanide	Weigh benefits vs risk	Breastfeeding not recommended; excretion in milk unknown	C
Ethacrynic acid	Use only if clearly needed	Breastfeeding not recommended; excretion in milk unknown	B
Furosemide	Weigh benefits vs risk	Breastfeeding not recommended; drug excreted in breast milk	C
Torsemide	Use only if clearly needed	Breastfeeding not recommended; excretion in milk unknown	B
Thiazides			
Bendroflumethiazide	Weigh benefits vs risk	Breastfeed with caution; drug excreted in breast milk	C
Benzthiazide	Weigh benefits vs risk	Breastfeed with caution; drug excreted in breast milk	C
Chlorothiazide	Use only if clearly needed	Breastfeed with caution; drug excreted in breast milk	B
Chlorthalidone	Use only if clearly needed	Breastfeeding not recommended; drug excreted in breast milk	B
Hydrochlorothiazide	Use only if clearly needed	Breastfeed with caution; drug excreted in breast milk	B
Hydroflumethiazide	Weigh benefits vs risk	Breastfeeding not recommended; drug excreted in breast milk	C
Indapamide	Use only if clearly needed	Breastfeeding not recommended; drug excreted in breast milk	B
Methyclothiazide[b]	Use only if clearly needed	Breastfeeding not recommended; drug excreted in breast milk	B
Metolazone	Use only if clearly needed	Breastfeeding not recommended; drug excreted in breast milk	B
Polythiazide	Weigh benefits vs risk	Breastfeed with caution; drug excreted in breast milk	D
Quinethazone	Weigh benefits vs risk	Breastfeed with caution; drug excreted in breast milk	D

Potassium-Sparing

Drug	Recommendation	Breastfeeding	Category
Amiloride	Use only if clearly needed	Breastfeeding not recommended; excretion in milk unknown	B
Eplerenone[c]	Use only if clearly needed	Breastfeeding not recommended; excretion in milk unknown	B
Spironolactone	Weigh benefits vs risk	Breastfeeding not recommended; drug excreted in breast milk	C
Triamterene	Use only if clearly needed	Breastfeeding not recommended; excretion in milk unknown	B
Endothelin Receptor Antagonists			
Ambrisentan	Contraindicated	Breastfeeding not recommended; excretion in milk unknown	X
Bosentan	Contraindicated	Breastfeeding not recommended; excretion in milk unknown	X
Sitaxsentan	Contraindicated	Breastfeeding not recommended; excretion in milk unknown	X
Human B-Type Natriuretic Peptide			
Nesiritide	Weigh benefits vs risk	Breastfeeding not recommended; excretion in milk unknown	C
Inotropic and Vasopressor Agents			
Digoxin	Weigh benefits vs risk	Breastfeed with caution; drug excreted in breast milk	C
Amrinone (Inamrinone)	Weigh benefits vs risk	Breastfeeding not recommended; excretion in milk unknown	C
Milrinone	Weigh benefits vs risk	Breastfeeding not recommended; excretion in milk unknown	C
Dobutamine	Use only if clearly needed	Breastfeeding not recommended; excretion in milk unknown	B
Dopamine	Weigh benefits vs risk	Breastfeeding not recommended; excretion in milk unknown	C
Isoproterenol	Weigh benefits vs risk	Breastfeeding not recommended; excretion in milk unknown	C
Epinephrine	Weigh benefits vs risk	Breastfeed with caution; drug excreted in breast milk	C
Metaraminol	Weigh benefits vs risk	Breastfeeding not recommended; excretion in milk unknown	C

(continued on next page)

Table 4
(continued)

Drugs	Pregnancy	Lactation	Pregnancy Category
Methoxamine	Weigh benefits vs risk	Breastfeeding not recommended; excretion in milk unknown	C
Midodrine	Weigh benefits vs risk	Breastfeeding not recommended; excretion in milk unknown	C
Norepinephrine	Weigh benefits vs risk	Breastfeeding not recommended; excretion in milk unknown	C
Phenylephrine	Weigh benefits vs risk	Limited absorption in GI tract; excretion in milk unknown	C
Lipid-Lowering Agents			
Bile Acid Sequestrants			
Cholestyramine	Weigh benefits vs risk	Breastfeed with caution; excretion in breast milk unknown	C
Colestipol	Weigh benefits vs risk	Breastfeed with caution; excretion in breast milk unknown	Not evaluated
Colesevelam	Use only if clearly needed	Breastfeed with caution; excretion in breast milk unknown	B
Cholesterol Absorption Inhibitor			
Ezetimibe	Weigh benefits vs risk	Breastfeed with caution; excretion in breast milk unknown	C
Fibric Acid Derivatives			
Fenofibrate	Weigh benefits vs risk	Breastfeeding not recommended; excretion in milk unknown	C
Fenofibric acid	Weigh benefits vs risk	Breastfeeding not recommended; excretion in milk unknown	C
Gemfibrozil	Weigh benefits vs risk	Breastfeeding not recommended; excretion in milk unknown	C
Nicotinic Acid	Weigh benefits vs risk	Breastfeed with caution; excretion in milk unknown	C
HMG-CoA Reductase Inhibitors			
Atorvastatin	Contraindicated	Breastfeeding not recommended; excretion in milk unknown	X
Fluvastatin	Contraindicated	Breastfeeding not recommended; drug excreted in breast milk	X

Drug	Pregnancy	Breastfeeding	Category
Lovastatin	Contraindicated	Breastfeeding not recommended; excretion in milk unknown	X
Pravastatin	Contraindicated	Breastfeeding not recommended; drug excreted in breast milk	X
Rosuvastatin	Contraindicated	Breastfeeding not recommended; excretion in milk unknown	X
Simvastatin	Contraindicated	Breastfeeding not recommended; excretion in milk unknown	X
Omega-3 Fatty Acids			
Omega-3-acid ethyl esters	Weigh benefits vs risk	Breastfeed with caution; excretion in milk unknown	C
Neuronal and Ganglionic Blockers			
Guanadrel	Use only if clearly needed	Breastfeeding not recommended; excretion in milk unknown	B
Guanethidine	Weigh benefits vs risk	Breastfeeding not recommended; drug excreted in breast milk	C
Mecamylamine	Weigh benefits vs risk	Breastfeeding not recommended; excretion in milk unknown	C
Reserpine	Weigh benefits vs risk	Breastfeeding not recommended; drug excreted in breast milk	C
Trimethaphan	Not recommended	Breastfeeding not recommended; excretion in milk unknown	D
Phosphodiesterase 5 Inhibitors			
Sildenafil	Use only if clearly needed	Breastfeed with caution; excretion in milk unknown	B
Tadalafil	Use only if clearly needed	Breastfeed with caution; excretion in milk unknown	B
Renin Inhibitor			
Aliskiren	Not recommended	Breastfeeding not recommended; excretion in milk unknown	C (first trimester) D (second and third trimesters)
Vasodilators			
Cilostazol	Weigh benefits vs risk	Breastfeeding not recommended; excretion in milk unknown	C
Diazoxide	Weigh benefits vs risk	Breastfeeding not recommended; excretion in milk unknown	C

(continued on next page)

Table 4
(continued)

Drugs	Pregnancy	Lactation	Pregnancy Category
Epoprostenol	Use only if clearly needed	Breastfeeding not recommended; excretion in milk unknown	B
Fenoldopam	Use only if clearly needed	Breastfeeding not recommended; excretion in milk unknown	B
Hydralazine	Weigh benefits vs risk	Breastfeeding not recommended; drug excreted in breast milk	C
Iloprost	Weigh benefits vs risk	Breastfeeding not recommended; excretion in milk unknown	C
Isosorbide dinitrate	Weigh benefits vs risk	Breastfeeding not recommended; excretion in milk unknown	C
Isosorbide mononitrate	Weigh benefits vs risk	Breastfeeding not recommended; excretion in milk unknown	C
Isoxsuprine	Weigh benefits vs risk	Breastfeeding not recommended; excretion in milk unknown	C
Minoxidil	Weigh benefits vs risk	Breastfeeding not recommended; drug excreted in breast milk	C
Nitroglycerin	Weigh benefits vs risk	Breastfeeding not recommended; excretion in milk unknown	C
Nitroprusside	Weigh benefits vs risk	Breastfeeding not recommended; excretion in milk unknown	C
Papaverine	Weigh benefits vs risk	Breastfeeding not recommended; excretion in milk unknown	C

Pentoxifylline	Weigh benefits vs risk	Breastfeeding not recommended; drug excreted in breast milk	C
Tolazoline	Weigh benefits vs risk	Breastfeeding not recommended; excretion in milk unknown	C
Vasopressor			
Vasopressin	Weigh benefits vs risk	Breastfeeding not recommended; excretion in milk unknown	C
Vasopressin Receptor Antagonists			
Conivaptan	Weigh benefits vs risk	Breastfeeding not recommended; excretion in milk unknown	C
Tolvaptan	Weigh benefits vs risk	Breastfeeding not recommended; excretion in milk unknown	C

Pregnancy Categories/US Food and Drug Administration Pregnancy Risk Classification: B, Either animal reproduction studies have not shown an adverse effect (other than a decrease in fertility). However, there are no controlled studies of pregnant women in the first trimester to confirm these findings and no evidence of risk in the later trimesters. C, Either animal studies have revealed adverse effects (teratogenic or embryocidal), but there are no confirmatory studies in women, or studies in both animals and women are not available. Because of the potential risk to the fetus, drugs should be given only if justified by potentially greater benefits. D, Evidence of human fetal risk is available. Despite the risk, benefits from use in pregnant women may be justifiable in select circumstances (eg, if the drug is needed in a life-threatening situation and/or no other safer acceptable drugs are effective). An appropriate warning statement appears on the labeling. X, Studies in animals and humans have demonstrated fetal abnormalities and/or evidence of fetal risk based on human experience. Thus, the risk of drug use and consequent fetal harm outweighs any potential benefit, and the drug is contraindicated in pregnant women. An appropriate contraindicated statement appears on the labeling.

Abbreviations: ACE, angiotensin-converting enzyme; HMG-CoA, hydroxymethylglutaryl-coenzyme A.

[a] Only diltiazem and verapamil are indicated for arrhythmias.

[b] The pregnancy category of methyclothiazide has ranged from B to D.

[c] This drug is usually classified as an aldosterone receptor antagonist rather than a potassium-sparing diuretic.

Data from Cheng-Lai A, Frishman WH. Appendix 3: Guide to cardiovascular drug use in pregnancy and with nursing. In: Frishman WH, Sica DS, editors. Cardiovascular pharmacotherapeutics. 3rd edition. Minneapolis (MN): Cardiotext; 2011.

and tenecteplase, are used for clot dissolution in the treatment of venous thromboembolic disease. They all cause a systemic fibrinolytic and antico-agulant effect with severely impaired hemostasis. In pregnancy, administration of a thrombolytic agent during the first 18 weeks of pregnancy may increase the risk of premature separation of the placenta because fetal attachment compo-nents at this time are mainly composed of fibrin. However, this problem has not been reported in patients treated with streptokinase and urokinase during the first 2 trimesters. Other reports on the use of thrombolytic agents to treat massive pulmo-nary embolism in pregnant women also described no placental bleeding with good maternal and fetal outcome.[164,165]

SUMMARY

A summary of the recommendations regarding the use of cardiovascular drugs during pregnancy and lactation is presented in **Table 4**.

REFERENCES

1. Loebstein R, Lalkin A, Koren G. Pharmacokinetic changes during pregnancy and their clinical rele-vance. Clin Pharmacokinet 1997;33:328–43.
2. Parbhoo SP, Johnston ID. Effects of oestrogens and progestogens on gastric secretion in patients with duodenal ulcer. Gut 1966;7:612–8.
3. Parker WA. Effects of pregnancy on pharmacoki-netics. In: Benet LZ, editor. Pharmacokinetic basis for drug treatment. New York: Raven Press; 1984.
4. Qasqas SA, McPherson C, Frishman WH, et al. Cardiovascular pharmacotherapeutic consider-ations during pregnancy and lactation. Cardiol Rev 2004;12:201–21, 240–61.
5. Krauer B, Krauer F, Hytten F. Drug prescribing in pregnancy. Edinburgh (United Kingdom): Churchill Livingstone; 1984.
6. Burrow GN, Duffy TP, Kersey R, editors. Medical complications during pregnancy. 5th edition. Phila-delphia: Saunders; 1999.
7. Metcalfe J, McAnulty JH, Ueland K. Burwell and Metcalfe's heart disease and pregnancy: physi-ology and management. 2nd edition. Boston: Little, Brown; 1986. p. 11–54.
8. Cole PL, Sutton MS. Normal cardiopulmonary adjustments to pregnancy: cardiovascular evalua-tion. Cardiovasc Clin 1989;19:37–56.
9. Herngren L, Ehrnebo M, Boreus LO. Drug binding to plasma proteins during human pregnancy and in the perinatal period. Studies on cloxacillin and al-prenolol. Dev Pharmacol Ther 1983;6:110–24.
10. Wood M, Wood AJ. Changes in plasma drug binding and a1-acid glycoprotein in mother and newborn infant. Clin Pharmacol Ther 1981;29:522–6.
11. Ralston DH. Perinatal pharmacology. In: Snider SM, Levinson G, editors. Anesthesia for obstetrics. Balti-more (MD): Williams & Wilkins; 1987. p. 50–8.
12. Rotmensch HH, Elkayam U, Frishman W. Antiar-rhythmic drug therapy during pregnancy. Ann Intern Med 1983;98:487–97.
13. Elkayam U, Gleicher N. Hemodynamics and cardiac function during normal pregnancy and the puerperium. In: Elkayam U, Gleicher N, editors. Cardiac problems in pregnancy. 3rd edition. New York: Wiley-Liss; 1998. p. 3–19.
14. Dunlop W. Serial changes in renal haemodynamics during normal human pregnancy. Br J Obstet Gy-naecol 1981;88:1–9.
15. Wadelius M, Darj E, Frenne G, et al. Induction of CYP2D6 in pregnancy. Clin Pharmacol Ther 1997; 62:400–7.
16. Levy G. Pharmacokinetics of fetal and neonatal ex-posure to drugs. Obstet Gynecol 1981;58(Suppl 5): 9S–16S.
17. Potondi A. Congenital rhabdomyoma of the heart and intrauterine digitalis poisoning. J Forensic Sci 1967;11:81–8.
18. Okita GT, Gordon RB, Geiling EM. Placental trans-fer of radioactive digitoxin in rats and guinea pigs. Proc Soc Exp Biol Med 1952;80:536–8.
19. Saarikoski S. Placental transmission and foetal distribution of 3H-ouabain. Acta Pharmacol Toxicol 1980;46:272–82.
20. Steinberg I, Mitani GM, Harrrison EC, et al. Digitalis glycosides in pregnancy. In: Elkayam U, Gleicher N, editors. Cardiac problems in pregnancy. 3rd edition. New York: Wiley-Liss; 1998. p. 426–31.
21. Gewitz M, Woolf P, Frishman WH, et al. Pediatric cardiovascular pharmacology. In: Frishman WH, Sica DA, editors. Cardiovascular pharmacothera-peutics. 3rd edition. Minneapolis (MN): Cardiotext; 2011. p. 519–46.
22. Spinnato JA, Shaver DC, Flinn GS, et al. Fetal supraventricular tachycardia in utero therapy with digoxin and quinidine. Obstet Gynecol 1984;64: 730–5.
23. Johnson WH, Dunnigan A, Fehr P, et al. Association of atrial flutter with orthodromic reciprocating fetal tachycardia. Am J Cardiol 1987;59:374–5.
24. Whelan AJ. Pregnancy and medical therapeutics. In: McKenzie CR, Ewald GA, editors. Manual of medical therapeutics. 28th edition. Boston: Little, Brown; 1995. p. 15.
25. Shotan A, Hurst A, Widerhorn J, et al. Antiar-rhythmic drugs during pregnancy and lactation. In: Elkayam U, Gleicher N, editors. Cardiac prob-lems in pregnancy. 3rd edition. New York: Wiley-Liss; 1998. p. 373.

26. Shaxted EJ, Milton PJ. Disopyramide in pregnancy: a case report. Curr Med Res Opin 1979;6:70–2.

27. Biehl D, Shnider SM, Levinson G, et al. Placental transfer of lidocaine: effects of fetal acidosis. Anesthesiology 1978;48:409–12.

28. Juneja MM, Ackerman WE, Kaczorowski DM, et al. Continuous epidural lidocaine infusion in the parturient with paroxysmal ventricular tachycardia. Anesthesiology 1989;71:305–8.

29. Tucker GT, Boyes RN, Bridenbaugh PO, et al. Binding of anilide-type local anesthetics in human plasma. II. Implications in vivo, with special reference to transplacental distribution. Anesthesiology 1970;33:304–14.

30. Gregg AR, Tomich PG. Mexiletine use in pregnancy. J Perinatol 1988;8:33–5.

31. Lownes HE, Ives TJ. Mexiletine use in pregnancy and lactation. Am J Obstet Gynecol 1987;157:446–7.

32. Doig JC, McComb JM, Reid DS. Incessant atrial tachycardia accelerated by pregnancy. Br Heart J 1992;67:266–8.

33. Wagner X, Jouglard J, Moulin M, et al. Coadministration of flecainide acetate and sotalol during pregnancy: lack of teratogenic effects, passage across the placenta, and excretion in human breast milk. Am Heart J 1990;119:700–2.

34. Wren C, Hunter S. Maternal administration of flecainide to terminate and suppress fetal tachycardia. BMJ 1988;296:249.

35. Allan LD, Chita SK, Sharland GK, et al. Flecainide in the treatment of fetal tachycardias. Br Heart J 1991;65:46–8.

36. Perry JC, Ayres NA, Carpenter RJ Jr. Fetal supraventricular tachycardia treated with flecainide acetate. J Pediatr 1991;118:303–5.

37. Vautier-Rit S, Dufour P, Vaksmann G, et al. Fetal arrhythmias: diagnosis, prognosis, treatment; apropos of 33 cases. Gynecol Obstet Fertil 2000;28:729–37.

38. Joglar JA, Page RL. Treatment of cardiac arrhythmias during pregnancy: safety considerations. Drug Saf 1999;20:85–94.

39. Frishman WH. Alpha- and beta-adrenergic blocking drugs. In: Frishman WH, Sica DA, editors. Cardiovascular pharmacotherapeutics. 3rd edition. Minneapolis (MN): Cardiotext; 2011. p. 57–85.

40. Eliahou HE, Silverberg DS, Reisin E, et al. Propranolol for the treatment of hypertension in pregnancy. Br J Obstet Gynaecol 1978;85:431–6.

41. Sandstrom B. Adrenergic beta-receptor blockers in hypertension of pregnancy. Clin Exp Hypertens 1982;B1:127–41.

42. Rashba EJ, Zareba W, Moss AJ, et al. Influence of pregnancy on the risk for cardiac events in patients with hereditary long QT syndrome. Circulation 1998;97:451–6.

43. Sherif IH, Oyan WT, Bosairi S, et al. Treatment of hyperthyroidism in pregnancy. Acta Obstet Gynecol Scand 1991;70:461–3.

44. Turner GM, Oakley CM, Dixon HG. Management of pregnancy complicated by hypertrophic obstructive cardiomyopathy. BMJ 1968;4:281–4.

45. Teuscher A, Bossi E, Imhof P, et al. Effect of propranolol on fetal tachycardia in diabetic pregnancy. Am J Cardiol 1978;42:304–7.

46. Bott-Kanner G, Schweitzer A, Reisner SH, et al. Propranolol and hydralazine in the management of essential hypertension in pregnancy. Br J Obstet Gynaecol 1980;87:110–4.

47. Ngo A, Frishman WH, Elkayam U. Cardiovascular pharmacotherapeutic considerations during pregnancy and lactation. In: Frishman WH, Sonnenblick EH, editors. Cardiovascular pharmacotherapeutics. New York: McGraw-Hill; 1997. p. 1309–46.

48. Hurst AK, Hoffman K, Frishman WH. The use of β-adrenergic blocking agents in pregnancy and lactation. In: Elkayam U, Gleicher N, editors. Cardiac problems in pregnancy. 3rd edition. New York: Wiley-Liss; 1998. p. 357–69.

49. Livingstone I, Craswell PW, Bevan EB, et al. Propranolol in pregnancy: three year prospective study. Clin Exp Hypertens 1983;2:341–50.

50. Taylor EA, Turner P. Antihypertensive therapy with propranolol during pregnancy and lactation. Postgrad Med J 1981;57:427–30.

51. Gladstone GR, Hordof A, Gersony WM. Propranolol administration during pregnancy: effects on the fetus. J Pediatr 1975;86:962–4.

52. Tunstall MB. The effect of propranolol on the onset of breathing at birth. Br J Anaesth 1969;41:792.

53. Pruyn SC, Phelan JP, Buchanan GC. Long-term propranolol therapy in pregnancy: maternal and fetal outcome. Am J Obstet Gynecol 1979;135:485–9.

54. Blake S, MacDonald D. The prevention of the maternal manifestations of pre-eclampsia by intensive antihypertensive treatment. Br J Obstet Gynaecol 1991;98:244–8.

55. Smith MT, Livingstone I, Hooper WD, et al. Propranolol, propranolol glucuronide, and naphthoxylactic acid in breast milk and plasma. Ther Drug Monit 1983;5:87–93.

56. O'Hare MF, Murnaghan GA, Russell CJ, et al. Sotalol as a hypotensive agent in pregnancy. Br J Obstet Gynaecol 1980;87:814–20.

57. Sonesson SE, Fouron JC, Wesslen-Eriksson E, et al. Foetal supraventricular tachycardia treated with sotalol. Acta Paediatr 1998;87:584–7.

58. Lisowski LA, Verheijen PM, Benatar AA, et al. Atrial flutter in the perinatal age group: diagnosis, management and outcome. J Am Coll Cardiol 2000;35:771–7.

59. Penn IM, Barrett PA, Pannikote V, et al. Amiodarone in pregnancy. Am J Cardiol 1985;56:196–7.

60. Valensise H, Civitella C, Garzetti GG, et al. Amiodarone treatment in pregnancy for dilatative cardiomyopathy with ventricular malignant extrasystole and normal maternal and neonatal outcome. Prenat Diagn 1992;12(9):705–8.

61. Strunge P, Frandsen J, Andreasen F. Amiodarone during pregnancy. Eur Heart J 1988;9(1):106–9.

62. Robson D, Jeeva RM, Storey GC, et al. Use of amiodarone during pregnancy. Postgrad Med J 1985;61:75–7.

63. DeWolf D, DeSchepper J, Verhaaren H, et al. Congenital hypothyroidism goiter and amiodarone. Acta Paediatr Scand 1988;77:616–8.

64. Widerhorn J, Bhandari AK, Bughi S, et al. Fetal and neonatal adverse effects profile of amiodarone treatment during pregnancy. Am Heart J 1991; 122:1162–5.

65. Laurent M, Betremieux P, Biron Y, et al. Neonatal hypothyroidism after treatment by amiodarone during pregnancy. Am J Cardiol 1987;60:142.

66. Magee LA, Downar E, Sermer M, et al. Pregnancy outcome after gestational exposure to amiodarone in Canada. Am J Obstet Gynecol 1995;172: 1307–11.

67. De Catte L, De Wolf D, Smitz J, et al. Fetal hypothyroidism as a complication of amiodarone treatment of persistent fetal supraventricular tachycardia. Prenat Diagn 1994;14(8):762–5.

68. Frishman WH, Sica DA. Calcium channel blockers. In: Frishman WH, Sica DA, editors. Cardiovascular pharmacotherapeutics. 3rd edition. Minneapolis (MN): Cardiotext; 2011. p. 99–120.

69. Byerly WG, Hartmann A, Foster DE, et al. Verapamil in the treatment of maternal paroxysmal supraventricular tachycardia. Ann Emerg Med 1991;20: 552–4.

70. Klein V, Repke JT. Supraventricular tachycardia in pregnancy: cardioversion with verapamil. Obstet Gynecol 1984;63(Suppl 3):16S–8S.

71. Orlandi C, Marlettini MG, Cassani A, et al. Treatment of hypertension during pregnancy with the calcium antagonist verapamil. Curr Therap Res 1986;39:884–93.

72. Belfort MA, Anthony J, Buccimazza A, et al. Hemodynamic changes associated with intravenous infusion of the calcium antagonist verapamil in the treatment of severe gestational proteinuric hypertension. Obstet Gynecol 1990;75:970–4.

73. Belfort M, Akovic K, Anthony J, et al. The effect of acute volume expansion and vasodilatation with verapamil on uterine and umbilical artery Doppler indices in severe preeclampsia. J Clin Ultrasound 1994;22:317–25.

74. Ulmsten U. Inhibition of myometrial hyperactivity by Ca antagonists. Dan Med Bull 1979;26:125–6.

75. Kanzaki T, Murakami M, Kobayashi H, et al. Hemodynamic changes during cardioversion in utero: a case report of supraventricular tachycardia and atrial flutter. Fetal Diagn Ther 1993;8: 37–44.

76. Kleinman CS, Copel JA, Weinstein EM, et al. Treatment of fetal supraventricular tachyarrhythmias. J Clin Ultrasound 1985;13:265–73.

77. Holbrook RH Jr, Gibson RN, Voss EM. Tocolytic and cardiovascular effects of the calcium antagonist diltiazem in the near-term pregnant rabbit. Am J Obstet Gynecol 1988;159:591–5.

78. Downing SJ, Edwards D, Hollingsworth M. Diltiazem pharmacokinetics in the rat and relationship between its serum concentration and uterine and cardiovascular effects. Br J Pharmacol 1987; 91(4):735–45.

79. Childress CH, Katz VL. Nifedipine and its indications in obstetrics and gynecology. Obstet Gynecol 1994;83:616–24.

80. Nootens M, Rich S. Successful management of labor and delivery in primary pulmonary hypertension. Am J Cardiol 1993;71:1124–5.

81. Pirhonen JP, Erkkola RU, Ekblad UU, et al. Single dose of nifedipine in normotensive pregnancy: nifedipine concentrations, hemodynamic responses, and uterine and fetal flow velocity waveform. Obstet Gynecol 1990;76:807–11.

82. Maigaard S, Forman A, Andersson KE, et al. Comparison of the effects of nicardipine and nifedipine on isolated human myometrium. Gynecol Obstet Invest 1983;16:354–66.

83. Leffler S, Johnson DR. Adenosine use in pregnancy: lack of effect on fetal heart rate. Am J Emerg Med 1992;10:548–9.

84. Report of the National High Blood Pressure Education Program Working Group on high blood pressure in pregnancy. Am J Obstet Gynecol 2000; 183:S1–22.

85. Lenfant C. Management of hypertension in pregnancy. J Clin Hypertens 2001;3:71–2.

86. Chobanian AV, Bakris GL, Black HR, et al. The seventh report of the Joint National Committee on Prevention, Detection, Evaluation, and Treatment of High Blood Pressure. The JNC 7 Report. JAMA 2003;289:2560–72.

87. Awad K, Ali P, Frishman WH, et al. Pharmacologic approaches for the management of systemic hypertension in pregnancy. Heart Dis 2000;2:124–32.

88. Brown MA, Hague WM, Higgins J, et al. The detection, investigation and management of hypertension in pregnancy: executive summary. Consensus statement from the Australasian Society for the Study of Hypertension in Pregnancy. Aust NZ J Obstet Gynaecol 2000;40:133–8.

89. Rey E, LeLorier J, Burgess E, et al. Report of the Canadian Hypertension Society consensus

conference: 3. Pharmacologic treatment of hypertensive disorders in pregnancy. CMAJ 1997;157: 1245–54.

90. Koch-Weser J. Drug therapy: hydralazine. N Engl J Med 1976;295:320–3.

91. Naden RP, Redman CW. Antihypertensive drugs in pregnancy. Clin Perinatol 1985;12:521–38.

92. Michael CA. Use of labetalol in the treatment of severe hypertension during pregnancy. Br J Clin Pharmacol 1979;8(Supp 2):211S–5S.

93. Lamming GD, Symonds EB. Use of labetalol and methyldopa in pregnancy induced hypertension. Br J Clin Pharmacol 1979;8(Supp 2):217S–22S.

94. Pickles CJ, Pipkin FB, Symonds EM. A randomized placebo controlled trial of labetalol in the treatment of mild to moderate pregnancy induced hypertension. Br J Obstet Gynaecol 1992;99:964–8.

95. Olsen KS, Beier-Holgersen R. Fetal death following labetalol administration in preeclampsia. Acta Obstet Gynecol Scand 1992;71:145–7.

96. Haraldsson A, Geven W. Severe adverse effects of maternal labetalol in a premature infant. Acta Paediatr Scand 1989;78:956–8.

97. Bowman ML, Bergmann M, Smith JF. Intrapartum labetalol for the treatment of maternal and fetal thyrotoxicosis. Thyroid 1998;8:795–6.

98. el-Qarmalawi AM, Morsy AH, al-Fadly A, et al. Labetalol vs. methyldopa in the treatment of pregnancy-induced hypertension. Int J Gynaecol Obstet 1995; 49:125–30.

99. Walker JJ, Greer I, Calder AA. Treatment of acute pregnancy-related hypertension: labetalol and hydralazine compared. Postgrad Med J 1983; 59(Suppl 3):168–70.

100. Willoughby JS. Sodium nitroprusside, pregnancy, and multiple intracranial aneurysms. Anaesth Intensive Care 1984;12:351–7.

101. Paull J. Clinical report of the use of sodium nitroprusside in severe preeclampsia. Anaesth Intensive Care 1975;3:72.

102. Stempel JE, O'Grady JP, Morton MJ, et al. Use of sodium nitroprusside in complications of gestational hypertension. Obstet Gynecol 1982;60: 533–8.

103. Ellis SC, Wheeler AS, James FM III, et al. Fetal and maternal effects of sodium nitroprusside used to counteract hypertension in gravid ewes. Am J Obstet Gynecol 1982;143:766–70.

104. Lieb SM, Zugaib M, Nuwayhid B, et al. Nitroprusside induced hemodynamic alteration in normotensive and hypertensive pregnant sheep. Am J Obstet Gynecol 1982;139:925–31.

105. Naulty J, Cefalo RC, Lewis PE. Fetal toxicity of nitroprusside in the pregnant ewe. Am J Obstet Gynecol 1981;139:708–11.

106. Hood DD, Dewan DM, James FM, et al. The use of nitroglycerin in preventing the hypertensive response to tracheal intubation in severe preeclamptics. Anesthesiology 1985;63:329–32.

107. Peng ATC, Gorman RS, Shulman SM, et al. Intravenous nitroglycerin for uterine relaxation in the post partum patient with retained placenta. Anesthesiology 1989;71:172–3.

108. Fasseas P, Dharia N. Acute myocardial infarction in pregnancy. Cardiol Rev 1998;15:23.

109. Calvin SE. Use of vasodilators during pregnancy. In: Elkayam U, Gleicher N, editors. Cardiac problems in pregnancy. 3rd edition. New York: Wiley-Liss; 1998. p. 391–7.

110. O'Grady JP, Parker RK, Patel SS. Nitroglycerin for rapid tocolysis: development of a protocol and a literature review. J Perinatol 2000;20:27–33.

111. von Dadelszen P, Ornstein MP, Bull SB, et al. Fall in mean arterial pressure and fetal growth restriction in pregnancy hypertension: a meta-analysis. Lancet 2000;355:87–92.

112. Wagner SJ, Barac S, Garovic VD. Hypertensive pregnancy disorders: current concept. J Clin Hypertens 2007;9:560–6.

113. Lindheimer MD, Taler SJ, Cunningham FG. ASH position paper: hypertension in pregnancy. J Clin Hypertens 2009;11:214–55.

114. Sibai BM. Caring for women with hypertension in pregnancy. JAMA 2007;298:1566–8.

115. Seely EW, Ecker J. Chronic hypertension in pregnancy. N Engl J Med 2011;365:439–46.

116. deSwiet M. Material blood pressure and birthweight. Lancet 2000;355:81–2.

117. Magee LA, Ornstein MP, von Dadelszen P. Management of hypertension in pregnancy. BMJ 1999;318:1332–6.

118. Horvath JS, Phippard A, Korda A, et al. Clonidine hydrochloride - a safe and effective antihypertensive agent in pregnancy. Obstet Gynecol 1985; 66:634–8.

119. Pipkin FB, Turner SR, Symonds EM. Possible risk with captopril during pregnancy: some animal data. Lancet 1980;2:1256.

120. Broughton-Pipkin F, Symonds EM, Turner SR. The effect of captopril (SQ 14,225) upon mother and fetus in the chronically cannulated ewe and in the pregnant rabbit. J Physiol 1982;323:415–22.

121. Ferris TF, Weir EK. Effect of captopril on uterine blood flow and prostaglandin E synthesis in the pregnant rabbit. J Clin Invest 1982;71: 809–15.

122. Keith IM, Will JA, Weir EK. Captopril: association with fetal death and pulmonary vascular changes in the rabbit (41446). Proc Soc Exp Biol Med 1982;170:378–83.

123. Broughton-Pipkin F, Wallace CP. The effect of enalapril (MK-421), an angiotensin-converting enzyme inhibitor, on the conscious pregnant ewe and her foetus. Br J Pharmacol 1986;87:533–42.

124. Minsker DH, Bagdon WJ, MacDonald JS, et al. Maternotoxicity and fetotoxicity of an angiotensin-converting enzyme inhibitor, enalapril, in rabbits. Fundam Appl Toxicol 1990;14:461–70.

125. Broughton-Pipkin F, Baker PN, Symoonds EM. Angiotensin-converting enzyme inhibitors in pregnancy. Lancet 1989;2:96–7.

126. Duminy PC, Burger PD. Fetal abnormalities associated with the use of captopril during pregnancy [letter]. S Afr Med J 1982;60:805.

127. Guignard JP, Burgener F, Calame A. Persistent anuria in neonate: a side effect of captopril. Int J Pediatr Nephrol 1981;2:133.

128. Fiocchi R, Lijnen P, Fagard R, et al. Captopril during pregnancy. Lancet 1984;2:1153.

129. Lindheimer MD, Katz A. Hypertension in pregnancy (current concepts). N Engl J Med 1985;313:675–80.

130. Nightingale SL. Warning on the use of ACE inhibitors in second and third trimester of pregnancy. JAMA 1992;267:2445.

131. Shotan A, Widerhorn J, Hurst A, et al. Risks of angiotensin-converting enzyme inhibition during pregnancy: experimental and clinical evidence, potential mechanisms, and recommendations for use. Am J Med 1994;96:451–6.

132. Cohen E, Garty M. Diuretics in pregnancy. In: Elkayam U, Gleicher N, editors. Cardiac problems in pregnancy. 3rd edition. New York: Wiley-Liss; 1998. p. 351–6.

133. Drug Information for the Health Care Professional, USP DI, vol. 1, 16th edition. Rockville (MD): United States Pharmacopeial Convention; 1996.

134. Kassamali R, Sica DA. Acetazolamide: a forgotten diuretic agent. Cardiol Rev 2011;19:276–8.

135. Merlob P, Litwin A, Mor N. Possible association between acetazolamide administration during pregnancy and metabolic disorders in the newborn. Eur J Obstet Gynecol Reprod Biol 1990;35:85.

136. Devoe LD, O'Dell BE, Castillo RA, et al. Metastatic pheochromocytoma in pregnancy and fetal biophysical assessment after maternal administration of alpha-adrenergic, beta-adrenergic, and dopamine antagonist. Obstet Gynecol 1986;68(Suppl):15s–8s.

137. Rubin PC, Butters L, Low RA, et al. Clinical pharmacological studies with prazosin during pregnancy complicated by hypertension. Br J Clin Pharmacol 1983;16:543–7.

138. Lecarpentier E, Morel O, Fournier T, et al. Statins and pregnancy. Between supposed risks and theoretical benefits. Drugs 2012;72:773–88.

139. Cox JL. Lipid-lowering drugs in pregnancy and lactation. In: Elkayam U, Gleicher N, editors. Cardiac problems in pregnancy. 3rd edition. New York: Wiley-Liss; 1998. p. 445–9.

140. National Cholesterol Education Program (NCEP) Expert Panel on Detection, Evaluation, and Treatment of High Blood Cholesterol in Adults (Adult Treatment Panel III). Third Report of the National Cholesterol Education Program (NCEP) Expert Panel on Detection, Evaluation, and Treatment of High Blood Cholesterol in Adults (Adult Treatment Panel III): final report. Circulation 2002;106:1343–421.

141. Frishman WH, Aronow WS. Lipid-lowering drugs. In: Frishman WH, Sica DA, editors. Cardiovascular pharmacotherapeutics. 3rd edition. Minneapolis (MN): Cardiotext; 2011. p. 323–75.

142. Hall JG, Pauli RM, Wilson KM. Maternal and fetal sequelae of anticoagulation during pregnancy. Am J Med 1980;68:122–40.

143. Ginsberg JS, Hirsh J, Turner DC, et al. Risks to the fetus of anticoagulant therapy during pregnancy. Thromb Haemost 1989;61:197–203.

144. Dahlman T, Hellgren MS, Blomback M. Thrombosis prophylaxis in pregnancy with use of subcutaneous heparin adjusted by monitoring heparin concentration in plasma. Am J Obstet Gynecol 1989;161:420–5.

145. Ginsberg JS, Greer I, Hirsh J. Use of antithrombotic agents during pregnancy. Chest 2001;119:122s–31s.

146. Forestier F, Daffos F, Rainaut M, et al. Low molecular weight heparin (CY 216) does not cross the placenta during the third trimester of pregnancy. Thromb Haemost 1987;57:234.

147. Andrew M, Boneu B, Cade J, et al. Placental transport of low molecular weight heparin in the pregnant sheep. Br J Haematol 1985;59:103–8.

148. Pettifor JM, Benson R. Congenital malformations associated with the administration of oral anticoagulants during pregnancy. J Pediatr 1975;86:459–62.

149. Vitale N, De Feo M, De Santo LS, et al. Dose-dependent fetal complications of warfarin in pregnant women with mechanical heart valves. J Am Coll Cardiol 1999;33:1637–41.

150. Howe AM, Lipson AH, de Silva M, et al. Severe cervical dysplasia and nasal cartilage calcification following prenatal warfarin exposure. Am J Med Genet 1997;71:391–6.

151. Haushka PV, Reid ML, Lian JB. Probable vitamin K dependence of gamma-carboxyglutamate formation in bone. Fed Proc 1976;35:1354.

152. Sherman S, Hall BD. Warfarin and fetal abnormality. Lancet 1976;1:692.

153. Holzgreve W, Carey JC, Hall BD. Warfarin-induced fetal abnormalities. Lancet 1976;2:914–5.

154. Olthof E, De Vries TW, Touwen BC, et al. Late neurological, cognitive and behavioral sequelae of prenatal exposure to coumarins: a pilot study. Early Hum Dev 1994;38:97–109.

155. Meschengieser SS, Fondevila CG, Santarelli MT, et al. Anticoagulation in pregnant women with mechanical heart valve prostheses. Heart 1999; 82:23–6.

156. Sbarouni E, Oakley CM. Outcome of pregnancy in women with valve prostheses. Br Heart J 1994;71: 196–201.

157. Salazar E, Izaguirre R, Verdejo J, et al. Failure of adjusted doses of subcutaneous heparin to prevent thromboembolic phenomena in pregnant patients with mechanical cardiac valve prosthesis. J Am Coll Cardiol 1996;27:1698–703.

158. McGehee W. Anticoagulation in pregnancy. In: Elkayam U, Gleicher N, editors. Cardiac problems in pregnancy. 3rd edition. New York: Wiley-Liss; 1998. p. 407–17.

159. Chan WS. What is the optimal management of pregnant women with valvular heart disease in pregnancy? Haemostasis 1999;29(Suppl S1): 105–6.

160. Turpie AGG, Gent M, Laupacis A, et al. A comparison of aspirin with placebo after heart valve replacement. N Engl J Med 1993;329:524–9.

161. Frishman WH, Lerner RG, Desai H. Antiplatelet and other antithrombotic drugs. In: Frishman WH, Sica DA, editors. Cardiovascular pharmacotherapeutics. 3rd edition. Minneapolis (MN): Cardiotext; 2011.

162. Imperiale TF, Stollenwerk PA. A meta-analysis of low-dose aspirin for the prevention of pregnancy-induced hypertensive disease. JAMA 1991;266: 260–4.

163. CLASP Collaborative Group. CLASP: a randomised trial of low dose aspirin for the prevention and treatment of pre-eclampsia among 9,364 pregnant women (CLASP: Collaborative Low Dose Aspirin Study in Pregnancy). Lancet 1994;343:619–29.

164. Baudo F. Emergency treatment with recombinant tissue plasminogen activator of pulmonary embolism in a pregnant woman with AT III deficiency. Am J Obstet Gynecol 1990;163:1274–5.

165. Flossdorf T, Breulmann M, Hopf HB. Successful treatment of massive pulmonary embolism with recombinant tissue plasminogen activator in a pregnant woman with intact gravidity and preterm labour. Intensive Care Med 1990;16:454–6.

Index

Note: Page numbers of article titles are in **boldface** type.

Cardiol Clin 30 (2012) 493–500
doi:10.1016/S0733-8651(12)00074-4
0733-8651/12/$ – see front matter © 2012 Elsevier Inc. All rights reserved.

Moving?

Make sure your subscription moves with you!

To notify us of your new address, find your **Clinics Account Number** (located on your mailing label above your name), and contact customer service at:

Email: journalscustomerservice-usa@elsevier.com

800-654-2452 (subscribers in the U.S. & Canada)
314-447-8871 (subscribers outside of the U.S. & Canada)

Fax number: 314-447-8029

**Elsevier Health Sciences Division
Subscription Customer Service
3251 Riverport Lane
Maryland Heights, MO 63043**

*To ensure uninterrupted delivery of your subscription, please notify us at least 4 weeks in advance of move.

Printed and bound by CPI Group (UK) Ltd, Croydon, CR0 4YY

03/10/2024

01040354-0008